"Palmer's impressive work is truly encyclopedic. Highly recommended."

—*Library Journal*

"This book is a must-read for solid, easy-to-understand information about liver diseases, how they are treated, and how to live a healthier lifestyle if you have been diagnosed with a chronic form of hepatitis."

—*Hepatitis* magazine

"The book provides an excellent and thorough review of liver disease. It is well written, up-to-date, and . . . will be a useful resource to all patients with liver disease and their family members."

—Kris V. Kowdley, M.D., FACP, Professor of Medicine,
Division of Hepatology and Gastroenterology,
University of Washington, Seattle

"This book is an invaluable service to people with hepatitis or other liver diseases. The American Liver Foundation uses it as a resource."

—Alan Brownstein, President/CEO,
American Liver Foundation

"This comprehensive guide to liver disease is a must-read for general practitioners and patients."

—Lewis Teperman, M.D., FACS, Director of Transplantation and
Liver Transplantation, New York University

"This book is an informative, detailed, yet easy-to-understand guide. It is useful not only for people with liver disease but also their families, friends, nurses, and other allied health professionals."

—Jennifer Jones, R.N., liver transplant coordinator, Mount Sinai Hospital

Dr. Melissa Palmer's Guide to

Hepatitis &
Liver Disease

What You Need to Know

REVISED EDITION

MELISSA PALMER, M.D.

AVERY

a member of Penguin Group (USA) Inc.

New York 2004

a member of
Penguin Group (USA) Inc.
375 Hudson Street
New York, NY 10014
www.penguin.com

Library of Congress Cataloging-in-Publication Data
Palmer, Melissa.
Dr. Melissa Palmer's guide to hepatitis and liver disease / Melissa Palmer.
p. cm.
Includes index.
ISBN 1-58333-188-3
1. Liver—Diseases—Popular works. 2. Hepatitis—Popular works.
I. Title: Dr. Melissa Palmer's guide to hepatitis and liver disease.
II. Title: Guide to hepatitis and liver disease. III. Title.
RC845.P27 2004   2003063905
616.3'62—dc22

Printed in the United States of America
13 15 17 19 20 18 16 14

Acknowledgments

To my husband, Alan Pressman, my heartfelt gratitude for the countless hours of unselfish time you spent re-working my writing into publishable prose. I am lucky to have had such a talented writer transforming my rough draft into a clear and easy-to-understand gem. A superb effort once again!

To Rags, Augie, Snooper, Ivan, and Chumley, my supportive companions into the wee hours of the night, you were invaluable throughout the entire process of writing this book. You guys are the cutest creatures on the planet.

To my mother, Harriet Palmer, thank you for being a sounding board, for your continuous encouragement and support, and for always being there when I needed you.

To Eileen Bertelli and Kristen Jennings, my sincere thanks for your invaluable assistance in editing and fine-tuning this book. Your editorial skills have greatly enhanced its word flow and its comprehensibility.

To the rest of the staff at Avery, much thanks for your many helpful suggestions, and especially your patience.

This book is dedicated to all of the patients in my practice, without whom this book would not have been possible.

This book is also dedicated to all individuals with liver disease worldwide—and to all healthcare professionals engaged in the fight against liver disease.

Contents

Part III: Understanding and Treating Other Liver Diseases

Part IV: Treatment Options and Lifestyle Changes

Introduction

I f you're like most people, you've never really thought much about your liver. After all, you can't feel it the way you can feel your heart beating. Your liver doesn't groan with hunger like your stomach, nor does it gurgle during digestion like your intestines. But now your doctor has told you there's something wrong with your liver, and you've suddenly become very much aware of its presence. Perhaps you're recovering from a lifetime of alcoholism and you have alcoholic liver disease, or maybe you've never had an alcoholic drink in your life. Maybe you've been diagnosed with liver cancer, or perhaps you're suffering from a genetic liver disorder. Or maybe—like approximately 4 million other Americans—you've been told that you have just become part of the hepatitis C epidemic sweeping the nation, or that you are one of the almost 400 million chronic carriers, worldwide, of the hepatitis B virus.

The diagnosis of these conditions can have a tremendous impact on the daily lives of many individuals and their loved ones. How do I know this? Because I personally take care of thousands of people with hepatitis and liver disease each year. Who am I? I am a hepatologist (liver specialist), and I have perhaps the largest private solo practice devoted to hepatitis and liver disease in the United States.

Over the past fifteen years, I have spent much of my time educating the lay and medical communities about hepatitis and liver disease through lectures and publications. I have been active in many voluntary societies devoted to the study, prevention, and treatment of liver disease. These nonprofit organizations include the American Liver Foundation (ALF), where I sit on the medical advisory board of the New York chapter, as well as on the nutrition education subcommittee of the national chapter. I run liverdisease.com, an Internet website devoted to liver disease. I have appeared on numerous television and radio programs, both locally and nationally, to discuss various aspects of hepatitis and liver disease, as well as the latest available treatments. I have appeared in videos and CD-ROMs aimed at educating the public and healthcare professionals about hepatitis and its treatment.

1

I have also actively participated in research studies of the most promising experimental drugs for the treatment of hepatitis. I have been interviewed on various issues pertaining to liver disease for many mainstream publications such as *Time, Cosmopolitan, Prevention,* and the *Los Angeles Times.* I also serve as a liver disease consultant to five prominent pharmaceutical companies.

I've often been told by family, friends, colleagues, and even my patients that I live my life in overdrive. And maybe they are right. While in the midst of my training in hepatology and gastroenterology, I decided to become a competitive bodybuilder. After a few years of training, I won the title of Ms. Northern States, appeared on multiple segments of the television show *MuscleSport USA,* and twice had my picture on the inside front cover of the magazine *Female Bodybuilding.* By then it was time to start my medical practice, so I gave up my short-lived career as a competitive bodybuilder. But I got a whole lot more out of the experience than just a few trophies. I learned a great deal about nutrition and exercise—two powerful tools that many doctors overlook in their treatment of illness. By combining what I learned as a bodybuilder with what I learned in medical school, I have been highly successful in keeping my patients healthy. In fact, I've learned so much about the effects of diet and exercise on liver disease that I am now considered one of the nation's experts on the subject.

You have a lot of questions. Is this disease serious? Am I putting my loved ones in danger? What treatments are available? What are the alternatives to conventional medicine? What medications should I avoid? Will I be able to have children? Is there a diet and exercise program that I can follow to help me get better? This book will help you answer all these questions and more. You'll learn how the liver works to neutralize poisons, to help digest the foods you eat, to combat infection, to control bleeding, and to regulate energy levels. You'll read about the differences between the various kinds of liver diseases and how each affects your body. You'll come to understand why it's critical to fight liver disease as soon as it's diagnosed, even though you may feel fine. You'll also learn what new treatments are available. If you're exploring alternative medicine, you'll learn which herbs, vitamins, minerals, and natural remedies may aggravate your liver disease and which ones may help.

And, if you are a loved one or a friend of someone who has liver disease, you will gain valuable information about how you can actively participate in his or her road to recovery. Plus, you will learn if there are any special measures or precautions you personally need to take in order to reduce your chances of also developing liver disease.

This book's first edition was for people with liver disease and their loved ones. Since the publication of the first edition, I have learned that many people—ranging from nurses to physician assistants and from liver transplant coordinators to doctors—have used this book to assist them in caring for their liver disease patients. I just want to say that I am touched and gratified by the tremendous amount of positive feedback that I have received from the lay public and medical community—and this has spurred me to produce the updated version, which you are about to read.

An updated version of this book makes sense for many reasons. Since the first edition was published, I have been relentlessly striving to learn even more about hepatitis and liver disease. This quest has taken the form of activities such as participating in trials of the most promising experimental medications; a three-year stint on the American Association for the Study of Liver Disease's (AASLD's) Practice Guidelines Committee (whose purpose it is to guide physicians worldwide on the diagnosis and treatment of liver disease); attending many conferences and lectures with other preeminent liver disease experts, enabling me to exchange ideas; and reading every article and published study on liver disease that I could get my hands on. Most important, much of the additional knowledge that I have gained since the publication of the first edition is experience-based—that is, knowledge acquired from my personal involvement in treating (typically with great success!) thousands of liver disease patients over the course of the past several years. I am excited about sharing this knowledge with you!

There is so much good news to share. Since the publication of the first edition, many remarkable advances have occurred in the field of hepatitis and liver disease. The most significant ones will be discussed in detail in this book. For more information on resource groups and websites on liver disease, as well as the extensive bibliography for this book, visit my website, www.liverdisease.com.

This book will introduce you to and help you understand the latest liver-related treatments and advances. It will enable you or your loved one, in conjunction with a specialist, to make educated decisions about the treatment of liver disease. In part 1, you'll learn what you need to know in order to increase your understanding of, and decrease your fears about, liver disease. In part 2, you'll read about viral hepatitis and its treatment. In part 3, you'll learn about some common liver disorders occurring in the United States today. Several of the chapters in this book unfold with stories about ordinary people whose lives were changed upon learning of their condition, but who are now benefiting from the latest treatments. (These case studies are composites based on actual people whose names and occupations were changed to protect confidentiality.) Part 4 discusses what steps liver disease patients can take to help manage their recovery and what effect this illness may have on their personal lives. In this part, you'll also read about transplantation and alternatives to conventional medical therapy.

(Note: A person with liver disease or hepatitis can be either male or female. The same holds true for a doctor. To avoid using the awkward "he/she" when not referring to a group, and still give equal time to both sexes, the masculine pronouns are used in parts 1 and 3 and the feminine pronouns are used in parts 2 and 4. This has been done in the interest of simplicity and clarity.)

In writing this book, I've drawn from information that I've obtained during more than fifteen years of extensive research on every aspect of liver disease, and from my firsthand experiences treating thousands of patients with liver disease.

In the introduction to the first edition of *Dr. Melissa Palmer's Guide to Hepatitis & Liver Disease,* I stated that my mission was to break through the wall of helplessness that at times surrounds liver disease and to provide people with the genuine hope that they can get better. Well, one objective of this revised edition is to encourage all people with hepatitis and liver disease to continue to fight on! Some very effective treatments are available, and the fight can be won!

Remember, you only have one liver. Liver disease can be treated. But you must play an active role in the process. This book, while not a substitute for a doctor's care, can be a guide on the road back to health. (Please note: A person with liver disease is advised to use this book in conjunction with the direct guidance of a liver specialist.)

Melissa Palmer, M.D.

Part One

The Basics

One

A LITTLE BACKGROUND ON THE LIVER

Tom, a forty-nine-year-old salesman, was feeling somewhat fatigued. He figured that this was to be expected. He was, after all, working ten-hour shifts in addition to coaching his son's Little League team. Moreover, he was going to be fifty years old in two months. Perhaps this explained his feeling tired all the time. But, at the insistence of his wife, Tom made an appointment with his family physician for a checkup.

At the doctor's office, Tom told his doctor that he was feeling less energetic than he used to. After asking some questions about Tom's history and conducting a physical exam, the doctor said, "You look fine. But we could use some additional information. I'm going to have my nurse draw some blood from you. Call me in a week to discuss the results of your blood tests."

Tom felt relieved. But when he called for the results of his tests a week later, he heard some hesitation in the doctor's voice. "Tom, you need to come back to the office for further testing. Your blood tests detected a possible problem with your liver."

"My liver?!" Tom responded with some disbelief. "What does this mean? There must be some mistake. What could be wrong with my liver?"

Tom's reaction to finding out there may be a problem with his liver is common among people with liver disease. But what exactly is liver disease? Most people know that drinking too much alcohol is bad for the liver and that it can lead to alcoholic liver disease. But few people know that there are viruses, genetic factors, medications, herbs, and *vitamins*—among other variables—that can adversely affect the liver. Even having too much body fat can cause liver damage. Also, few people know that without a healthy liver, you would not have the energy to work or do simple daily chores; or that if you cut yourself shaving, you would not be able to stop bleeding; or that if you were exposed to toxic chemicals, your body could not filter out these dangerous, potentially life-threatening substances; or that if approximately 85 percent of the liver stops functioning, practically every other organ in the body would eventually deteriorate.

In order to understand liver disease, you must first learn about the structure and functions of the liver—nature's most miraculous life-giving machine. To help you do this, this chapter discusses the anatomy of the liver and the liver's many functions. It finishes up by explaining exactly what liver disease is.

THE LOCATION AND STRUCTURE OF THE LIVER

The *liver* is a wedge-shaped gland located on the upper right side of the body lying beneath the rib cage, which functions as its personal protective barrier. (See figure 1.1.) Making up about 2 to 3 percent of the body's total weight, the liver is the largest organ in the body. The liver is made up of two major sections, known as lobes. The left lobe is only one-fifth the size of the right lobe. The liver is crisscrossed by a densely packed web of blood vessels and special passageways called bile ducts. This organ's blood supply is a complicated superhighway with two main "thoroughfares" allowing blood to enter the liver—one called the *portal vein* and the other called the *hepatic artery* (note that *hepatic* means "liver"). Blood exits the liver through the *hepatic vein.* The cells that make up the liver are known as *hepatocytes.*

Nestled beneath the liver lies a pear-shaped organ called the *gallbladder.* Its main function is to store and concentrate bile. The liver and the gallbladder are connected by *bile ducts.* The bile ducts, as their name suggests, carry *bile*—a bitter, greenish mixture of acids, salts, and other substances—into the intestines. The liver is strategically located in the body so that it can communicate efficiently with all of the other organs, in addition to performing numerous vital functions essential to daily living.

THE LIVER'S MANY FUNCTIONS

The brain thinks. The heart beats. The stomach digests. But there's no single active verb to describe what the liver does. This is because the liver has so many different jobs to perform. In fact, if you were to write a classified ad that covered all the liver's responsibilities, it might read something like this:

> **WANTED**—One highly reliable, extremely flexible organ that can act as watchdog, grocer, housekeeper, bodybuilder, energy plant supervisor, and sanitation engineer. Will be required to process and sort gallons of digested food from the stomach and intestines each day. Must discriminate among fats, proteins, and carbohydrates and send

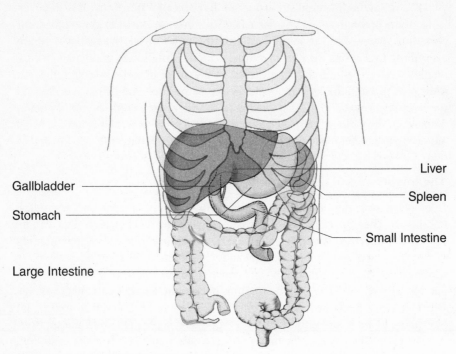

Figure 1.1. Location of the Liver

them wherever they are needed in the body. Must be able to detoxify thousands of substances—ranging from alcohol to bug spray to turpentine fumes—that may be ingested with food and drink, absorbed through the skin, or breathed in the air. Should be able to dismantle old, worn-out blood cells and recycle whatever parts are salvageable and prepare the rest for elimination. Must transform cholesterol into steroid hormones, such as androgens and estrogens, and share responsibility with the kidneys to control thyroid hormones, which influence metabolism. Must regulate sugar levels for proper energy management and create clotting factors that stop bleeding from cuts or other wounds. Additional duties will include—but are not limited to—building reserves of vitamins A, D, E, K, and B_{12} as well as iron and copper. Must be able to accomplish all of the above without weighing more than 3 to 4 pounds.

That's a pretty tall order. But the liver accomplishes it all silently, working in the background, never advertising its presence. Sometimes, when a part of the liver is damaged or removed, it is even called upon to perform the incredible task of "regenerating" itself! (See the inset "The Myth of the Regenerating Liver" on page 10.)

The following material discusses the liver's many functions. It also covers some of the problems that can arise when liver disease exists. In general, it is important to always keep in mind two basic functions of the liver. First, virtually everything that enters the digestive tract—foods, drinks, and medicines, for example—and everything that is breathed in the air or absorbed through the skin must pass through the liver in an attempt to be purified and detoxified. Second, the liver ensures that the other organs in the body are supplied with sufficient amounts of the various fuels, such as carbohydrates, proteins, and vitamins, which are necessary to get a person successfully through each day.

The Importance of Bile, Bilirubin, and Bile Acids

Bile does double-duty both as an aid in the digestion of fats and as a neutralizer of poisons. The importance of bile was recognized as far back as 400 B.C., in the days of Hippocrates, who suggested that an imbalance of the four body humors, or fluids—blood, phlegm, black bile, and yellow bile—signified disease. Bile is formed in hepatocytes (liver cells) and consists mainly of *bile acids* and pigments; cholesterol; *electrolytes,* such as sodium, potassium, and calcium; and proteins. Bile is released from the liver cells into the *duodenum*—the first part of the small intestine—to aid in digestion. The liver's bile ducts collect the bile and transport it to the gallbladder. There, the bile is concentrated and stored until the cells along the inside lining of the small intestine send a hormonal signal that some fatty food, say a double-fudge brownie, has entered the digestive system. A muscle surrounding the gallbladder contracts, and a little bile is squirted into the intestines through the bile ducts. In much the way detergent helps to lift grease off a dirty plate, bile surrounds the fats and helps to break them apart so that the body can digest them. Pretty soon that brownie starts to dissolve into clumps that are small enough to pass through the rest of the intestines and out of the body. Therefore, when liver disease exists, there may be trouble digesting fatty foods. Simi-

The Myth of the Regenerating Liver

The liver is commonly known by its remarkable ability to regenerate itself. But this statement is somewhat misleading. The liver does not really regenerate itself the way in which a starfish re-grows a missing arm. If an individual has up to 80 percent of a healthy liver removed, the remaining portion of the liver will expand to fill the empty space until its original weight is achieved. In this scenario, the liver will be fully functioning. However, if the remaining portion of a liver is permanently and severely scarred (*decompensated cirrhosis*), this expansion process may not occur, and "regeneration" would therefore be impossible.

lar to its action on fat, bile envelops some poisons in a protective barrier until they can be safely carted out of the body in the feces.

The yellow color that is commonly associated with bile is mainly due to one of its components, known as *bilirubin.* Bilirubin is actually a waste product of worn-out, old, red blood cells. When the bilirubin level rises in the blood from hepatitis or liver disease, an individual becomes *jaundiced.* This is noted as a yellow tint to the skin and eyes. Jaundice is discussed more in chapters 2 and 3.

Bile acids are a major component of bile and are closely involved in both the production and elimination of cholesterol. Most people associate cholesterol with something that you do not want to have too much of. This is partly correct, as virtually everyone knows that too much cholesterol clogs the arteries. However, what many people do not realize is that cholesterol also is a significant component of all living tissues and is involved in the processing of vitamins and hormones. If a person's diet contains an excess of cholesterol-containing foods, it is the job of the bile acids to scavenge this surplus of cholesterol particles and eliminate them from the body. Some types of liver disease are marked by abnormally high cholesterol levels. This will be discussed in detail in chapter 15.

The Liver's Role in Processing Vitamins and Minerals

The liver is a warehouse for the storage of many vitamins and *minerals,* including vitamins A, B_{12}, D, E, and K; copper; and iron. For example, a normal liver contains approximately a two years' requirement of vitamin A. Centuries ago, Asian physicians were known to remove the livers from wild animals and place them on the eyes of people complaining of vision problems. While this may sound barbaric, it is now known that vitamin A may help alleviate night blindness—a condition resulting from vitamin A deficiency. Since the liver stores these vitamins and minerals, beware of overloading its storage capabilities. For instance, people who supplement their diets with too much vitamin A or iron can actually damage their livers. This can occur even in people who have normally functioning livers. So, you can imagine what too much of a good thing could do to someone who already has liver disease. Don't add insult to injury! The toxic effects of too much iron are also demonstrated in the liver disease hemochromatosis—a disorder of iron overload. See chapter 18 for more on this disorder.

You may already know that the body uses fats as a kind of storehouse for excess calories. But did you know that fats are also necessary for the absorption of vitamins A, D, E, and K? These vitamins can exist only in a fatty solution. So if the bile ducts are blocked, as sometimes happens in liver disease, the body cannot digest the fats it needs to absorb these vitamins. This is particularly serious in the case of vitamin K, which the body needs to make the blood clot. It's one reason why some people with liver disease have a pronounced tendency to bleed. Unfortunately, the liver is such a complicated organ that simply taking more vitamin K doesn't correct this problem. For more information on vitamins and minerals and your liver, see chapter 23.

The Liver's Role in Attacking Poisons

It's one thing to break down fats and help absorb vitamins. It's quite another, however, to neutralize poisons. You might be surprised at just how vigilant the liver can be in this regard. Everything from aspirin to herbs to chemical solvents to recreational drugs is considered potentially dangerous. Therefore, in addition to the actions of bile, some cells in the liver are individually equipped to dismantle potentially toxic molecules piece by piece or to alter them in such a way that they can be more easily eliminated from the body. That is why many people compare the liver to a giant filter that helps keep your insides clean. If that filter should ever get broken or damaged by a liver disorder, the rest of your body would slowly turn into the biological equivalent of a toxic dump.

The Liver's Role in Building Muscles

You don't have to be Arnold Schwarzenegger to appreciate the liver's role as a bodybuilder. All the muscles in the body are made up of compounds called *proteins,* which are in turn composed of *amino acids* linked together like paper clips in a chain. It's up to the liver to produce enough of the right type of amino acids for the body to build good, healthy muscles. Without these building blocks, your body would have trouble maintaining your muscles, such as those in your arms, legs, neck, and even your heart. In fact, if your liver is too damaged to metabolize proteins correctly, your muscles may literally waste away. This makes you prone to bone fractures, as bones easily become brittle when their protective muscle lining is diminished. For more information on how you can slow, or possibly even prevent, this process, see chapter 23.

The Liver's Role in Regulating Energy

A car runs on gasoline. A computer depends on electricity. The body uses its own special kind of fuel, a carbohydrate molecule called *glucose.* The liver's job is to keep the right amount of glucose in the blood and to keep it flowing to the organs that need it at all times. One of the ways it does this is by storing excess glucose in the form of another carbohydrate called *glycogen.* Whenever the body runs low on glucose, it can tap the glycogen in the liver for a little extra energy boost. If your liver is inflamed or damaged, your body will have trouble regulating the glucose levels in your blood. This is one of the reasons that many people with liver disease tire so easily.

The Liver's Role in Maintaining Hormonal Balance

The liver also has an intricate relationship with hormones, including steroid and thyroid hormones. Did you know that the hormones that give us feminine and masculine traits—that is, *estrogens* and *androgens*—are actually made from cholesterol? Since it's the liver's job to regulate the production and breakdown of these substances, liver disease can lead to hormonal imbalances. One effect of such an imbalance is the appearance of feminine characteristics in men, such as *gynecomastia* (breast enlargement). See chapter 2 for more information on physical abnormalities and liver disease.

The Liver's Role in Processing Drugs

Most drugs that are taken orally must be processed by the liver in order to be absorbed and used efficiently by the body. Those drugs that are best absorbed by the body have the characteristic of being fat soluble. Drugs that are not fat soluble are known as water-soluble drugs. Water-soluble drugs are poorly absorbed when swallowed, have difficulty getting into the bloodstream, and are promptly eliminated from the body. Thus, most drugs are fat soluble. When a fat-soluble pill or tablet is swallowed, it is readily absorbed by the fat (lipid) cells lining the walls of the stomach and intestines and is able to easily gain access into the bloodstream. A drug must enter the bloodstream in order for it to have its desired effect. After a drug has produced its effect, it must be eliminated from the body. Fat-soluble drugs circulate through the bloodstream, either attached to proteins or trapped by fat cells. They are not easily eliminated. In order to eliminate these drugs from the body, they must be converted into water-soluble products. This job is efficiently accomplished by the liver.

The liver is the only organ in the body whose blood vessels contain wide-open holes, called *fenestrations*. This unique characteristic allows the entrance of most drugs and other substances through these blood vessel holes and into the liver cells. Once inside the liver cells, fat-soluble drugs are converted into water-soluble drugs with the help of a complex group of specialized enzymes known as the *cytochrome P450 system*. Once this has been done, the drug, now rendered water soluble, is excreted back into the bloodstream and is capable of being efficiently eliminated by the body.

When the liver has been damaged, the *metabolism* (breakdown) of certain drugs and medications may be altered. Dangerous levels of these drugs may accumulate in the body, potentially causing serious adverse consequences. Therefore, it is essential that a person who has liver disease inform his doctor of the drugs and medicines he is taking, including any over-the-counter drugs or herbal preparations.

The Liver's Role in Having a Clear Mind

Ammonia is a harmful chemical that is produced in the body from certain foods (mainly animal proteins) during the process of digestion. It is the liver's job to convert ammonia into a nontoxic substance known as urea, which can easily be eliminated from the body via the kidneys. If the liver is damaged and cannot perform this function, ammonia can build up in the blood and brain. This can cause a condition referred to as "brain fog" or *encephalopathy,* which is a state of mental confusion (please refer to chapter 6 for more details about encephalopathy).

CONCLUSION

So far you've learned that the liver is an extraordinarily complex organ that controls virtually every aspect of your body's daily functions and that it accomplishes this feat efficiently and quietly. So what exactly is liver disease? Unfortunately, due to the complexities of the liver, this question cannot be answered in just a few simple sentences. Instead, it will take an entire book to explain the intricacies of liver disease. Fortunately, you're reading the right book! In chapter 2, the first symptoms, signs, and other clues that something is wrong with the liver will be discussed. In addition, some of the physical manifestations that indicate that a person has liver disease will be described in detail.

Two

SIGNS, SYMPTOMS, AND OTHER CLUES OF A LIVER PROBLEM

In chapter 1, we met Tom, whose feeling of fatigue was the first clue that something was wrong with his health. This prompted him to make an appointment with his family doctor. Through the process of taking a history, performing a physical exam, and drawing some routine blood work, Tom's doctor was able to determine that his problem was liver related. Tom's wife was wise to urge him to see his doctor so quickly. Since liver disease can sometimes exist for a long time without exhibiting any obvious symptoms, Tom may have continued to remain unaware of his condition.

Of all the organs in the body, the liver is truly the strong, silent type. Whether it's fighting a viral infection or struggling under the burden of excess scar tissue, the liver rarely complains. It just keeps performing its many functions the best it can. That is why liver disease can progress for years before it's noticed. In fact, in most cases of liver disease, the first clues that something is wrong are virtually imperceptible. It is often when the liver is on the verge of collapse and can no longer perform its duties that its deterioration becomes apparent.

So how do most people find out they have liver disease? Well, sometimes—as in Tom's case—there is a subtle clue that something is wrong, such as feeling fatigued. But even these warnings may be so vague and may evolve so gradually that they go unnoticed by the person with the disease, as well as the people he comes in contact with on a daily basis. In fact, sometimes an infrequent acquaintance will be the first to detect a change in a person's appearance or personality. In other cases, a doctor may recognize the physical manifestations of liver disease while performing a routine physical examination. Or, through eliciting specific information from the patient, the doctor will make a connection between his responses and liver disease.

This chapter discusses some of the symptoms associated with liver disease—

symptoms that may result in a visit to the doctor's office. It explains what to expect at the doctor's office during the initial visit; what the doctor is looking for during the exam; and the significance of what he may find.

SYMPTOMS OF LIVER DISEASE

Symptoms of liver disease are very nonspecific. There is no distinct symptom that accurately indicates that something is wrong with the liver, or what kind of liver disease someone has, or how serious the problem might be. In fact, many people with liver disease have absolutely no symptoms whatsoever. That's right! Sometimes even in the advanced stages. This is known as being *asymptomatic,* or as having a "silent disease." So feeling fine doesn't always mean that nothing is wrong.

Often the first clues that something is wrong with the liver include fatigue, pain, fever, flu-like symptoms, jaundice, altered mental status, itching, abdominal distention, and weight gain. Any one of these symptoms may prompt someone to make a doctor's appointment. In general, a person may encounter some or all of these symptoms at any time during his disease—either intermittently or consistently. To learn about the treatments for these symptoms, see chapter 20.

Fatigue

Fatigue is a symptom characterized by a diminished ability to exert oneself, usually associated with a feeling of being tired, bored, weak, and/or irritable. Fatigue is probably the most common and debilitating symptom of liver disease. It is universal to all types and stages of liver disease. In some people, fatigue begins several years after the liver disease diagnosis has been made. In others, it is the primary reason for seeking medical attention in the first place. Oftentimes, multiple visits are made to a variety of different types of doctors in search of the cause of the fatigue before it is connected with liver disease. Some people even seek psychiatric evaluation since depression often accompanies fatigue.

Fatigue may occur at any time of day, but it is most common in the morning. Often, little more than an hour after awakening, a person may already feel the exhaustion of having worked an entire day. Others describe weakness and lack of energy throughout the whole day. Their usual "pep" is gone. Even little tasks become more trying, and around 4:00 P.M., they simply must lie down to take a nap.

Fatigue can be caused by the liver disease itself or from disorders—such as thyroid disease or vitamin deficiencies—often associated with liver disease. The doctor must carefully look at all of the factors possibly contributing to his patient's feeling of fatigue, as some factors can be easily corrected.

Pain

Most people with liver disease expect to feel pain over their liver. This type of pain is known as *right upper quadrant pain or tenderness (RUQT).* However, RUQT is rarely due to chronic liver disease. RUQT occurs most commonly in the acute stages of liver disease, such as in acute viral hepatitis. It may occasionally occur when one experiences a flare-up of a chronic liver disease, although these flare-ups are uncommon. It is most often caused by acute inflammation, irritation, and distention of the liver's surface. Otherwise, the liver is rarely tender.

If pain in the region of the liver is experienced, other causes must be considered. For example, it may indicate *gallstones,* which happen to be associated with many liver diseases. Or it may indicate *liver cancer*—also known as *hepatoma* or *hepatocellular carcinoma (HCC).* Scar tissue from prior abdominal surgery known as *adhesions* is also a cause of abdominal pain. Intestinal pain must also be considered, as the right side of the large intestine lies in close vicinity to the liver (see figure 1.1 on page 9). Many people claim that although they do not actually feel pain in the liver region, they experience a rather vague sense of "fullness" or an "awareness" of the liver. The cause for this is unclear. If a person experiences abdominal pain associated with swelling of the abdomen, *ascites*—the accumulation of fluid in the abdomen—must be considered. Ascites is associated with advanced liver disease and is discussed in chapter 6. Other causes of abdominal pain include those related to the stomach, such as peptic ulcer disease and gastritis, which are not necessarily indicative of liver disease and are readily treatable when discovered.

Fever

Fever is seen in some people with acute viral hepatitis—especially hepatitis A— and in some people with alcoholic hepatitis. These forms of hepatitis will be discussed in chapters 8 and 17, respectively. Fever is also experienced by some people with medication-induced hepatitis, which will be discussed in chapter 24. However, this symptom is uncommon in people with chronic liver disease.

If fever occurs in a person who has ascites, an infection of this fluid may be present. This is a serious condition known as *spontaneous bacterial peritonitis (SBP)* and will be discussed in chapter 6. *Cholangitis* is an infection in the bile ducts and can occur, for example, in a person with gallstones, or in connection with a liver disease known as primary sclerosing cholangitis (which will be discussed in chapter 15).

Flu-like Symptoms

During the acute stages of liver disease, a person may experience symptoms similar to those of the flu. These symptoms, which include fever, muscle and joint aches, decreased appetite, nausea, rashes, headaches, weight loss, and generalized weakness, may last anywhere from several days to several weeks before they are completely resolved. In a person who has chronic liver disease, these symptoms are not as common but may occur intermittently throughout the course of the disease. If any of these flu-like symptoms are constant in a person with chronic liver disease, a cause other than a liver problem should be investigated by a doctor.

Jaundice

Jaundice—noted by a yellow tint to the skin and eyes—is not actually a symptom but a sign of liver disease, which is usually detected during a physical exam. It becomes apparent when the bilirubin rises to a level greater than 2.5 milligrams per deciliter (2.5 mg/dl). (A normal bilirubin level is lower than 1.5 mg/dl.) When a person's bilirubin level is elevated, stools may become a light clay color and urine may become a dark tea color.

Many people think that if they have never been jaundiced, then they have never had and do not currently have liver disease. This is far from the truth. In fact, many people who have liver disease never experience jaundice. But in others, it may be the first clue that something is wrong. In these cases, jaundice may occur as a manifestation of acute hepatitis or it may be an ominous sign of deteriorating liver disease. It is important to keep in mind that jaundice can be due to myriad causes, some of which are not even related to the liver. These causes are discussed in more detail in chapter 3.

Altered Mental Status

For some people, the first clue that something is wrong may be *encephalopathy*—altered mental status. A person experiencing a mild, chronic form of encephalopathy may constantly forget simple things, such as where he placed his glasses or whether he already took his medication. Or he may get irritable over insignificant things or experience other behavioral changes. A person experiencing a more severe, acute form of encephalopathy may forget major information, such as what year it is or even his own name and address. Or the person may react in a strangely inappropriate or even violent manner. Encephalopathy is a sign of severe liver deterioration. It is discussed in more detail in chapter 6.

Itching

Pruritus is the medical term for itching. It is commonly the first clue that something is wrong in people with primary biliary cirrhosis, which will be discussed in chapter 15. Pruritus can also occur in any liver disease complicated by *cholestasis*—impairment or failure of bile flow—such as in people with cirrhosis complicated by jaundice. Pruritus is a symptom that can be extraordinarily annoying and extraordinarily difficult to treat. It can range in intensity from being so mild that it does not interfere with daily activities to being so intense that it inhibits a person from sleeping at night or even holding down a regular job. The itching can occur all over the body or be limited to specific areas, such as the palms of the hand or the upper back. Some people describe this sensation as a tingling or burning sensation beneath the skin, which is not relieved by any amount of scratching. Sometimes itching can become so severe that patients will resort to scratching themselves with sharp objects, thereby causing permanent scars.

Abdominal Distention and Weight Gain

One liver-related symptom that often leads a person to seek evaluation from a doctor may be abdominal distention associated with an unexplained weight gain. As discussed previously, abdominal distention may be due to ascites—the accumulation of fluid in the abdomen. This is a sign of severe deteriorating liver disease and must be clearly distinguished from other causes of abdominal distention.

Many patients with liver disease become bloated due to *malabsorption* or *maldigestion*—impaired or inadequate absorption or digestion of certain foods. Abdominal distention will result as the digestive tract fills with gas. This is a readily reversible condition treatable by specific food avoidance, but, to the untrained eye, it may look like ascites.

Nonalcoholic fatty liver disease (NAFLD) is another condition leading to abdominal distention and liver abnormalities. In people with NAFLD due to being overweight, a distended abdomen is due solely to excessive *adipose* (fatty) *tissue*. This condition, which is discussed in chapter 16, is sometimes reversed with weight loss.

Other Symptoms

Other symptoms that can be the first clues that something is wrong with the liver include altered sleeping habits, joint aches, a persistent rash, and/or depression. These symptoms are not specific to liver disease, and, as always, a full evaluation should be conducted by a doctor in order to specifically determine their causes.

THE INITIAL VISIT TO THE DOCTOR

The initial visit to the doctor consists of a consultation and a physical exam. Typically, blood is drawn for testing. During the consultation, the doctor will ask the patient a variety of questions. Some of the responses may provide the doctor with clues that something is wrong with the patient's liver. After the consultation, the doctor will perform a physical exam to look for other clues that may indicate a liver-related disorder. Blood tests that provide additional information will be discussed in chapter 3.

The Consultation—Questions, Questions, Questions

So many things can go wrong with the liver that the doctor must ask many questions to accurately assess the cause and severity of the liver problem, as well as what type of treatment may be necessary. The list below details potential questions that the doctor may ask at the initial office visit to help determine the nature of the liver disorder. This list is provided so that the patient will know what to expect at the consultation and will be prepared to answer these questions during the visit. Answering these questions may also help trigger the patient's memory of past incidents or family history of liver disease and, as such, may provide some insight as to why he has a liver disorder.

- What symptoms brought you here? When did they start? Are they getting worse?

- Have you ever been told that something is wrong with your liver?

- Have any of your family members ever been told they have liver disease?

- To what extent have you been sexually promiscuous?

- Have you ever had sex with someone of the same gender?

- Have you ever used recreational drugs like cocaine or heroin? Have you ever shared an intravenous needle? A cocaine straw?

- Have you ever had any tattoos or are any of your body parts pierced?

- Have you ever received or donated blood or blood products?

- Did you serve in the military?

- What is your occupation?

- Where were you born?

- How much alcohol do you drink?

- What's your usual diet like? Has your appetite changed recently?

- Have you recently eaten shellfish or wild mushrooms?

- Have you gained or lost weight in the past few months?

- Have you recently traveled outside the United States?

- What is your past medical and surgical history, including any anesthesia you might have received?

- Do you have a bleeding problem or excessive bleeding?

- Do you use paint thinners, pesticides, or other toxic substances as part of your job or around the house?

It is a good idea for the patient to provide the doctor with a list of any over-the-counter medications, herbal remedies, and vitamins or diet pills that he may be taking. Although these substances do not require a prescription and are not thought of as dangerous, they can adversely affect the liver in some cases.

As indicated by the above list, the patient should expect to answer some highly personal questions. It is extremely important for the patient to tell the doctor the whole truth—whether it happened in the past or is occurring in the present. Of course we all have done things we would rather forget. It is convenient to think that certain episodes from the past don't count anymore, but with diagnosing liver disease, everything counts, even if it occurred a very long time ago. Remember, all patient records are kept strictly confidential. The patient must sign a written, witnessed authorization before any information is released to anyone. Therefore, keeping the doctor in the dark about past events can only hurt the chances for getting better. (Please see chapter 4 to learn more about the patient privacy act, known as HIPAA—Health Insurance Portability and Accountability Act of 1996.)

The Physical Exam—Signs of Liver Disease

After the consultation, a thorough physical examination will be performed in order to look for *signs*—the physical clues or findings—of liver disease. Keep in mind that the liver is so adept at hiding what's wrong—especially in the earliest stages of the illness—that even a doctor can't always tell from a physical exam that something is wrong with the liver, let alone what specific type of liver disease a patient has, or how damaged the liver is. Consequently, many patients with liver disease, even those with cirrhosis, pass their physical exams with flying colors.

If liver disease is so hard to detect, why does the doctor bother examining the patient? First, it gives the doctor a baseline against which to compare any future changes. Second, although there are no obvious outward signs in the earliest stages of chronic liver disease, there are some subtle changes in appearance that may be present when someone has developed cirrhosis, changes that an astute doctor will detect. Third, there are a few physical findings that are actually suggestive of specific types of liver disease. These will be discussed below. Last, and most important, there are numerous physical clues that are associated with a more serious outcome—cirrhosis and liver failure.

The Baseline Exam

The doctor will commence the exam by assessing the patient's overall appearance. Are there signs of chronic weight loss, or do the muscles appear to be withering away? How's the blood pressure, pulse, and breathing? Is there a fever? Does the breath smell of alcohol? Is there any mental confusion? Are there track marks from intravenous drug use? Are there any rashes, lesions, or unusual masses? Is the skin or are the eyes jaundiced? Do the hands and nails have signs of liver disease? (By the way, the brown spots on the back of the hands that many people call *liver spots* actually have nothing to do with the liver.) Are there signs of fluid retention, such as *pedal edema* (swollen ankles) or ascites? Is the liver hard and nodular (a sign of trouble) or is its texture smooth (a sign of health)? If the liver is either too big or too small, disease may be indicated. An enlarged liver is known as *hepatomegaly*.

Now that the doctor has assessed the general appearance of the patient, let's discuss the physical findings suggestive of cirrhosis. Three points must be stressed.

First, a person with *cirrhosis* may manifest one, none, all, or any combination of these signs. Second, some of these signs may occur in people with liver disease, who have not yet progressed to cirrhosis. And third, many of these signs are present in people without liver disease at all.

Signs That Suggest Cirrhosis

When the liver becomes *cirrhotic*—severely scarred and damaged—it cannot properly execute its many important functions, which were discussed in chapter 1. This may become apparent during the physical exam. As the liver struggles to manufacture proteins, there may be evidence of general deterioration in a person's health—predominantly noted by the loss of muscle mass known as *muscle wasting*. This is usually most prominent on the upper body and arms.

The spleen may enlarge to compensate for the decreased functional abilities of the damaged liver. This is known as *splenomegaly*. The *spleen* is an organ lying directly opposite the liver under the rib cage on the left side of the body. The spleen plays a role in the storage of *platelets*. Platelets are blood cells that help blood to clot. Thus, an enlarged spleen is often associated with *thrombocytopenia*—a low platelet count. This is discussed in chapter 3.

Many abnormalities may become evident due to the failure of the liver to metabolize endocrine hormones properly as a consequence of cirrhosis. *Liver palms* (*palmar erythema*) is characterized by bright red coloring of the palms, particularly at the base of the thumb and pinky. It may be associated with some throbbing or warmth of the hands. Enlarged blood vessels found on the upper chest, back, face, and arms, resembling little red spiders, are known as *spider angiomatas.* They characteristically *blanch* (turn white) if light pressure is applied to their centers. Body hair patterns may change. Men note that they need to shave less often. Hair becomes sparse on the chest, face, and pubic region. Women may have decreased underarm hair. *Gynecomastia* (breast enlargement) may become noticeable in men, and breasts may also feel tender.

There are other manifestations of cirrhosis that do not have a clear explanation. These include *Terry's nails,* a condition in which the normal pinkish color of the nail bed turns completely white and the half-moon circles at the base of the nails disappear; and *paper money skin,* a condition in which the upper body is covered with numerous thin blood vessels that resemble the silk threads in a U.S. dollar bill.

Signs That Suggest a Specific Liver Disease

Most manifestations of liver disease are universal to all liver diseases, independent of their cause. However, there are a few findings that may suggest a specific liver disease. *Xanthomas* (an irregular yellow nodule or patch usually found on the ankles, elbows, and knees) and *xanthelasmas* (a yellow nodule or patch on the eyelids) are associated with very high cholesterol levels and are found in people with primary biliary cirrhosis (see chapter 15). These irregular patches can be very disfiguring and painful. These nodules can also be found in other liver diseases and in other diseases associated with elevated cholesterol levels.

People with cirrhosis due to alcoholic liver disease will likely have many readily visible physical signs. *Dupuytren's contracture* is a puckering of the palm that prevents a person from totally straightening out his hand. The severity of this deformity may correlate with the quantity of alcohol consumed. *Parotid gland enlargement* may also occur. The parotid gland is a gland on the face located under the ear. When it becomes enlarged, it causes the earlobes to protrude at right angles to the jaw. In addition to gynecomastia, the testicles may shrink, a condition known as *testicular atrophy*. Testicular atrophy may also be a manifestation of hemochromatosis.

A *hepatic bruit,* a harsh, musical sound heard when a stethoscope is placed over the liver, is suggestive of *liver cancer (hepatoma)*.

Signs That Suggest Liver Failure

Liver failure is defined as the cessation of normal liver function. It can occur in a previously healthy individual with no prior evidence of liver disease. This is known as *acute* or *fulminant liver failure*. Or it may occur as the end result of cirrhosis. Signs of liver failure foreshadow a poor outcome and are the most ominous findings of a physical exam.

Encephalopathy, which was discussed on page 18, virtually always accompanies liver failure. Sometimes, people with encephalopathy are initially seen by a doctor in a hospital setting after a family member discovers them unconscious in a coma. *Fetor hepaticus* is a foul, sweetish, or feceslike smell on the breath (often compared to that of a "dead mouse" or "corpse"). This can be a sign of either acute or chronic liver failure and often precedes encephalopathy. *Asterixis,* which occurs with encephalopathy, is an uncontrollable flapping of the hands that becomes noticeable when a patient stretches out his arms, palms out, as if stopping traffic.

Scleral icterus is the yellow discoloration of the sclera (whites of the eyes), and jaundice, as you've learned, is the yellow discoloration of the skin and eyes. Both of these conditions are manifestations of an elevated bilirubin level. Ascites is the accumulation of excess fluid in the abdomen. When ascites is associated with fever and abdominal pain, *spontaneous bacterial peritonitis (SBP)* may be present. If there is a massive amount of ascites, one may even have a protrusion of the umbilicus (belly button), known as an *umbilical hernia*. In severe cases, the belly button can actually burst open, causing a massive leak of ascitic fluid. Dilated blood vessels can snake out from the belly button—an appearance appropriately termed *caput medusa*. *Edema* is fluid accumulation in the legs, especially the ankles (pedal edema). Immediate evaluation and treatment of these manifestations of liver failure—which will be addressed in chapters 6 and 20—are crucial.

CONCLUSION

After reading this chapter, you should know what to expect when you or your loved one goes to the doctor for an evaluation of a liver-related problem. Also, you are now more knowledgeable about the symptoms and signs of liver disease. Depending upon which signs and symptoms a patient mentions or displays at the time of the initial evaluation, the doctor may have a general idea of what is wrong with his liver. On the other hand, the doctor still may not be able to determine whether a liver disorder actually exists. In either case, the next step is to perform some routine blood tests to obtain additional diagnostic information. Chapter 3 will introduce you to the basic blood tests and imaging studies that doctors utilize in their efforts to diagnose individuals who have liver disease.

Three

BLOOD TESTS AND IMAGING STUDIES—LEARNING WHAT YOU NEED TO KNOW

After consulting with Tom and conducting a physical exam, Tom's doctor decided that some blood tests were needed in order to gather additional information. Included in all or most routine panels of blood are tests pertaining to the liver. These tests are commonly referred to as liver function tests (LFTs). *Some of Tom's LFTs were abnormal, which led his doctor to the conclusion that there was a problem with Tom's liver. Tom also had a sonogram of his liver, which was normal. He assumed that since his liver sonogram was normal that there was nothing wrong with his liver. Tom subsequently learned that this was not necessarily the case.*

The significance, usefulness, and limitations of liver function tests (LFTs) are discussed in this chapter. Unfortunately, LFTs cannot identify a specific liver problem. However, there are some additional specialized blood tests, which are not included in routine blood work, that can be ordered if a certain liver disease is suspected. (The table on page 33 details these special blood tests.) In addition, this chapter discusses the various imaging studies, such as sonograms, CT scans, and MRIs, that are used to visualize the liver.

UNDERSTANDING LIVER FUNCTION TESTS (LFTs)

Wouldn't it be nice if your liver came equipped with a dashboard, like the one in your car that tells you when the oil needs changing, that the engine's overheating, or you need to find a gas station in a hurry? Since it doesn't, doctors have come to rely on a number of blood tests—known as *liver function tests (LFTs)*—to give them some indication of what's going on inside the liver. But don't be fooled by this name. While LFTs are commonly used to reflect how well the liver is working, this name can be misleading, as it is impossible for any blood test to accurately assess all of the liver's varied functions. Thus, like the indicator lights and gauges in a car, the LFTs are not a perfect indication of exactly what's wrong. They can, however, alert the doctor that something is amiss with the liver. Furthermore, they can help determine which additional tests are necessary. And, when used in conjunction with these additional tests, LFTs give the doctor a better idea of what is wrong with the liver and how well the liver is working. By keeping track of the results from the LFTs over the months and years ahead, both the patient and the doctor may—in some cases—have an idea whether the liver condition has stabilized, improved, resolved, or worsened; whether a specific treatment is working or if something different needs to be tried; and whether it is time to refer the patient for a liver transplant evaluation.

LFTs consist of many different blood tests that check the levels of liver enzymes (transaminases and cholestatic liver enzymes); bilirubin; and the liver proteins. The following is a discussion of these tests.

Liver Enzymes

Four separate liver enzymes are included on most routine laboratory tests. They are *aspartate aminotransferase (AST or SGOT)* and *alanine aminotransferase (ALT or SGPT),* which are known together as *transaminases;* and *alkaline phosphatase (AP) and gamma-glutamyl transferase (GGTP),* which are known together as *cholestatic liver enzymes.* Elevations of these enzymes can indicate the presence of liver disease.

AST and ALT (Transaminases)

AST and ALT are associated with inflammation and/or injury to liver cells, a condition known as *hepatocellular liver injury.* Damage to the liver typically results in a leak of AST and ALT into the bloodstream.

Because AST is found in many other organs besides the liver, including the kidneys, muscles, and heart, having a high level of AST does not always (but often

---

A Word About Normal Reference Ranges

When laboratory test results are reported to the doctor, they are typically compared to values obtained from a group of healthy people. The range of these "normal values" is known as the *reference range* or *reference interval.* The high and low ends of the interval are commonly referred to as the upper and lower limits of normal. This reference range may differ slightly from one time to the next and from one laboratory to the next. Your doctor will take this information into consideration when interpreting a single isolated laboratory result.

does) indicate that there is a liver problem. For example, even vigorous exercise may elevate AST levels in the body. On the other hand, because ALT is found primarily in the liver, high levels of ALT almost always indicate that there's a problem with the liver. (However, a normal ALT level does not necessarily mean that the liver is definitely normal. More about this later.)

Despite what one might expect, high levels of transaminases in the blood don't always reveal just how badly the liver is inflamed or damaged. This is an extremely important point to keep in mind. The normal ranges for AST and ALT are 0 to 40 IU/l and 0 to 45 IU/l, respectively. (IU/l stands for international units per liter and is the most commonly accepted way to measure these particular enzymes.) But someone who has an ALT level of 50 IU/l is not necessarily in better condition than someone with an ALT level of 250 IU/l! This is because these blood tests measure inflammation and damage to the liver at an isolated point in time. For instance, if the liver is inflamed on the day that blood was drawn—let's say, if a patient consumes an alcoholic drink a few hours prior to blood being drawn—the levels of the transaminases may be much higher than if alcohol had not been consumed. Following the same reasoning, if the liver was damaged years before—by excessive alcohol use—the results of a blood test done today may be normal, but a damaged liver may still be present.

To confuse issues even further, there are many other factors besides liver injury that could affect the levels of AST and ALT. For example, males have higher transaminase levels than females, and African-American men have higher AST levels compared with Caucasian men. Even the time of day that a blood sample is drawn may influence the level of transaminase elevation; people appear to have higher transaminase levels in the morning and afternoon than in the evening. Food intake does not appear to have a significant effect on transaminase levels. Thus, levels do not significantly differ in the fasting and nonfasting state. Also, transaminase levels may vary from day to day.

The ratio of the ALT and AST may also provide useful information regarding the extent and cause of liver disease. Most liver diseases are characterized by greater ALT elevations than AST elevations with two important exceptions. Both cirrhosis and alcohol abuse are associated with higher AST levels than ALT levels, often in a ratio of approximately 2:1.

Elevations of the transaminases occur as a result of so many causes that they give the doctor only a vague clue of the diagnosis. Additional testing is required in order to determine more precisely what is wrong with the liver. Some possible causes of elevated transaminase levels include the following:

- Viral hepatitis

- A fatty liver

- Alcoholic liver disease

- Drug/medication-induced liver disease

- Autoimmune hepatitis

- Herbal toxicity

- Genetic liver diseases

- Liver tumors

- Heart failure

- Strenuous exercise

GGTP and AP (Cholestatic Liver Enzymes)

High levels of GGTP and AP hint at a possible blockage of the bile ducts or possible injury to, or inflammation of, the bile ducts. This type of problem is characterized by an impairment, or failure, of bile flow, which is known as *cholestasis*. This type of liver injury is known as *cholestatic liver injury*, and this type of liver disease is known as *cholestatic liver disease*. (Primary biliary cirrhosis, discussed in chapter 15, is an example of a cholestatic liver disease.) *Intrahepatic cholestasis* refers to bile duct blockage or injury within the liver. Intrahepatic cholestasis may occur in people with primary biliary cirrhosis or liver cancer (see chapter 19), for example. *Extrahepatic cholestasis* refers to bile duct blockage or injury occurring outside the liver. Extrahepatic cholestasis may occur in people with gallstones.

When a blockage or inflammation of the bile ducts occurs, the GGTP and AP can overflow like a backed-up sewer and seep out of the liver and into the bloodstream. These enzymes typically become markedly elevated—approximately ten times the upper limit of normal.

GGTP is found predominantly in the liver. AP is mainly found in the bones and the liver but can also be found in many other organs, such as the intestines, kidneys, and placenta. Therefore, elevated levels of AP will indicate that something is wrong with the liver only if the amount of GGTP is raised as well. Keep in mind that GGTP can be elevated without AP being elevated, as GGTP is a sensitive marker of alcohol ingestion and certain *hepatotoxic* (liver toxic) drugs. It should be noted that for unclear reasons, people who smoke cigarettes appear to have higher AP and GGTP than nonsmokers. Also, levels of AP and GGTP are most accurate after a twelve-hour fast. You are beginning to get an inkling of the complexities that arise when evaluating abnormal LFTs!

Normal levels of AP range from 35 to 115 IU/l, and normal levels of GGTP range from 3 to 60 IU/l. Some causes of elevated AP and/or GGTP include the following:

- Primary biliary cirrhosis

- Primary sclerosing cholangitis

- Nonalcoholic fatty liver disease (NAFLD)

- Alcoholic liver disease

- Liver tumors

- Drug-induced liver disease

- Gallstones

Bilirubin

Bilirubin is the yellow-colored pigment that the liver produces when it recycles worn-out red blood cells. Normal bilirubin levels are less than 1 mg/dl (milligram per deciliter). When levels become elevated, eyes and skin may turn yellow (jaundice), urine may appear a dark-tea color, and stools may look like light-colored clay. Elevated bilirubin, while not the most common abnormality in blood tests pertaining to the liver, is quite obvious on a physical exam, and it is the liver-related abnormality most familiar to the general public.

A phrase doctors often hear from their patients is, "I can't have liver disease, I'm not yellow." People are often surprised to discover that most people with liver disease will never become yellow. In fact, many bilirubin elevations are not even related to liver disease at all. Bilirubin metabolism is very complex and consists of many steps. A problem with any one of these steps results in an abnormally high level of bilirubin. As it pertains to the liver, an elevated bilirubin level is usually associated with worsening liver disease or with bile duct blockage (cholestasis). Some possible causes of a high bilirubin level include the following:

- Primary biliary cirrhosis

- Primary sclerosing cholangitis

- Alcoholic hepatitis

- *Hemolysis*—red blood cell (RBC) destruction

- Drug-induced liver disease

- *Choledocholithiasis* (gallstones in the bile duct)

- Liver failure or general worsening of liver disease

- Tumors affecting the liver, bile ducts, or gallbladder

- Viral hepatitis

- Benign familial disorders of bilirubin metabolism, such as Gilbert's syndrome

Bilirubin elevations are often associated with GGTP and AP level elevations. When elevated levels of bilirubin, GGTP, and AP occur concurrently, a person is referred to as being cholestatic. However, if the bilirubin level remains normal and the GGTP and AP remain elevated, the person is known as having *anicteric cholestasis.* Diseases marked by elevations of bilirubin, GGTP, and AP are known as *cholestatic liver diseases.*

Liver Proteins

Albumin, prothrombin (factor II), and *immunoglobulins* are proteins that are made primarily by the liver. Abnormal levels of these proteins can help determine whether there is a serious liver disorder present.

Albumin

Normal blood levels of albumin are about 4 g/dl (grams per deciliter). When the liver becomes severely damaged, it loses its ability to make albumin. People with chronic liver disease accompanied by cirrhosis often have levels of albumin below 3 g/dl. A low albumin level in general is an indicator of poor health and nutrition and is not specific to liver disease.

Prothrombin Time

The liver manufactures most of the clotting factors that the body uses to stop bleeding. The time it takes to produce a clot, called the *prothrombin time (PT),* generally runs from nine to eleven seconds. Vitamin K is an important factor in the blood-clotting process. If the liver is very seriously damaged or if a vitamin K deficiency is present (as sometimes occurs in cholestatic liver diseases such as primary biliary cirrhosis), the PT will run much longer than normal, thereby in-

---

A Word About Gilbert's Syndrome

Gilbert's syndrome is a very common, albeit benign, inherited disorder of bilirubin breakdown (metabolism). It occurs in approximately 4 to 9 percent of the population. It is characterized by intermittently elevated bilirubin levels. The presence of Gilbert's syndrome is usually discovered when blood tests are routinely performed, when they are performed for the evaluation of an unrelated problem, or for preemployment or preinsurance screening. Bilirubin levels usually rise to about 3 mg/dl, but rarely do they go any higher than 5 mg/dl. Levels typically increase during periods of fasting, stress, menstruation, or during the course of an unrelated illness or infection. Jaundice is the only abnormality found on physical exam. Some people complain of nonspecific symptoms such as abdominal discomfort, nausea, or fatigue; however, some experts feel that these symptoms are due to anxiety. All other LFTs are normal. Imaging studies, such as a liver sonogram and liver biopsy, are not indicated, but should be normal if performed. No long-term complications arise from this harmless syndrome and no therapy is required.

creasing the risk of excessive bleeding. In some cases, injections of vitamin K can help the PT return to normal. Improvement of the PT with a vitamin K injection indicates that the liver is still functioning. When the PT does not normalize after a vitamin K injection, a condition known as a *coagulopathy* (a tendency to bleed excessively), severe liver damage, and/or liver failure may exist. To adjust for variation among laboratories in calibrating the PT, the *international ratio (INR)* is often used.

Immunoglobulins

Immunoglobulins are proteins associated with the immune system, some of which are made by the liver and some of which are made by *leukocytes*—white blood cells (WBCs). A variety of immunoglobulins are increased in many people who have chronic liver disease. Elevations of the immunoglobulins A, G, and M (IgA, IgG, and IgM) can be suggestive of specific liver diseases (see table 3.1).

Platelets

Platelets are blood cells that help the blood form clots. The spleen plays a role in the storage of platelets. In people with cirrhosis, the spleen works overtime to compensate for the decreased functional abilities of the damaged liver. This is associated with an enlarged spleen (*splenomegaly*) and a low platelet count, known as *thrombocytopenia*. A normal platelet count is 150 to 450 x 10^3/microliter. If a patient has a value lower than 150 x 10^3/microliter, thrombocytopenia is said to be present, and cirrhosis should be contemplated as a diagnosis.

Ammonia (NH$_3$)

Ammonia is a product of amino acid breakdown. Increased levels of ammonia may be a sign of encephalopathy. Some doctors use ammonia levels to monitor the course of people with encephalopathy, but some studies have demonstrated a poor correlation between ammonia levels and degree of encephalopathy, and its use for this purpose is controversial. Measurement of the ammonia level in people with liver disease is not recommended, as mild increases may occur with any liver disease and are not diagnostic of encephalopathy. Finally, there are multiple factors that can artificially elevate ammonia levels, thereby skewing interpretability, including cigarette smoking, certain medications such as valproic acid (a medication used to treat seizures), accidentally mixing the patient's perspiration with their blood sample during the blood draw, and laboratory delay in analyzing the blood sample.

Some Final Thoughts on Blood Work

Remember, an isolated group of blood test results cannot be used to predict the future of a person with liver disease. The actual numbers themselves may have little significance. Their meaning is only important in conjunction with a multitude of other factors, each of which must be carefully interpreted by a doctor. In other words, don't get too hung up about the individual numbers. Each is just one piece of a very large puzzle. In most cases, the numbers are just a clue that something is wrong—only the first step toward a correct diagnosis.

After the routine blood tests are evaluated, more specific blood work is usually required in order to pinpoint an exact cause of liver abnormalities. Table 3.1 on page 33 lists the blood tests that are used to diagnose specific liver diseases. These blood tests will be discussed in more detail throughout the book. Usually, the laboratory provides the doctor with the results of routine blood work within a day or two; but the results of more specific blood tests may take up to two weeks, depending on the laboratory. The waiting period may not be easy (try to be a patient patient).

UNDERSTANDING IMAGING STUDIES

After the blood tests have been performed, the doctor will want to visualize the liver as a whole. Therefore, the next step is a trip to the radiologist's office to obtain one or more imaging studies of the liver.

There are several methods that can be used to obtain an image of the liver. They include taking a *sonogram,* also known as an *ultrasound* or *sono;* a *computerized axial tomography scan,* also known as a *CT* or *CAT scan;* or a *magnetic resonance image (MRI)*. All of these imaging scans are *noninvasive* (no surgery required), they do not hurt, and they can be done while the patient is awake and lying on his back. One or more of these imaging studies are usually performed to make sure the liver is located where it is supposed to be in relation to the other organs; to determine if there are any abnormal masses in the liver; to assess whether the liver is enlarged or shrunken; and/or to find out if gallstones are present in the gallbladder.

Sonograms

While a sonogram is most commonly thought of as the imaging study used to see the fetus in a pregnant woman, it is, in fact, the most frequently used imaging study to visualize the liver. A sonogram is a fast and inexpensive way to get a look at this organ. Although it is performed in a radiologist's office, no radiation is actually used—sound waves produce the image.

Sonograms are usually performed on a patient with an empty stomach. This allows the gallbladder to remain full of bile, which makes it easier to spot gallstones. In fact, more than 95 percent of all gallstones are discovered during a sonogram. Sonograms are also used to detect masses on the liver, which can be either *benign* (noncancerous) or *malignant* (cancerous), but they cannot definitively distinguish between the two. Furthermore, sonograms can estimate the size of a detected mass. However, even if a sonogram appears normal, it doesn't mean

Table 3.1. Blood Tests Used to Diagnose Specific Liver Diseases

Liver Disease	Blood Test	Chapter Reference
Hepatitis A	Hepatitis A Antibody IgM and IgG	8
Hepatitis B	• Hepatitis B core Antibody (HbcAb)	9
	• Hepatitis B surface Antigen (HbsAg)	
	• Hepatitis B surface Antibody (HBsAb)	
	• Hepatitis B e Antibody (HBeAb)	
	• Hepatitis B e Antigen (HBeAg)	
	• Hepatitis B viral DNA (HBV DNA)	
Hepatitis C	• Hepatitis C Virus Antibody (HCVAb)	10
	• Hepatitis C Virus Ribonucleic Acid (HCV RNA)	
	• Elevated Immunoglobulin G (IgG)	
Autoimmune Hepatitis	• Antinuclear Antibody (ANA)	14
	• Smooth Muscle Antibody (SMA)	
	• Antiliver/Kidney Microsomal Antibody (LKMAb)	
	• Elevated Immunoglobulin G (IgG)	
Primary Biliary Cirrhosis	• Antimitochondrial Antibody (AMA)	15
	• Elevated Immunoglobulin M (IgM) (PBC)	
Alcoholic Liver Disease	• Blood Alcohol Level	17
	• Elevated Immnoglobulin A (IgA)	
	• Mean Corpuscular Volume (MCV) > 95 fl	
	• Vitamin B_{12} and Folate Deficiency	
	• Desialylated Transferrin Level	
Hemochromatosis	• Iron (Fe)	18
	• Ferritin	
	• Percent Transferrin Saturation	
	• Total Iron Binding Capacity (TIBC)	
	• Gene Testing—Histocompatibility Leukocyte Antigens (HLA-H) and DNA Probe Analysis by PCR	
Liver Cancer (Hepatoma)	• Alpha-Fetoprotein (AFP) > 400ng/dl	19

that there is no problem with the liver. In fact, many people who have liver disease have had sonograms that look perfectly fine, as Tom's did in the beginning of this chapter. Therefore, don't be surprised if the doctor orders more tests after the sonogram.

CT Scans and MRIs

CT scans and MRIs provide more comprehensive views of the liver in relation to its adjacent organs. They are most often utilized to further evaluate a mass found on a sonogram. CT scans utilize gamma radiation by transmitting an X-ray beam through the liver. Any abnormal masses will stop the X-ray beam in its tracks, and an image will be recorded. With an MRI, electromagnetic radiation creates a picture of the liver. MRIs are useful in detecting a fatty liver, iron overload, and *hemangiomas*—a benign blood tumor (see chapter 19).

Some Final Thoughts on Imaging Studies

Many exciting breakthroughs have been made that have enhanced the diagnostic accuracy of these imaging studies. However, even these advanced techniques don't tell the whole story of what's going on with the liver. It is very important to understand that the liver is a master of camouflage. Even people with severe liver disease and cirrhosis may have normal imaging studies. This is a key point to remember, and it bears repeating. Sonograms, CT scans, and MRIs can look totally normal at any stage of liver disease. That is why doctors have come to rely on the liver biopsy, which will be discussed in chapter 5, as the gold standard for evaluating liver disease.

CONCLUSION

After reading this chapter, you should now understand that blood tests and imaging studies may give some important clues, but don't always determine exactly what is wrong with the liver. Also, they may not help in assessing the degree of inflammation or damage that has occurred. A liver biopsy is the only test that can accurately provide this information. Chapter 5 is devoted to discussing this procedure in detail. But first, it is crucial to find a specialist who is skilled in determining when a liver biopsy should be performed and has the expertise to accurately interpret the results and who can most effectively apply them to the treatment of the patient. The next chapter discusses the different types of doctors that a person may choose for his specialized care and assists him in choosing the right one. It also explains what qualifications to look for in a specialist and where and how to obtain this information.

Four

CHOOSING THE RIGHT DOCTOR

*Tom's doctor advised him to consult a specialist for further evalua-
tion of his liver disorder and referred him to a gastroenterologist. At
the gastroenterologist's office, Tom noticed that the waiting room
was chockful of pamphlets and other literature on stomach and intestinal disorders, but there was nothing on liver disease.*

*Tom was taken into the consultation room by the receptionist.
There, the gastroenterologist asked Tom some questions about his
health before leading him to another room for the physical exam. At
the end of the exam, the gastroenterologist said, "You look healthy,
Tom. I've reviewed your blood work and the sonogram report from
your doctor. Since your LFTs are only slightly elevated, you don't
need further evaluation with a liver biopsy and you don't need to
start on any treatment. See me again in six months and we'll repeat
the tests. But if you start to feel worse, call me."*

"Why do I feel so fatigued?" Tom asked. "What should I do?"

*"Get more rest and just take it easy for a while," was the gastroen-
terologist's reply.*

*Tom left with mixed emotions. On the one hand, he was relieved
that the doctor thought he didn't need a biopsy. On the other hand,
Tom recalled reading an article stressing the importance of liver
biopsies and early treatment of liver disease. Tom felt a little uneasy.
"Does this gastroenterologist really focus his practice on liver disease? Is there a specialist in my town whose practice is concentrated
on liver disease? And can I find such a doctor?"*

*Looking for answers, Tom searched the Internet (which had
many websites devoted to liver disease), called several nonprofit organizations, and even conducted some research at his local library.*

*He also asked people he knew to recommend a liver specialist. Tom's
hard work led him to a hepatologist—a liver specialist—in his area.
At the initial visit, the hepatologist strongly recommended a liver
biopsy to further evaluate Tom's condition and began to discuss possible treatment options. Tom was surprised at how different the two
doctors' opinions were.*

For a person with liver disease, finding the right doctor is no simple task. It
may require both time and effort. In many instances, someone with chronic
liver disease will be under the care of the same doctor for many years or
possibly his entire life. Therefore, choosing the right specialist is a decision of
extraordinary importance. But finding "Dr. Right," unfortunately, is not always
so easy.

This chapter takes you step-by-step through the process of finding a qualified specialist in liver disease. It discusses the differences in expertise among the
various types of doctors who treat liver disease. It explains what qualifications to
look for in a specialist and where and how to obtain information regarding the
specialist's qualifications and credentials. It will also cover what a patient should
expect from the doctor's office and the office staff, and what to do if a specialist
does not participate in the patient's insurance plan. Finally, included are some
tips on how to prepare for, and get the most out of, the initial consultation with a
specialist.

WHAT KINDS OF DOCTORS TREAT LIVER DISEASE?

There are many different kinds of doctors who evaluate and treat people with
liver disorders. First, there is the family physician or internist. These doctors are
also referred to as primary care physicians (PCPs). They are often the first ones
to discover that something is wrong with the liver. From there, the patient is customarily referred to a specialist—either a gastroenterologist, hepatologist, or infectious disease specialist—for further evaluation and treatment. This specialist
may be in a practice located at an academic institution or in a private practice
located in a community setting. The difference between the various types of doctors a patient with liver disease encounters may sometimes be confusing. Hopefully, this section will clarify these differences in order to eliminate any future
confusion.

The Medical Doctor (MD)

Medical doctors (MDs) are physicians who have successfully completed four
years of medical school training. After graduating from medical school, these
doctors must complete a minimum of one additional year of training in a hospital in what is known as an internship. They must then pass a state-licensing exam
in order to practice medicine in that state. After obtaining their license, they have

the right to practice medicine in that state. However, many doctors choose to continue their training in a hospital by undergoing a residency—typically an additional two years.

After completing their residency, these doctors must take an exam in order to become board certified in a specialty, such as family medicine or internal medicine. Doctors may practice medicine whether or not they pass this exam. Doctors who become family doctors or internists have general knowledge in all areas of medicine including the heart, lungs, kidneys, stomach, intestines, and liver. At this time, a doctor may decide to undergo additional specialty training, known as a fellowship, in a specific area of internal medicine, such as gastroenterology, hepatology, or infectious diseases, in order to become an expert in these areas.

The Doctor of Osteopathy (DO)

Doctors of osteopathy (DOs) are commonly referred to as osteopaths. These are doctors who graduated from a four-year osteopathic school. They must also complete a one-year internship in a hospital in order to be eligible to obtain a license to practice medicine. Osteopaths can also choose to undergo an additional two-year residency and may thereafter undergo specialty training in a specific area of medicine.

Osteopaths tend to focus on treating "the body as a whole," particularly on the body's ability to heal itself. Osteopaths typically center their treatment on the musculoskeletal system, the muscles and bones, often using techniques such as bone manipulation and a form of massage.

The Family Physician

A family physician is a doctor—either an MD or a DO—who has been trained to prevent, diagnose, and treat medical conditions in people of all ages. The family physician takes care of the general health of the patient and his entire family. Their training is not limited to internal medicine but includes some training in psychiatry, obstetrics, gynecology, and surgery. These are the "Marcus Welby" doctors, seemingly able to handle almost any general problem.

There is a separate board certification examination specifically for family practitioners. This is known as the family practice boards. Specializing in family practice medicine requires an additional three years' training beyond medical school. The amount of exposure to and degree of expertise in liver disease vary among family practitioners. However, family physicians have not undergone additional specialized training in liver disease.

The Internist

An internist is a doctor—an MD or a DO—who is trained to prevent, diagnose, and treat medical conditions in adolescents and adults, including the elderly. Internists have received some basic training in subspecialty areas of internal medicine, including gastroenterology, hepatology, and infectious diseases. Internists are trained to treat both straightforward and complex problems of the internal organs. They are also trained in emergency medicine and critical care medicine. There is a separate board certification examination specifically for internists. It is known as the internal medicine boards. Specializing in internal medicine requires an additional three years' training beyond medical school.

The amount of exposure to and degree of expertise in liver disease vary among internists. Internists have the option of continuing their training in a subspecialty of internal medicine. This requires applying for, and being accepted into, a fellowship in the subspecialty of their choice. Gastroenterology, hepatology, and infectious diseases are among the many subspecialties of internal medicine.

The Gastroenterologist

A gastroenterologist is an internist who has completed specialty training in the treatment of digestive disorders. Digestive disorders include disorders of the esophagus, stomach, small and large intestines, pancreas, gallbladder, and liver. In order to become board certified in gastroenterology, the doctor must first become board certified in internal medicine. In order to become eligible to even take the examination for board certification in gastroenterology, a gastrointestinal (GI) fellowship lasting an additional two to three years beyond an internal medicine residency must be completed.

During the course of their two to three years of training in gastroenterology, some gastroenterologists have little exposure to patients with liver disease. On the other hand, some gastroenterologists have a great deal of exposure to patients with liver disease during the course of their gastroenterology specialty training. Thus, the level of experience and expertise among gastroenterologists in diagnosing and treating liver disease varies greatly. It is important for the patient to determine the gastroenterologist's level of expertise in liver disease prior to establishing a long-term medical relationship with this type of doctor. This will be discussed on page 42.

The Hepatologist

A hepatologist is the most experienced and qualified type of doctor to treat people with liver disease. Since there is currently no separate board certification examination in the field of hepatology, there is no official definition of a hepatologist. However, there are specialized training programs for doctors who are focused solely on liver disease. These are known as hepatology fellowships and typically last from one to two years. Over the course of a hepatology fellowship, a doctor receives comprehensive training in the diagnosis and treatment of liver disease. This specialty training typically includes extensive exposure to all liver diseases, including those that are rare and infrequently seen. This intense training in liver disease is rarely matched in a gastroenterology fellowship.

A physician who successfully completes a hepatology fellowship is considered a hepatologist. Most hepatologists, although not all, are also gastroenterologists. These doctors have successfully completed both a hepatology and a gastroenterology fellowship. Occasionally, gastroenterologists who have not completed a fellowship in hepatology nonetheless focus their medical practice primarily on the diagnosis and treatment of people with liver disease. While these physicians do not have a separate diploma in the field of liver disease, they may also be considered hepatologists.

For many reasons, it is to the patient's advantage to choose a hepatologist to treat his liver disease. The patient can be virtually assured that the hepatologist will have substantial experience in the diagnosis and treatment of the full range of liver diseases. Furthermore, hepatologists are likely to be the first to learn about the most up-to-date therapies—both FDA-approved and experimental—and to incorporate them into their practices. However, whether someone chooses to see a gastroenterologist or a hepatologist, it is important to find a doctor who is willing to work with him as an equal partner in the healing process.

Infectious Disease Specialists

An *infectious disease specialist* is an internist who has completed a specialty fellowship in infectious diseases of all types. Many infectious disease specialists treat people with liver disease caused by infections, such as hepatitis B and C (both of which are caused by viruses). During the course of their two years of training in infectious diseases, some infectious disease specialists have little exposure to patients with viral hepatitis. On the other hand, some infectious disease specialists receive a great deal of exposure to patients with viral hepatitis during the course of their specialty training. Thus, the level of expertise among infectious disease specialists in diagnosing and treating viral hepatitis varies greatly. It is important for the patient to determine the infectious disease specialist's level of expertise in treating hepatitis B or C prior to establishing a long-term medical relationship with this type of doctor. It should be stressed that infectious disease doctors have no special expertise treating liver diseases that are not caused by infections such as alcoholic liver disease or autoimmune hepatitis.

Academic Physicians Versus Private Practitioners

People searching for a doctor should be aware of the differences between academic physicians and private practitioners. Each type of doctor has pros and cons that must be carefully weighed by the patient as part of the process of choosing a physician.

The Academic Physician

An academic physician is a doctor who has accepted a faculty position on staff at a hospital. Often, though not always, the hospital will be associated with a medical school. These doctors spend a portion of their time teaching medical students and physicians-in-training (interns, residents, and fellows) about their specialty—in this case, hepatology. Also, some academic physicians spend a considerable percentage of their time conducting research, as opposed to treating patients. Although some of this research is performed in a laboratory, some is within the context of clinical trials involving patients. (See chapter 11 for a discussion of clinical trials.)

These physicians are usually, but not always, board certified in their specialty, and some have contributed significantly to the advancement of the medical profession in their specialty. However, this is not always the case. Academic physicians carry a title such as assistant professor, associate professor, or professor. This title is based on a number of factors, including, but not limited to, how long they have been practicing in their specialty, their leadership skills, their teaching skills, and the contributions made by them in their specialty. No one should ever assume that the qualifications of a given academic physician are superior to those of a given private practitioner merely based on the academic physician's title or employment by a hospital. This may even hold true of the department chairman.

Academic physicians are generally expected to stay abreast of the newest developments in their field. Such a physician may have initiated or prompted the investigation of a new drug or may have played a significant role in the development of a new medical procedure. Frequently, but not always, academic physicians are involved in conducting investigational trials on the most promising experimental drugs. However, the requirements of entering a study at an academic center may be very rigid and typically involve a risk that the patient will be given a *placebo* (dummy drug).

Doctors at an academic institution usually allot some time to patient care. However, since these physicians must also teach, the patient will sometimes be evaluated and treated primarily by a doctor-in-training rather than the more experienced faculty member he was expecting. Although these doctor trainees must discuss the patient with the academic physician, the patient will have no assurance of ever meeting with the academic physician. Sometimes the patient will only briefly meet with the academic doctor whose credentials prompted his visit in the first place. This may occur on the initial consultation and/or on subsequent visits. Thus, the patient may experience but cannot count on a close personal relationship with this doctor. Therefore, it is important for a patient making an appointment with a physician who is on staff at a hospital to inquire whether he will be seeing the doctor in a clinic setting or in some type of private office. And whether he will be seeing the doctor he is requesting the appointment with, opposed to his associates or staff, both for the initial consultation and follow-up visits.

Finally, since academic physicians are typically based within a hospital, their office hours are often limited. Rarely, if ever, will these physicians make themselves available for routine appointments after 5:00 P.M., before 8:00 A.M., or on weekends. And since these doctors have so many other duties in the hospital, such as meetings, teaching, and lecturing, typically only two or three days at most will be devoted to seeing patients, and then only for a limited number of hours. The result of such limited hours is that usually the patient will only be able to book an appointment several weeks, if not months, in advance. Furthermore, hospital-based physicians are typically away from their practice many weeks out of the year attending meetings and lecturing.

The Private Practitioner

A private practitioner is a physician who typically focuses his career on patient care. Usually, but not always, private practitioners take care of people who are admitted to local hospitals in their communities. That is, these private practitioners have either admitting or consulting privileges at one or more local hospitals. Some private practitioners may also be affiliated with an academic institution, where they also treat patients and occasionally teach. And some private practitioners do not see patients in a hospital setting at all but only in their office for consultations.

Private practitioner physicians may be in solo practice, wherein only one doctor is running the practice; in a partnership, wherein two or more physicians share the responsibilities of the practice; or in a group practice, wherein several doctors are affiliated across an array of different medical specialties. As compared with an academic setting within a large hospital, a personal relationship with the physician is more likely to develop in a private-practice setting (although this is not always the case). If the physician is not a solo practitioner, the patient should inquire whether he will be seen by the same physician on each visit. Similarly, all patients in the process of choosing a physician should inquire whether they will be seen by an actual doctor, as opposed to a nurse or physician's assistant (PA), on each visit.

Private practitioners typically have much longer and more flexible office hours than physicians who are hospital staff members. Thus, early morning as well as evening and weekend hours are often available. Of course, the actual hours of availability vary considerably among private practitioners. Also, as compared with hospital-based physicians, private practitioners are less likely to be away from their offices for extended periods of time. Thus, it is possible to obtain an appointment with a highly qualified hepatologist in private practice much more quickly (usually within a few weeks) than with an academic hepatologist of similar stature.

A person doesn't necessarily have to be treated at an academic institution in order to enroll in a clinical trial of an experimental drug. Some private practitioners conduct clinical studies as part of their practice, in the same manner as would an academic physician. However, this is not especially common and generally applies only to the most knowledgeable privately practicing hepatologists. This is an important area to inquire about prior to making an appointment with the doctor. Typically, studies run in a private practitioner's office are less rigid in terms of criteria for including or excluding subjects and are less likely to involve the use of a placebo as compared with those conducted at an academic institution. It is important to thoroughly research the credentials of the physician conducting the study, whether the study is conducted in a private-practice setting or at an academic institution. This will be discussed in further detail in chapter 11.

Finally, many people with liver disease incorrectly assume that if they are treated by an academic physician who is affiliated with a transplant center, this will automatically increase their chances of obtaining a new liver, should one be required. This is a total misconception, as all people are subject to identical rules, regulations, and criteria for liver transplantation—regardless of whether the patient is being treated within an academic or private-practice setting. (See chapter 22 for more about liver transplantation.)

WHAT TO LOOK FOR IN A SPECIALIST

Now that you are familiar with the different kinds of doctors, the next step is to find out about the specialist you have chosen and how he runs his office.

What questions should be asked to determine the doctor's experience treating people with liver disease?

Determining the Doctor's Experience with Liver Disease

It is essential to find a doctor who has a significant amount of experience in taking care of people who have liver disease. Information about hepatitis and liver disease rapidly changes. Thus, unless the doctor deals with these diseases multiple times a day, it is unlikely that he will be up to date with information. Even most textbooks are two to three years out of date by the time they are published. In this regard, the patient should pose some basic questions to the doctor. See the sample questions that follow. Also, there is no guarantee that the doctor will be totally forthcoming about his level of experience. It's very important to remember that just because the doctor's business card or door sign says liver disease, it shouldn't be assumed that his practice focuses on liver disease. The printer and the sign maker do not verify the doctor's qualifications and credentials.

Did your specialty training include a liver fellowship?

As discussed above, a doctor may have trained in the general specialty of gastroenterology, which includes some training in liver disease, or the doctor may have additional training specifically in liver disease. Doctors typically, but not always, hang their diplomas on the wall. Therefore, simply looking at the doctor's wall to see if there are two separate diplomas—one for liver disease and the other for gastroenterology—will answer this question in many instances.

Approximately what percentage of your practice is devoted to liver disease, and about how many liver disease patients are you presently treating?

Some doctors have a very large practice but treat very few individuals with liver disease. Other doctors have a relatively small practice, but it may be one that is devoted primarily to taking care of people with liver disease. And some doctors—despite being well known in the field of hepatology—have not actually treated many people with liver disease. These doctors, who often work at large, well-respected hospitals, have devoted their careers to liver disease research rather than patient care.

It is important to know how experienced the doctor is in treating patients with liver disease. However, while you may be tempted to ask the doctor his age or how long he has been in practice, these questions are of debatable usefulness. Though most people would prefer not to be treated by a doctor who has just completed specialty training, the actual amount of years in practice may not be a reliable indicator of the doctor's experience with liver disease. For example, a doctor who has been in practice for thirty years may treat only ten individuals with liver disease each week. While another doctor, who may have been in practice for ten years, treats thirty people with liver disease each week. Who is more qualified? The answer is they both may be sufficiently qualified. The bottom line is that the age of the physician and the actual number of years he has been in practice are not reliable criteria by which to judge a doctor's level of experience.

Are you involved in liver disease research?

It is advisable to ask the doctor whether he has participated in or is currently conducting research devoted to liver disease. For example, a doctor may be involved in experimental trials to evaluate a promising new form of diet or drug therapy for liver disease or may be involved in evaluating a new method of diagnosing liver disease. A doctor involved in such investigations will afford the patient the opportunity not only to learn firsthand about the most up-to-date therapies, but also may enable the patient to begin using a promising form of therapy before it becomes readily available to the public.

Have you written any articles on liver disease? Have you written or contributed to any books on liver disease?

A patient should feel free to inquire about the doctor's medical research experience and also about whether the doctor has authored any publications on liver disease. Many of the most knowledgeable hepatologists have published articles in well-respected peer-review medical publications, such as *Hepatology, Gastroenterology,* or *Seminars in Liver Disease.* This can be independently checked by accessing MEDLINE on the Internet or by asking for a copy of the article. Doctors are usually more than happy to comply with such a request. Remember, however, that articles appearing in medical publications are written for other physicians and other members of the medical community. These articles will, therefore, contain technical medical terminology. Some doctors have written articles on liver disease for the general public. These may appear in local newspapers, general circulation magazines, specialty publications, such as *Hepatitis* magazine, or publications such as the American Liver Foundation newsletters and pamphlets.

Some of the doctors who are the most dedicated to liver disease have demonstrated their dedication by writing book chapters, book forewords, or entire books on the subject of liver disease—either for the medical or lay community. The patient should feel free to inquire about any of these publications.

What is your knowledgeability regarding alternatives to conventional medical therapies?

While a liver specialist is primarily involved in prescribing mainstream medical treatments, he should also be knowledgeable about the available alternatives to conventional medical therapy. Extensive evaluation of any alternative treatment is essential before its effectiveness can be assessed. How familiar is the doctor with the alternative therapy in question? How is the doctor basing his recommendations as to the alternative in question? How many of the doctor's patients tried this alternative treatment, and what were the results?

If a doctor is going to treat your liver disease, it is important that he be knowledgeable as to the most popular alternative treatments for liver disease. While the doctor may not necessarily recommend their usage, it is important that he be conversant with their pros and cons.

THE DOCTOR'S OFFICE AND STAFF

In addition to the qualifications of the doctor, there are several important factors that a prospective patient should consider when choosing a liver specialist. It is important to search for a practice in which the doctor has attempted to make the practice convenient, available, and private. This section discusses some additional issues to consider when finding a doctor to treat your liver disease.

Office Staff

Often, the patient can get a baseline impression of the doctor by observing how the office is run. Take note of whether the office staff seems to be knowledgeable about liver disease. A person telephoning the office may not always be able to contact the doctor immediately. Does the doctor have a nurse, medical assistant, or office manager who can promptly and accurately answer questions in the doctor's absence?

Office Availability

What is the availability of the doctor and the doctor's staff? How many days a week is the office open? Are the doctor's hours flexible? Are evening and weekend appointments available? How long must the patient wait to get an appointment? A doctor may not have an appointment available the same day a patient calls, but no matter how busy the doctor's practice is (even in the busiest of practices), a patient should be able to schedule an appointment within three or four weeks—at most.

How long does the patient have to wait once in the doctor's office? If on every visit, the patient is left waiting for more than two hours in the waiting room, then there is something wrong with the doctor's method of scheduling. But a long wait on occasion should not be cause for concern. Emergencies sometimes arise and can result in delays.

Office Privacy

It is important to be treated by a medical practice that respects your privacy. In fact, it's the law. Is the nurse's and office reception area enclosed with a window or door, or is it open, thereby allowing patients' names and personal information to be overheard? Does the doctor or his staff discuss other patients' information (e.g., on the phone) while in your presence? Can you rely on the doctor and his staff to take the necessary steps to protect your medical information? Is the doctor's practice in compliance with the Health Insurance Portability and Accountability Act of 1996 (HIPAA)?

Office Services

People with liver disease generally need frequent assessment of their blood work. Therefore, it is important to find out whether blood will be drawn at the doctor's

---

What Is HIPAA?

The *Health Insurance Portability and Accountability Act* of 1996 *(HIPAA)* was developed by the Department of Health and Human Services (HHS). This law applies uniformly to all areas of the United States effective as of April 15, 2003. These laws are a national standard. No doctor's office or hospital in any area of the country is exempt from this law. The HIPAA law is designed to protect the security and confidentiality of patients' *protected health information (PHI)* whether it is on paper, in computers, or communicated orally. PHI is any information that the doctor's office possesses about the patient that identifies the patient and relates to their past, current, and future physical and/or mental health condition, and the healthcare products and services that have been provided. Under this law your medical records and conversations with the doctor and doctor's staff are not readily available to anyone without your written authorization.

All doctors' offices must provide written notice to their patients describing their rights under this law. Patients typically will be asked to sign, initial, or otherwise acknowledge that they received this notice. Furthermore, a notice must also be posted in the doctors' office describing the basic features of this law. An office that does not display an HIPAA notice is in violation of their patients' privacy rights and is subject to both civil and criminal penalties. The same applies to an office that does not provide you with a written notice describing your rights under HIPAA.

office or whether the patient will be sent to a laboratory to have blood drawn. Obviously, it is a great convenience to have blood drawn in the doctor's office at the time of the visit.

Often the patient with liver disease will need evaluation of his digestive system for a variety of reasons. The evaluation will typically include an upper endoscopy and a colonoscopy. An *upper endoscopy* is a flexible tube with a light at the end and is performed to evaluate the *esophagus* for possible *esophageal varices,* and the stomach for possible ulcers or infection. A *colonoscopy* is a flexible tube with a light at the end of it and is done to evaluate the lower intestines (colon) for polyps or rectal bleeding, for example. Some doctors perform these tests in the comfort, privacy, and convenience of their office. Other doctors perform these tests at the local hospital, which is invariably more time consuming for the patient, as well as less convenient.

Who Will the Patient Actually Be Seeing?

It is crucial for the patient to find out whether he will be seeing the same doctor on the initial as well as subsequent visits or a doctor's representative such as a nurse, physician's assistant (PA), or medical assistant (MA). For many doctors, their standard procedure is to conduct only the initial evaluation of the patient, and all subsequent visits, phone calls, or other contacts with the patient are handled by a doctor's representative, also called a *physician extender.* In such practices, the doctor is directly involved with the patient's care only in the event of a serious complication. However, in many practices, every patient is managed personally by the doctor at all stages. A patient should also find out how many doctors there are in the practice and whether you will be seeing the same doctor at each visit. It is in the best interest of the patient to establish a relationship with one doctor. This way, the doctor's familiarity with the patient's medical history and special needs will be maximized. This is likely to lead to the highest rate of success in treatment of the patient's liver disease.

THE WAYS DOCTORS HELP PATIENTS OUTSIDE THEIR PRACTICES

Treating each person individually is the standard way a doctor helps patients get better. But there are additional ways that a doctor can help people—ways in which he can reach out to large groups of people with liver disease and to their loved ones all at once.

If a doctor spends his spare time involved in activities relating to liver disease, such as writing articles, lecturing, making radio or television appearances, creating instructional videos, or running a website devoted to liver disease, it's pretty obvious that this doctor is dedicating his career, as well as his free time and spare energy, to helping people with liver disease. Patients should not hesitate to ask their doctors if they are involved in any of these worthy activities.

Publications

A doctor who writes articles on liver disease can reach a large number of people. The article can be contributed to a local newspaper, a health-related magazine, or the newsletter or brochure of a support group or a nonprofit organization devoted to liver disease, such as the American Liver Foundation (ALF) or Hepatitis Foundation International (HFI). Similarly, many pharmaceutical companies involved in the treatment of liver disease have literature concerning the disease and its treatment. The patient should find out if the doctor has contributed to any of these publications. Doctors who have had articles published will often have copies available at their offices that the patient can take home to read.

Lecturing

Does the doctor give lectures on liver disease, either within the local community or nationally? Lectures are regularly sponsored by nonprofit organizations such as ALF or HFI. The general public is normally invited to attend these lectures, either free of charge or for a very minimal fee. A knowledgeable doctor should be able to inform the patient of the date and location of scheduled lectures in the community or nearby areas. The patient should find out if the doctor is invited to speak at these lectures. A doctor who is involved in lecturing to the public will gladly tell the patient when the next lecture is scheduled, so that the patient may attend if he wishes. Or the doctor will describe to the patient the most recent lecture that he has given.

Media Appearances

The media is a means by which the doctor can reach out to many people with liver disease and their loved ones all at the same time. By communicating to the public through the media, the doctor is able to spread information about liver disease to thousands, if not millions, of people. Health topics are frequently discussed on news programs and talk shows. Often, local or cable television stations devote entire programs to liver disease, and radio programs often have short segments related to health topics. The patient should find out if the doctor has appeared on television or radio shows concerning liver disease, or if the doctor has participated in the production of any videotapes devoted to liver disease. A doctor who has appeared on television, radio, or videotape will probably be able to provide the patient with a taped copy of the show or, at the very least, provide information about how to obtain a copy.

Internet Websites

There are numerous liver-related websites on the Internet. The patient should find out if the doctor is involved in running one of these websites. The doctor should be able to direct the patient to some informative, accurate Internet websites related to liver disease. This topic will be discussed in more detail later in this chapter on page 49.

Associations and Foundations

Methods for the diagnosis and treatment of liver disease change rapidly on an ongoing basis. It is important to be treated by a doctor who is familiar with the most up-to-date developments. There are many professional organizations that keep doctors abreast of the most recent information on liver disease. The most prominent of these organizations in the field of liver disease is the American Association for the Study of Liver Disease (AASLD). A doctor who has been elected to membership in the AASLD is most likely to be actively involved in liver disease. The AASLD is an association of physicians and scientists who are dedicated to the advancement and application of knowledge of liver disease.

There are also numerous lay (nonprofessional) organizations that are dedicated to increasing the awareness of liver disease. Perhaps the best known of these is the American Liver Foundation (ALF), a voluntary nonprofit organization whose membership consists of doctors, patients, and any other individuals interested in liver disease. The ALF's major goals include educating the public about liver disease and fostering the prevention and treatment of liver disease. A doctor may be involved with the ALF to varying degrees, ranging from being a member to running a support group to lecturing to the public on a topic pertaining to liver disease. Doctors who have demonstrated exceptional dedication to the cause of helping individuals with liver disease are often invited to serve as a board member of the ALF, either at the national or local level. A patient can contact the ALF to inquire about a doctor's level of activity in this organization.

INSURANCE AND HMO PLANS

A full discussion of insurance plans, including HMOs, POSs, and PPOs, is beyond the scope of this book. However, all patients should be aware that if the doctor they decide they would like to consult is not included in their plan, most insurance plans will pay for a visit if—and this is an important if—the doctor offers special or unique services that no other doctor in the plan offers. For example, some liver specialists offer a wealth of experience treating people with liver disease, which greatly exceeds that of any other doctors who are currently listed on the plan, or they are offering treatment options that are not available through any of the other doctors on the plan. In these circumstances, an appeal letter or even a phone call to the appropriate insurance company representative explaining the situation often results in the patient being granted coverage for a consultation with the desired specialist. Also, the patient may want to ask the doctor personally if he would consider joining his health plan.

LIVER DISEASE SPECIALISTS AND THE INTERNET

The Internet may be considered a double-edged sword when it comes to liver disease. It is an ocean of both information and misinformation. Surf with caution. The number of Internet websites continues to grow at an explosive rate. Despite the relative newness of the Internet, there are already thousands of Internet websites devoted to liver disease and hepatitis. It can be difficult for the layperson to determine which information is correct and which is not. It is most important for the patient using the Internet to determine who is sponsoring the website.

Is a pharmaceutical company maintaining the website? For example, Schering-Plough, Roche, and Intermune, three major drug companies that manufacture and distribute pharmaceuticals used in the prevention or treatment of liver disease, all maintain Internet websites. Each of these websites contains useful information, but keep in mind that these companies also are promoting their products. Is it a well-respected hepatologist who maintains the website? For example, I maintain a regularly updated Internet website, and there are a number of other excellent hepatologists who also maintain websites devoted to liver disease. Or, is it a health-care professional who is not a hepatologist? Does a well-established not-for-profit organization maintain the website? For example, ALF and HFI, in addition to many other groups, maintain helpful websites. Is it a knowledgeable patient eager to help others who maintains the site? Or is it a not-so-knowledgeable patient who is giving false and possibly dangerous information? Be careful.

Some websites provide referrals to doctors who purportedly specialize in liver disease. Unfortunately, it is often impossible to ascertain what criteria were used in selecting the referred doctors. Some sites merely require a doctor to pay a fee in order to be listed. While it may be difficult to obtain accurate information from searching the Internet, one generality may be relied on: If the doctor has a website devoted to liver disease, it is likely his practice is focused on taking care of people with liver disease.

CONSULTING WITH THE SPECIALIST

Now that the patient has located a specialist, there are a few tips to follow, which will help make the appointment as smooth and efficient as possible for both the patient and the doctor. It is normal to be nervous about seeing a specialist. So much new and crucial information will be provided to the patient during this visit. It is to be expected that after the initial consultation is over, the patient will not recall a significant amount of what the doctor has said. For this reason, the patient should try to have a relative or close friend along for the consultation. Prior to the visit, the patient should make a list of all of the questions that he wants answered during this visit. The patient should bring this list to the consultation and should not leave the doctor's office until every question has been satisfactorily answered. It's perfectly okay to take short notes while the doctor is talking and to check off each question after the doctor has answered it. If necessary, the patient should request that the doctor write down unfamiliar technical medical terms used during the conversation.

The patient can make the initial consultation more productive for the specialist by bringing all prior records from other doctors to the visit. This will better enable the doctor to promptly and accurately assess the patient's condition on the initial visit. It is especially important to bring the doctor copies of all previously performed blood work, imaging studies, and liver biopsy reports or slides. Doing so will not only assist the doctor, but it can sometimes eliminate the necessity of repeating the tests and/or biopsy.

Remember, all prior records, reports, and slides legally belong to the patient. These records should never be difficult for the patient to obtain. However, most doctors' offices, hospitals, and medical facilities require a written request authorizing the release of the records to another doctor or hospital. Often there is a fee. Be aware that the maximum fee that by law can be charged for medical records is seventy-five cents per page.

Finally, the patient should always bring the doctor a list of all medications, including over-the-counter medications, vitamins, dietary supplements, and/or herbal remedies, that he is taking. The more comprehensive the information the patient provides, the more accurate the specialist's advice will be.

FINDING SECOND OPINIONS

If a patient is not comfortable with the advice he receives from a specialist, it is advisable to seek another opinion. Always make sure that a second opinion is provided by a doctor whose knowledge of liver disease is superior to, or at least equal to, that of the first specialist. However, patients should keep multiple opinions in perspective. Under no circumstances should patients ever make it their objective to shop around for opinions until they hear the diagnosis or prognosis that they are looking for. A game plan of this nature could only cause a serious illness to be left neglected, untreated, or treated inappropriately. It is natural for anyone to hope to hear that there is nothing wrong and that a liver biopsy and treatment aren't necessary. In some cases, these statements may in fact be accurate; however, if the patient has seen two or three well-respected liver specialists, all of whom concur that something is wrong, the patient must accept that he has a chronic illness that may require treatment.

CONCLUSION

It should be the goal of every patient to get the best medical care available. While everyone hopes that his specialist is supplying him with the most accurate and up-to-date information, it is the patient's responsibility to do more than just hope. Patients can and should independently research the expertise level and credentials of a doctor prior to making an appointment for the consultation. Although this is time consuming and requires some effort, there is no question that it is well worth it. Once the "right" specialist has been found, the patient will be proud to have enhanced his prospects for treatment and wellness. The patient can start down the road to recovery by feeling confident in the doctor's abilities and by concentrating on getting better. In the long run, this is actually the quickest route to follow. Don't wait years to find "Dr. Right." Start your search today! Now that you know what to look for in a doctor, the next chapter will tell you what to expect from a liver biopsy.

Five

WHAT YOU SHOULD KNOW ABOUT LIVER BIOPSIES

After a long search, Tom found a liver specialist about whom he felt confident. This specialist provided Tom with an abundance of additional information about liver disease. After reviewing the results of Tom's blood work and the sonogram of Tom's liver, the specialist recommended a liver biopsy. Tom was relieved that he would soon find out what condition his liver was in, but he was also a little nervous— what was undergoing a liver biopsy all about?

All of the aspects of liver biopsies, including exactly what a liver biopsy is, why a biopsy is often necessary for diagnosing a liver problem, and who should avoid having a biopsy are addressed in this chapter. You will also be taken step-by-step through the actual process of the biopsy and provided with information on what to do before and after the procedure has been performed. Although the risks of having a liver biopsy are very low, this chapter will also describe the potential complications of this procedure.

THE LIVER BIOPSY AND WHY IT'S NECESSARY

A *liver biopsy* is the removal of a tiny piece of liver tissue using a special needle. The fragment taken out resembles a one-inch piece of string or a tiny worm. Its removal does not disturb the functioning of the rest of the liver. The liver sample is sent to a laboratory, where it is carefully examined by a pathologist under a microscope. Hepatologists also have expertise in examining liver biopsy specimens and will customarily examine this sample in conjunction with the pathologist.

Microscopes have the capability of greatly magnifying the liver cells— allowing abnormalities to be seen that could not otherwise have been detected by the physical examination, the blood tests, or the imaging studies. The size of the biopsy is approximately 1 to 3 centimeters in length and approximately 1 to 2 millimeters in diameter. This represents about 1/50,000 of the total mass of the liver. Because most liver diseases affect the entire organ uniformly, this tiny sample is usually representative of the entire liver and provides a complete story. It is unlikely that this specimen would look better or worse than the rest of the liver, but it can happen—though very rarely. This uncommon occurrence is known as a *sampling error.*

The liver biopsy is the only diagnostic procedure that can really take the mystery out of liver disease. A biopsy can determine exactly what's wrong with the liver and exactly how badly the liver has been damaged. This information is crucial in order to outline a course of treatment, assess the response to treatment, and determine a prognosis. The information obtained through a liver biopsy cannot be as accurately obtained through any other method, including imaging studies and extensive blood work. Blood tests, such as FIBROSpect, and combinations of blood tests and clinical features, have been evaluated that may assist in the determination of the presence or absence of significant liver scarring without the need of a liver biopsy. However, until this or similar tests that are discussed in detail in the next chapter have been validated, a liver biopsy continues to be "the gold standard."

WHEN A LIVER BIOPSY ISN'T NECESSARY

The doctor and the patient must work together to determine all aspects of the patient's care, including the issue of undergoing a liver biopsy. The potential benefits of the biopsy must outweigh the potential risks. When the risks outweigh the benefits, other approaches to the patient's care are in order. There are two general groups of people who should not have a liver biopsy.

The first group includes individuals for whom a biopsy would lend no additional insight into their treatment or prognosis. For example, a person with acute hepatitis A (see chapter 8) would receive the same treatment regardless of the liver biopsy results. Also, a person with a suspected medication-induced liver disease (see chapter 24) may benefit from discontinuing the medication first and then assessing whether or not the liver-related abnormalities normalize. If they don't, a liver biopsy may then become necessary.

The second group includes people who are simply too ill to undergo a biopsy. For example, a patient who has cirrhosis complicated by ascites runs the risk of leakage of ascitic fluid through the liver biopsy incision site, in addition to multiple other complications such as excessive bleeding. Finally, if the patient is uncooperative—for example, unable to remain still or unwilling to sign a consent form—the biopsy should not be performed.

PREPARING FOR THE LIVER BIOPSY

There are many ways that a person can prepare for the biopsy to maximize the odds that things will go smoothly. Prior to scheduling the biopsy, the patient should make the doctor aware of any drug allergies or of pregnancy or possible pregnancy. Because the liver is packed full of blood vessels, the greatest (although still minimal) risk of complications stems from bleeding. Therefore, as discussed below, all blood-thinning substances should be avoided for at least one week to ten days prior to the biopsy. Also, the patient should ask the doctor for specific instructions on when, in relation to the biopsy, he should stop taking prescribed medications. The patient should also know that more blood work and perhaps a sonogram (if not already done) will be performed.

The doctor will usually request that a patient *fast*—abstain from eating or drinking—for at least eight hours prior to the biopsy. Some doctors, however, may permit a light breakfast in order to allow the gallbladder to empty.

Drugs and Other Substances to Avoid Prior to the Biopsy

Although it's important to keep in mind that bleeding occurs in only a small percentage of biopsies, it is vital that for at least one week to ten days prior to the biopsy and one week after the biopsy, the patient refrain from taking any drugs that interfere with the body's ability to form a clot. This will minimize the danger of excess bleeding. When in doubt as to whether a medication may be taken or not, always ask the doctor or the pharmacist at least ten days prior to the biopsy.

The drugs to be avoided include blood thinners such as Coumadin; antiplatelet medications such as Plavix; aspirin or any of the nonsteroidal anti-inflammatory drugs (NSAIDs) such as ibuprofen (Advil, Motrin, Pamprin, Nuprin, etc.), naproxen (Aleve); and the cyclooxygenase-2 (COX-2) inhibitors (Celebrex, Vioxx, and Bextra). Medications containing acetaminophen (Tylenol) are permissible in moderation. In fact, in doses of less than 4 grams of acetaminophen per day—eight pills or less of acetaminophen taken over a twenty-four-hour period of time—acetaminophen is quite safe for the liver. (Note: Each acetaminophen tablet or pill typically contains 500 mg of acetaminophen.)

Because vitamin E can enhance the effects of drugs like Coumadin and aspirin, it should also be discontinued a week prior to the biopsy. Multivitamin supplements usually contain vitamin E and therefore must also be avoided. Some herbs, such as ginkgo biloba, ginseng, and garlic have blood-thinning properties and should be avoided.

Blood Work and Sonogram

Blood work to assess the risk of bleeding during the procedure—prothrombin time and platelet count—will be performed by the doctor no more than one month but usually within a week or two prior to the biopsy. If one of these tests is very abnormal, a transfusion of fresh frozen plasma (FFP) or platelets may be necessary before proceeding with the biopsy. Alternatively, if the patient has a known bleeding disorder, such as hemophilia, the doctor may suggest having the biopsy done by a special method (see page 58) or avoiding the biopsy altogether.

It is standard procedure for the doctor to take a sonogram of the liver to assess the possible presence of any unusual anatomic abnormalities or the presence of any unsuspected liver masses prior to the biopsy. If an abnormality is detected, the doctor usually has the radiologist perform the biopsy while visualizing the liver with an imaging study (see page 57).

THE DAY OF THE BIOPSY

The patient will be required to make advance arrangements to be driven home from the hospital by a friend or relative on the day of the biopsy. Most biopsies are performed in either a hospital's radiology unit, its gastroenterology procedure suite, or its ambulatory (outpatient) unit. On the day of the biopsy, a consent form must be signed by the patient, formally giving permission for the procedure to take place. If the consent form raises any issues that the doctor hasn't already addressed, the patient should ask for clarification right away.

The patient will be asked to remove all clothing from the waist up and to put on a hospital gown. It's a good idea for the patient to use the restroom at this time. This is because he will not be allowed out of bed for two to six hours after the biopsy. The patient is then asked to lie down on the stretcher or hospital bed and place his right arm beneath his head, so that the doctor may have clear access to his liver.

It's normal to feel anxious prior to any procedure. Therefore, the patient should feel free to request a mild sedative. In this case, a small *intravenous (IV)* catheter will be inserted into a vein in the arm. A small amount of sedative medicine, such as Valium or Versed, will be administered to take the edge off. However, it is not advisable to be totally asleep. It's important for the patient to be alert enough to let the doctor know if there is any pain or other symptoms.

After the biopsy is over, the patient is instructed either to lie flat on his back or to lie on his right side for two to six hours. For most people, the hardest part of the biopsy is having to lie still for this length of time. However, it's an important precautionary measure. If anything is going to go wrong (see "Complications of a Liver Biopsy" on page 58), it is most likely to happen in the first few hours after the procedure has been completed. Fortunately, this waiting period usually turns out to be one long bore—it's a good idea to bring along a book or a personal stereo with earphones to while away the hours. During the waiting period, a nurse will come by regularly to monitor the pulse, blood pressure, breathing, and temperature. Usually, after a few hours have passed, the patient is given a light lunch. Then, two to six hours after the biopsy, it's time to go home.

TECHNIQUES FOR PERFORMING LIVER BIOPSIES

There are many different techniques used in performing a liver biopsy. The actual technique used is dependent upon the patient's overall health in addition to the expertise and preference of the doctor.

The Blind-Stick Method

The classic technique doctors use to perform a liver biopsy is commonly called the "blind percutaneous stick" method. But don't let this somewhat alarming nickname bother you. Although it's true the doctor cannot see the liver through the layers of skin, muscles, and fat that make up the abdomen, an experienced doctor can locate the liver by using a combination of sound and feel. The word *percutaneous* simply means "passage through the skin."

The doctor will begin by asking the patient to lie flat on his back with his right hand under his head and to remain as still as possible. In much the same way that a carpenter might tap a wall to find a hollow area, the doctor will tap the abdomen to determine where the liver is and where it isn't. The next step is to reduce the risk of infection by cleaning the skin with an antiseptic agent and by covering the biopsy site with sterile towels. The antiseptic may feel a bit cool to the touch. Then, the doctor will inject a local anesthetic agent, such as Lidocaine, into this area in order to numb the skin. The injection usually stings a little, but this mild discomfort generally disappears after a few seconds. Once the anesthetic has taken effect, the doctor will make a very tiny nick in the skin about the size of a pinhead over the area where he determined the liver to be. While some doctors instruct the patient to hold his breath at this point, others instruct the patient to just breathe normally.

The biopsy itself involves a quick jab with a special needle through the skin, into the liver, and out again. This jab literally takes no longer than one-tenth of a second. The needle will suction out one or two tiny slivers of liver, about one to one-and-a-half inches long. The procedure is now over! Remember, with the exception of the skin, the liver is the largest organ in the body; therefore, an experienced specialist should have little difficulty locating it by using the blind percutaneous stick method.

Occasionally, the liver sample isn't large enough, and the doctor may have to insert the biopsy needle a second time. This may happen if the liver has become so hardened by cirrhosis that the needle has difficulty penetrating the liver's surface or in cases where the patient is very obese.

The doctor will now put a bandage over the insertion point and will ask the patient to lie either flat or on the right side for the next two to six hours. At this point, most patients can't believe that the biopsy is over. They wonder what they were so nervous about in the first place. From start to finish, the entire procedure should take no longer than ten minutes.

The Ultrasound-Guided Biopsy

The ultrasound-guided biopsy has now become the most commonly used technique to perform a liver biopsy. The ultrasound-guided biopsy is performed either by the radiologist in the radiology suite or by the gastroenterologist or hepatologist after the radiologist has marked a safe area (via ultrasound) to guide the biopsy needle to the liver. Some gastroenterologists and hepatologists have been trained to mark his or her own site using the ultrasound. In any case, most studies suggest that there are less complications and less biopsy pain when ultrasound guidance is used.

A sonogram or a computerized tomography (CT)–guided biopsy may also be used in situations where more precision is required. Such cases arise when the doctor is uncertain about the location of an appropriate site to insert the needle or when the doctor wants to sample an abnormal growth found in one specific area of the liver. In rare cases, other organs, such as the gallbladder or the intestines, may be in the way of the liver, making it more difficult to find. Or, if the patient is extremely overweight, the liver may be surrounded by so many layers of fat that it can be difficult to locate. Or, if cirrhosis is present, the liver may have shrunk so much that some doctors need extra help in finding it. In any of these scenarios, or due to the personal preference of the doctor, the doctor may decide to use a sonogram or a CT scan to guide the biopsy needle to the liver.

Other Biopsy Methods

The other methods used to obtain a liver specimen are somewhat more complicated. In some special cases, a radiologist will be brought in to perform what is called a transvenous or transjugular liver biopsy. This technique is used if a patient has a problem with blood clotting, known as *coagulopathy,* which is defined as a prolonged prothrombin time of greater than 3 seconds; or if the patient has a platelet count of less than 60 x10^3/microliter, known as *thrombocytopenia;* or if the patient has *ascites,* an abnormal accumulation of fluids in the abdomen; or if the patient is morbidly obese.

A small tube is first inserted into a vein in the neck (the jugular vein) and is then directed into the vein that drains the liver (the hepatic vein). The biopsy needle is threaded through this tube and into the liver, and a sample of liver tissue is retrieved.

Another technique is known as the laparoscopic liver biopsy. It is usually performed in the operating room by a surgeon, but some liver specialists are trained in this procedure. It involves the insertion of a thin, lighted tube—a *laparoscope*—into a small incision made in the abdominal wall, in order to directly view the liver. A biopsy needle is inserted into this lighted tube, and a sample of liver tissue is retrieved.

Finally, if a patient is undergoing open abdominal surgery for an unrelated reason, a liver sample can be taken by the surgeon at that time.

COMPLICATIONS OF A LIVER BIOPSY

As with any invasive procedure, there are inherent risks involved. The good news is that in the hands of a qualified, experienced doctor, the incidence of problems resulting from a liver biopsy is extraordinarily rare and, if caught in time, can generally be corrected. In fact, complications from a liver biopsy have been reported in less than 1 percent of all individuals undergoing the procedure. And with ultrasound-guided liver biopsy the complication rate is even lower. Moreover, the risk of death from a liver biopsy is virtually unheard of—occurring in approximately 0.01 percent of patients, resulting from one of the complications discussed below.

The incidence of complications increases with the number of attempts to obtain a piece of liver, and most are evident within the first few hours after the procedure. This is the reason for the two- to six-hour waiting period after the procedure has been performed. Early recognition is the most important aspect in the treatment of any complications resulting from the biopsy. It is extremely important to contact the doctor if you suspect any problems have occurred as a result of the biopsy. The following are some potential complications that may occur as a result of this procedure.

Bleeding

Most incidents of bleeding after a liver biopsy are inconsequential and do not require treatment. If massive bleeding does occur, however, it can usually be treated with blood transfusions and close monitoring in the intensive care unit of a hospital. Only rarely will surgical intervention be required. Bleeding usually results from puncturing an enlarged blood vessel within the liver, which sometimes cannot be avoided. Bleeding is usually evident within the first few hours after a liver biopsy.

Puncture of Other Organs

Since the liver is surrounded by so many other organs, sometimes the kidney, colon, or lung may be punctured in error. The incidence of this may be reduced by having an ultrasound-guided biopsy performed. However, when this complication occurs, it rarely results in any serious problems, as the small puncture hole typically closes and heals on its own. However, a hospital stay is usually in order. An exception to this is the uncommon instance of puncturing the gallbladder or its bile ducts, which can result in leakage of bile into the abdomen, thereby causing *peritonitis*—an infection of the abdominal fluid. This is usually treated with intravenous antibiotics, admission to the hospital, and drainage of the bile with a small catheter. Since a sterile technique is used during a liver biopsy, other types of infection are rare, but when they occur, they are usually transient, mild, and easily treated with antibiotics.

Pain

Most people agree that their liver biopsy was relatively painless and much easier than they ever expected it to be. While not actually a complication, pain is the most common complaint after a biopsy. Approximately 30 percent of liver biopsy patients state that they felt as if someone had quickly punched them in the side, or they describe a dull, aching sensation in the right shoulder. Pain may also occur around the stomach and over the site of the needle stick, but is typically mild. Any discomfort is best remedied by taking one or two acetaminophen tablets. This discomfort will usually resolve within an hour. Remember, don't take any NSAIDs or aspirin-based products either a week before or after the biopsy, as they can increase the chance of bleeding.

If the patient finds that he is still in pain more than twenty-four hours after having left the hospital, or that the pain is getting worse, he should call his doctor immediately and return to the hospital's emergency room.

WHAT TO DO AFTER THE BIOPSY

After undergoing a biopsy, the patient should take it easy the first day. He should refrain from doing any heavy lifting or undertaking any strenuous activities. In addition, he should not drive for at least twenty-four hours or undertake any energetic activities, including dancing and sports. If severe pain, shortness of breath, abdominal distention, fever, or chills should occur, it is prudent to contact the doctor and return to the hospital. After twenty-four hours, he can remove the bandage and take a bath or a shower. If the patient has a physically demanding job, he should plan to stay out of work for at least forty-eight to seventy-two hours. People who have desk jobs may return to work the next day.

It may take as long as a week to obtain the results of the biopsy. It is best for the patient to make a follow-up appointment with the doctor to discuss these findings at length. It is also a good idea for the patient to bring a family member or close friend along to assist in asking questions concerning the results.

CONCLUSION

After reading this chapter, any fears a person has about undergoing a liver biopsy should be significantly, if not totally, alleviated. You should now feel confident that a liver biopsy is a very quick and relatively painless procedure with an extremely low complication rate when performed by an experienced doctor. In fact, recent advances, such as ultrasound-guided biopsies and the administration of a mild anesthetic during the biopsy, have made this procedure safer and more painless than ever. The most important purpose of undergoing a biopsy is to determine the degree of scarring that has occurred in the liver. Total scarring of the liver is known as cirrhosis. The next chapter discusses cirrhosis, which can occur as a result of a number of different liver diseases.

Six

A LOOK AT CIRRHOSIS

Tom's liver biopsy went smoothly. It was much easier than he had ex-
pected it to be. He made an appointment for the following week to
discuss the results with his specialist. Tom's wife went to the follow-
up appointment with him. When the receptionist led them into the
doctor's private consultation office, Tom's anxiety level rose. Once
the couple was seated, the doctor said, "Tom, the results from the
biopsy indicate that you have cirrhosis." "Cirrhosis?!" Tom ex-
claimed. "What is cirrhosis, and how did I get it?"

In this chapter, you are provided with an in-depth description of cirrhosis—
severe scarring of the liver. The symptoms and signs associated with cirrhosis are described and the diagnosis of cirrhosis is discussed. This chapter will
also address which liver diseases can lead to cirrhosis, and what the potential
complications of this condition are. Finally, this chapter will discuss some potential therapies that may reverse cirrhosis in its earliest stages.

WHAT IS CIRRHOSIS?

The liver is an incredibly resilient organ, but unfortunately it isn't indestructible.
Sometimes the damage that occurs as a result of excessive alcohol, a virus, or
some other chronic disease overwhelms the liver's capacity to function. Healthy
liver cells are destroyed and scarring occurs. Scarring, known as *fibrosis,* is the
liver's effort to keep the damage done by alcohol or the hepatitis C virus (HCV),
for example, contained. But scar tissue can block the blood flow through the liver,
resulting in an inability of the liver to perform its normal duties. If alcohol, or
HCV, is not eliminated from the body, scarring becomes extensive. The liver
becomes rock hard and nodular (lumpy). This condition is known as *cirrhosis.*
Although the presence of cirrhosis does not signify that health problems will

inevitably develop, a person with cirrhosis should be aware that he is at an increased risk of suffering many serious complications.

Cirrhosis is the end product of any one of a number of different liver diseases, which will be discussed briefly on page 63 and in more detail in later chapters. Regardless of the cause, the potential consequences of cirrhosis are the same. Whereas a healthy liver typically repairs and regenerates itself when injured, once cirrhosis has occurred, the damage may never be undone.

When I was a student at Mount Sinai Medical School in the early 1980s, I was taught that cirrhosis was irreversible. In fact, even as recently as the publication of the first edition of this book, the year 2000, it was still the gospel belief among most liver disease experts that, while cirrhosis could occasionally be slowed or even halted, it could never be reversed. However, some recent studies have shown that with removal of the cause of the underlying liver disease—alcohol or the hepatitis C virus (HCV), for example—and with effective treatment, cirrhosis can be reversed, at least in its very early stages, when scarring is minimal. Recent progress has been made in the control and reversal of cirrhosis. This is confirmed by the decline in the number of cirrhosis-related deaths in the United States over the last twenty years. Therapies such as interferon and ribavirin for chronic hepatitis C, and Epivir and Hepsera for chronic hepatitis B, have been shown to reverse cirrhosis in its early stages. There have been anecdotal reports of scarring being reversed after treatment in people with autoimmune hepatitis (chapter 14), primary biliary cirrhosis (chapter 15), and hemochromatosis (chapter 18). Thus, cirrhosis should no longer be considered an irreversible condition.

The point at which cirrhosis becomes irreversible is not clear. But there is a broad consensus among liver disease experts that once cirrhosis has advanced to its late stages—when complications from extensive scarring have occurred (known as *decompensated cirrhosis*), it can never be reversed. And cirrhosis continues to be the eighth most common cause of death overall in the United States and the fourth leading cause of death among Americans between the ages of thirty and sixty. But being diagnosed with cirrhosis is not necessarily a death sentence. Usually, when cirrhosis is fatal, it is because it has proceeded unchecked and untreated for many years. If, however, it is caught in its early stages, there will often be steps that the patient and doctor can take to control, and possibly even reverse, its progression.

Despite having cirrhosis, many people have lived well past the age of ninety. Of course, prevention remains the best medicine; therefore, most of the treatments doctors prescribe, as well as the nutrition and exercise tips discussed in chapter 23, are aimed at trying to keep the liver from progressing to cirrhosis in the first place.

LIVER DISEASES THAT CAN LEAD TO CIRRHOSIS

Not all liver diseases cause cirrhosis—only those that cause chronic, ongoing damage to the liver can lead to permanent scarring of liver tissue. For example, someone with hepatitis A will usually recover completely after a few weeks and, as such, will not be at risk for developing cirrhosis. But someone who has lived for decades with a chronic liver condition, such as hepatitis C or hemochromatosis, would be a prime candidate for cirrhosis.

Fortunately, in most cases, cirrhosis takes many years to develop. Therefore, just because a person is at risk for cirrhosis doesn't necessarily mean that he will definitely develop this condition over the course of a normal life span. Also, the slow pace at which cirrhosis develops allows a person to obtain treatment from a liver specialist before cirrhosis occurs.

Alcoholic liver disease and chronic hepatitis C are the two most common causes of cirrhosis in the United States. However, there are other circumstances that can give rise to permanent liver damage. Even some herbal remedies and medications can trigger massive scarring of the liver (see chapters 21 and 24, respectively). Although a discussion of every condition that has the potential to cause cirrhosis is beyond the scope of this book, some causes include the following:

- Viral hepatitis—hepatitis B, C, and D

- Autoimmune hepatitis

- Primary biliary cirrhosis

- Nonalcoholic fatty liver disease (NAFLD)

- Excess alcohol consumption

- Hemochromatosis

- Excessive intake of vitamins, such as vitamin A (see chapter 23)

- Certain herbal remedies, such as comfrey (see chapter 21)

- Certain medications, such as methotrexate, isoniazid, and Aldomet (see chapter 24)

- Primary sclerosing cholangitis (see chapter 15)

- Vascular anomalies—for example, Budd-Chiari syndrome (see chapter 21)

- Congestive heart failure (see your doctor for more information)

- *Wilson's disease,* a genetic disorder of copper overload (see your doctor for more information)

THE SYMPTOMS AND SIGNS OF CIRRHOSIS

The symptoms and physical signs of cirrhosis are essentially uniform regardless of its cause. The silent nature of liver disease, as discussed in chapter 2, means that it often leaves few obvious clues as to the extent of the damage being done.

Some people with cirrhosis feel perfectly normal or have vague symptoms, such as fatigue, decreased appetite, nausea, and loss of libido. These individuals are known as having *compensated cirrhosis*. People with compensated cirrhosis often live a normal life span with relatively few health-related consequences due to cirrhosis. However, they remain at risk for developing potentially fatal complications, such as internal bleeding, encephalopathy, and/or ascites. When one of these complications develops, it is known as *decompensated cirrhosis*. While the complications of decompensated cirrhosis can be controlled, the liver is now beyond the point of any possible repair, and a liver transplant must be considered. The potential complications of cirrhosis will be discussed in more detail on page 65. Liver transplantation is discussed in chapter 22.

DIAGNOSING CIRRHOSIS

As discussed in chapter 2, the doctor may be able to detect signs of cirrhosis on a physical exam. General signs of malnutrition, such as muscle wasting, will be looked for. The doctor will pay close attention to the texture and size of the liver. As opposed to the soft, smooth feel of a healthy liver, a cirrhotic liver feels hard and bumpy. This is because normal liver tissue has now been replaced by scar tissue and nodules.

The size of the liver is variable. Despite what most people think, a cirrhotic liver may stay the same size, shrivel up, or enlarge (a condition known as hepatomegaly). As discussed on page 22, the spleen may enlarge—a condition known as splenomegaly—to compensate for the decreased functional abilities of the damaged liver.

A digital rectal exam will be performed to check for signs of internal bleeding. Upper intestinal bleeding produces distinctive black, foul-smelling stools known as *melena*. A person experiencing such a condition should bring it to his doctor's immediate attention, as this may be a sign of decompensated cirrhosis and may require emergency treatment.

Some laboratory test results may suggest cirrhosis. These results include a low albumin level, an abnormally low cholesterol level, an elevated or prolonged prothrombin time, a decreased platelet count, and/or an elevated *alpha-fetoprotein (AFP)* level of 100 ng/ml (nanograms per milliliter). (See chapter 3 for a discussion of these tests.) Imaging studies of the liver may suggest, but cannot confirm, cirrhosis. Ultimately, the only way to confirm the suspicion of cirrhosis is through a liver biopsy. However, this may change in the future as new noninvasive methods involving combinations of blood tests are being developed as a possible way to diagnose cirrhosis without a liver biopsy. *FIBROSpect* is a blood test developed by Prometheus Laboratories that can differentiate among degrees of liver scarring in people with hepatitis C who are unable or unwilling to undergo a liver biopsy. The FIBROSpect blood test is undergoing testing for its validity in other liver diseases as well. Similarly, researchers from France have utilized another blood test known as the FIBROTest to predict the presence or absence of cirrhosis. And researchers from Spain have developed a fibrosis index based on age, GGT, platelet count, and cholesterol level that appears to be quite accurate in predicting the level of scarring. However, until these tests have been validated, a liver biopsy continues to be the the gold standard to determine the presence or absence of cirrhosis.

In general, cirrhosis looks pretty much the same, regardless of which type of liver disease caused it. As such, once cirrhosis has occurred, a physician will not be able to definitively identify which liver disorder caused it, even from a liver biopsy specimen.

THE POTENTIAL COMPLICATIONS OF CIRRHOSIS

Chapter 1 discussed the liver's varied functions—actions that are essential to our daily existence. Cirrhosis interferes with these everyday functions. Although the presence of cirrhosis does not signify that health problems will inevitably develop, a person with cirrhosis should be aware that he is at an increased risk of suffering many serious complications. These complications are discussed in detail below. Treatments for some of these potential complications will be discussed in chapter 20.

Bleeding Problems

A normally functioning liver makes numerous factors—known as *coagulation factors*—that help blood clot. When the liver becomes scarred, it can no longer effectively produce these factors. Therefore, some people with cirrhosis have difficulty clotting, which is manifested by a tendency to bleed excessively. This is known as *coagulopathy.* A person experiencing this complication may find that his daily routine has become a challenge—for such a person, simple activities, such as brushing one's teeth or shaving, may result in a severe bleeding episode.

The doctor can detect coagulopathy by performing a blood test. An elevated or prolonged prothrombin time (PT) (see chapter 3) will indicate the presence, but not the cause, of coagulopathy. Administration of vitamin K may correct coagulopathy if it is due to cholestasis. However, simply replenishing vitamin K stores in the body will not help if cirrhosis is the cause, as the liver will be too damaged to properly synthesize this vitamin. Transfusions of fresh frozen plasma (FFP) will temporarily stop bleeding and should be given in emergency situations or prior to undergoing any invasive procedure or surgery. Note that people usually do not have excessive bleeding unless the PT is prolonged for more than three seconds above normal values (normal being nine to eleven seconds).

Another cause of excessive bleeding in people with cirrhosis may be *thrombocytopenia,* a low platelet count (see chapter 3). Platelets are also intricately involved in helping blood to clot. The spleen plays an important role in the storage of platelets. An enlarged spleen (splenomegaly) often occurs in people with cirrhosis. This indicates that the spleen is working overtime, which often results in a diminished platelet count. Transfusions of platelets will temporarily stop bleeding and should be given in emergency situations or prior to undergoing any invasive procedure or surgery. Note that people usually do not have excessive bleeding unless the platelet count falls to under 25×10^3 (normal values being 150×10^3), but a transfusion of platelets is usually considered at a platelet count of 50 to 75×10^3 if a patient is undergoing surgery.

It is important for people with cirrhosis, especially those with bleeding tendencies, to avoid medications such as aspirin and other nonsteroidal anti-inflammatories. These may cause or worsen bleeding, as can herbs such as ginkgo and garlic, which have anticoagulant properties.

Kidney Problems

Damage to the body's largest filtering organ, the liver, puts a great deal of stress on the body's other major filtering organ—the kidneys. Many kidney disorders have been associated with cirrhosis. The most common of these is fluid retention, resulting in edema and ascites. This is usually treated with water pills, known as *diuretics,* and a special low-sodium (low-salt) diet.

The most serious complication associated with the kidneys is known as *hepatorenal syndrome (HRS).* HRS is defined as progressive deterioration of kidney function occurring in a person with advanced liver disease. This usually happens in patients who are already in the hospital due to other complications of cirrhosis. HRS can result in death unless a liver transplantation is performed. Since this complication is associated with lack of urination, kidney dialysis may be necessary as a time-gaining measure until liver transplantation can be performed. HRS can be prevented by avoiding the use of medications that can damage the kidneys, such as aminoglycosides (gentamycin, for example) or nonsteroidal anti-inflammatory drugs (NSAIDs such as Motrin and Advil) and by avoiding the overuse of diuretics used to treat fluid accumulation. Early recognition and prompt treatment of other complications of cirrhosis, such as infection and internal bleeding, may also prevent this syndrome from occurring.

Osteoporosis (Bone Loss)

Osteoporosis is a condition marked by decreased bone mass and density. This leads to a weakening of bones, thereby increasing the risk of bone fractures. People with any chronic liver disease are at increased risk for the development of osteoporosis due to a lack of activity resulting from excessive fatigue, poor nutritional habits, reduced muscle mass, and impaired production of hormones, known as *hypogonadism.* See chapter 20 for a full discussion of osteoporosis.

Hepatocellular Carcinoma (HCC)/Hepatoma (Liver Cancer)

Anyone who has cirrhosis—whether compensated or decompensated—is at risk for developing liver cancer, also known as *hepatocellular carcinoma (HCC)* or *hepatoma*. Risk varies with the cause of liver disease. *Prognosis* (the anticipated course of a disease without treatment) depends upon many factors. Liver cancer will be discussed in detail in chapter 19. It should be noted that if a person with cirrhosis has unexplained weight loss or abdominal pain, an extensive search for liver cancer should be undertaken.

Other Cancers

Aside from liver cancer, other types of cancer have been found to occur with above-average frequency in those with cirrhosis. These cancers include lung, larynx, pancreas, kidney, urinary bladder, pharynx, colon, and breast.

Some of these cancers are particularly prevalent in people with cirrhosis who drink excessive amounts of alcohol and smoke cigarettes. Whether cirrhosis leads to an increased risk of cancer or whether a person's lifestyle habits are the cause of the cancer is unknown. Most likely it is due to a combination of factors. In any case, people who have, or who are at risk for, cirrhosis are advised to avoid all use of alcohol and tobacco.

Portal Hypertension and Decompensated Cirrhosis

Most people are familiar with the word *hypertension*—the medical term for high blood pressure. But most people do not know that the liver can suffer from its own type of high blood pressure, which is known as *portal hypertension*. Due to extensive scarring of the liver that occurs in cirrhosis, the vessels associated with blood flow to and from the liver may become obstructed. This, in combination with increased blood flow to the liver, leads to elevated pressure in the portal circulation.

The liver—a very resourceful organ—attempts to adapt to the above situation by creating alternative routes that bypass this obstruction. These alternative passageways for blood flow are known as *collateral shunts* or simply *collaterals*. These shunts enable blood to be rerouted to and circulated throughout the rest of the body. Unfortunately, the formation of these shunts has its drawbacks, as they can give rise to serious and even life-threatening complications. Once any one of the complications associated with portal hypertension—ascites, esophageal varices, portal gastropathy, and encephalopathy—has occurred, it means that the body can no longer compensate for the extensive scarring that has occurred in the liver. Such a patient no longer has compensated cirrhosis. Rather, he is considered to have decompensated cirrhosis. People with any form of portal hypertension should be evaluated for liver transplantation. The following is a discussion of the complications of portal hypertension. The treatment of these complications will be discussed in chapter 20.

Ascites

Ascites is the most common complication of portal hypertension. Once ascites has developed, the patient now has decompensated cirrhosis. The chances of this person living one year drops from greater than 90 percent to less than 50 percent. Thus, the development of ascites is a serious complication that requires prompt evaluation and treatment. *Ascites* is a disorder characterized by massive accumulation of fluid in the *peritoneal cavity*—the space between the abdominal organs and the skin. In addition, the kidneys tend to retain sodium and water in people with portal hypertension, leading to further fluid accumulation. This accumulation results in abdominal swelling and distention. In most cases, the disorder is readily apparent to the doctor on a physical exam. In cases where the diagnosis of ascites is suspected but not obvious, an abdominal sonogram can be used to detect whether small amounts of ascitic fluid, often as little as 100 ml, have accumulated. A fever in a person with established ascites may indicate that an infection of this fluid is present. This is a serious, life-threatening condition known as *spontaneous bacterial peritonitis (SBP)* and needs to be treated with hospitalization and emergent intravenous (IV) antibiotics.

It is estimated that half of the people with compensated cirrhosis will develop ascites within approximately ten years. While the presence of ascites usually stems from cirrhosis, there are other causes of ascites unrelated to liver disease, such as kidney failure, heart failure, or ovarian cancer.

Varices

Varices are enlarged, distended blood vessels that result from the formation of collateral shunts in people with portal hypertension. (Think of varices as varicose veins that occur inside the body.) Approximately 45 (range 20 to 70) percent of people with cirrhosis have varices, and an individual with cirrhosis has approximately a 6 percent chance in a given year of developing varices. While varices may occur in many parts of the body, those occurring in the *esophagus* (food pipe) and upper portion of the stomach are the most likely to burst and hemorrhage, and large varices are more likely to bleed than small varices. Bursting occurs about one-third of the time and usually results in profuse, uncontrollable vomiting of bright-red blood. This is known as *hematemesis*. Hematemesis is a life-and-death emergency that requires immediate hospitalization and therapy. Approximately 30 percent of episodes of hematemesis from esophageal varices result in death.

An *upper endoscopy* is required for both diagnosis and treatment of bleeding esophageal varices. An upper endoscopy is a procedure in which a thin tube with a light at the end—somewhat like a flexible telescope—is inserted into the patient's mouth and passed into the esophagus, stomach, and duodenum. This simple procedure does not hurt and is usually done after the administration of intravenous conscious sedation—which means that the patient is given a mild sedative medication, such as Versed, Valium, or Demerol, through an IV. As a result, the procedure does not cause the patient to experience any pain. In fact, patients usually do not remember having the procedure performed at all. Most liver disease experts recommend that an upper endoscopy be performed every two to three years on patients with cirrhosis to determine the presence of esophageal varices and to assess the risk of bleeding.

Varices also can occur in the rectum, and in some cases these varices may bleed. The bleeding of rectal varices is sometimes mistaken for hemorrhoidal bleeding. Since these two conditions are unrelated and, as such, entail different treatments, it is important for the doctor to differentiate between them. Usually, bleeding from rectal varices is treated in much the same manner as esophageal variceal bleeding. Varices can also occur in other parts of the gastrointestinal tract—such as the large and small intestines—but bleeding is relatively infrequent from these areas. Therapies for varices will be discussed in greater detail in chapter 20.

Congestive Gastropathy

Up to 50 percent of people with cirrhosis are likely to bleed due to a buildup of pressure in the stomach known as *portal hypertensive gastropathy* or *congestive gastropathy*. This cause of bleeding must be distinguished from other causes of bleeding that can occur in people with cirrhosis. These other causes include esophageal or gastric varices, peptic ulcer disease, and *gastritis*—inflammation of the stomach. These disorders, as well as congestive gastropathy, are diagnosed by an upper endoscopy. Treatment depends on the source of bleeding.

Encephalopathy

Encephalopathy is an altered or impaired mental status, typically leading to coma, which can occur in people with cirrhosis. Encephalopathy is often associated with poor coordination, fetor hepaticus (foul-smelling breath), and asterixis (uncontrollable flapping of the hands (see chapter 2). The exact cause of encephalopathy is not known but is probably due to a combination of factors. Most researchers believe that it mainly has something to do with the ailing liver's inability to clear toxins—primarily ammonia—from the body. In fact, elevated blood levels of ammonia are found in approximately 90 percent of people with encephalopathy. When ammonia and other poisons begin to accumulate in the brain, a variety of mental disturbances occurs.

In mild cases—known as minimal hepatic encephalopathy—a person will develop subtle personality changes (such as irritability), a change in sleeping patterns, short-term memory loss, shortened attention span, apathy toward life, or poorly coordinated movements. People suffering from encephalopathy will commonly lose their tempers over minor incidents or have mood swings for no apparent reason. They also may repeatedly enter a room, forgetting what they needed from the room in the first place, or may continually misplace common objects such as reading glasses, only to find that the glasses were on top of their head the whole time! These people may also have an increased incidence of automobile accidents, as their reaction time may be somewhat impaired.

In more severe cases, total confusion associated with inappropriate behavior will occur. A person may become outright violent or may be so confused that he cannot properly identify the current year, season, or even his own family members. Sometimes a person will sleep all day and can only be partially aroused. This obviously is a more serious condition and requires hospitalization.

In most cases, encephalopathy is easily detected on a physical examination in a patient known to have cirrhosis. Whenever there is a question about the diagnosis, an imaging study, such as a CT scan or an MRI, of the brain should be performed in order to eliminate other potential causes, such as a brain tumor, blood clot, or meningitis (brain infection). The factors that can precipitate encephalopathy in the cirrhotic patient should be searched for and immediately addressed by the doctor. These factors as well as the treatment of encephalopathy will be discussed in chapter 20.

CONCLUSION

In this chapter, you learned that cirrhosis, originally believed to be an irreversible condition of scarring of the liver, can at times be reversed. This typically requires targeted and aggressive treatment in addition to removal of the specific cause of cirrhosis. You also learned that a person may live a long healthy life with compensated cirrhosis. However, once the disease has progressed to decompensated cirrhosis, the potentially fatal complications of portal hypertension can occur. Many of the liver diseases that can potentially lead to cirrhosis will be discussed throughout the remainder of this book. Part 2 of this book will discuss another term, which is often misused and misunderstood—*hepatitis*.

Part Two

Understanding and Treating Viral Hepatitis

Seven

AN OVERALL LOOK
AT HEPATITIS

The results of Tom's liver biopsy revealed that he had cirrhosis. But how did he get it? Tom wanted to know. The doctor told him that his cirrhosis—still in its early stages—was caused by hepatitis. Tom's doctor suggested that he start therapy, in an attempt to halt or slow the progression of his cirrhosis. But Tom was very confused and wondered to himself, "How did I get hepatitis? How can I have both hepatitis and cirrhosis? Did hepatitis lead to cirrhosis? Will I still be able to work? Can I infect my wife and son?" Tom's doctor answered all of his questions, putting his concerns to rest.

This chapter explains the concept of *hepatitis*—a medical term that is often misunderstood and misused. It outlines the differences between acute, chronic, and fulminant hepatitis, and also discusses the multiple causes of hepatitis. In addition, this chapter helps you to distinguish between viral hepatitis and other causes of hepatitis. The symptoms and physical signs associated with hepatitis are discussed, as well as the way in which a doctor arrives at a diagnosis. This includes a discussion of liver function test (LFT) abnormalities and the necessity of imaging studies and/or a liver biopsy. Treatment is briefly discussed but will be dealt with in greater detail in the respective chapters for each type of hepatitis. This chapter also provides a brief overview of the different types of viral hepatitis and helps to dispel some common misconceptions about viral hepatitis. Finally, this chapter provides a preview of the immune system—the body's personal army in the fight against viruses—and how it relates to viral hepatitis. The natural history of a disease (the course that a disease most likely will take if untreated) and the prognosis of a disease are discussed in the corresponding chapters on each type of hepatitis.

WHAT IS HEPATITIS?

Many people mistakenly believe that the medical term *hepatitis* is synonymous with the medical term *viral hepatitis,* and that all forms of hepatitis are contagious. Actually, the word *hepatitis* is a catchall term that refers to any inflammation (*-itis*) of the liver (*hepar*) and does not imply a specific cause or connote contagiousness. (Inflammation of the liver is defined as an irritation or swelling of liver cells.)

Hepatitis is a term that encompasses many different causes. Only hepatitis caused by a virus (viral hepatitis) is potentially infectious to others. Consequently, hepatitis from causes other than that of viruses cannot be spread through food or by interpersonal or sexual contact.

Hepatitis is generally described using two broad categories. One category refers to how long a person has hepatitis—acute, chronic, or fulminant. The other category refers to what factor caused the hepatitis—viral hepatitis, autoimmune hepatitis, nonalcoholic fatty liver hepatitis, alcoholic hepatitis, or toxin-induced hepatitis. For example, a person may be described as having acute hepatitis B or chronic hepatitis C. The next few pages will describe these categories in more detail.

DIFFERENCES BETWEEN ACUTE, CHRONIC, AND FULMINANT HEPATITIS

One way of categorizing hepatitis is by how long inflammation in the liver lasts. As such, hepatitis is divided into two broad types—acute hepatitis and chronic hepatitis. Another type of hepatitis, fulminant hepatitis, is an especially severe form of acute hepatitis, and thus may be considered the third type of hepatitis.

Inflammation of the liver that lasts less than six months is known as *acute hepatitis.* Within six months, many people with acute hepatitis, regardless of the cause, are completely healed. However, some people do progress from acute to chronic hepatitis, and some experience a particularly severe, potentially fatal form of acute hepatitis—fulminant hepatitis. In people with acute hepatitis who do not progress to chronic or fulminant hepatitis, the inflammation in the liver totally subsides. All of the symptoms, signs, and LFT abnormalities associated with this condition resolve. The liver typically self-repairs any short-term damage it may have suffered. No permanent damage is done to the liver, and the person does not suffer any long-term consequences.

Inflammation of the liver that lasts longer than six months is known as *chronic hepatitis.* People who progress from acute hepatitis to chronic hepatitis are at risk of developing cirrhosis and the complications of cirrhosis. Those with acute hepatitis who progress to chronic hepatitis typically have very mild or no symptoms, and it is not always possible for the doctor to identify who will progress to chronic hepatitis or suffer from fulminant hepatitis.

The third category of hepatitis is known as *fulminant hepatitis.* Fulminant hepatitis is a particularly serious form of acute hepatitis associated with jaundice, coagulopathy, and encephalopathy. In these people, liver failure occurs abruptly, usually within approximately eight weeks from the onset of symptoms or within approximately two weeks from the onset of jaundice.

THE CAUSES OF HEPATITIS

Hepatitis is also described by its cause. Although hepatitis is most frequently caused by viruses, other causes include autoimmune liver disease, obesity, alcohol, and some medications and herbs. Don't forget, the precise meaning of hepatitis is simply "inflammation of the liver." The following is a brief discussion of these causes, which will be discussed in more detail in later chapters.

Viruses

A *virus* is a tiny microorganism that is much smaller than bacteria. Its main activity and goal consist of reproducing more viruses. A virus is capable of growth and multiplication only once it has entered a living cell. The main goal of the hepatitis virus is to enter a liver cell, reproduce more hepatitis viruses, destroy the cell, and move on to attack the next liver cell.

At least five different viruses specifically attack the liver leading to viral hepatitis. These are known as hepatitis viruses. Each type of viral hepatitis is different, and they all have distinct characteristics. They are known by alphabetical names: hepatitis A through E. Four other viruses, hepatitis F (probably nonexistent), hepatitis G, the *transfusion-transmitted virus (TTV),* and S.E.N.-V (S.E.N. are the initials of the person in whom the virus was first isolated; "V" stands for virus) may also specifically attack the liver. When infection with one of these viruses causes inflammation of the liver, the resulting condition is known as viral hepatitis. (Other viruses, such as herpes simplex virus and Epstein-Barr virus, can also attack the liver. However, since the liver is not the principal organ damaged by these viruses, they are not considered hepatitis viruses and will not be covered in this book.) Hepatitis A, B and D, and C, will be discussed in detail in chapters 8, 9, and 10, respectively.

Autoimmunity

Autoimmune diseases occur when the body's immune system fails to recognize one of its own organs as belonging to itself. The immune system then attacks that organ in an attempt to remove the "foreign intruder" from the body. When the organ under attack fights back, it becomes inflamed. In a case when the immune system attacks the liver, the liver becomes inflamed as it fights back. This condition is known as *autoimmune hepatitis* and will be discussed in chapter 14.

Obesity

Many of the health risks of being overweight, such as heart disease, diabetes, and high blood pressure, are well known. But few people are aware of the extent to which being overweight can adversely affect the liver. Being overweight can cause excess fat to deposit in the liver, causing inflammation. This is known as *nonalcoholic fatty liver hepatitis,* since it occurs in people who do not drink excessive amounts of alcohol. Being overweight is just one component of fatty liver hepatitis, a disease that will be discussed in detail in chapter 16.

Alcohol

It is common knowledge that alcohol can be harmful to the liver. Drinking too much alcohol can lead to inflammation of the liver. This is known as *alcoholic hepatitis* and will be discussed in chapter 17. Many additional factors, such as being female, genetic vulnerability, diet, and infection with the hepatitis B or C virus, may worsen the effects of alcohol on the liver. This will be discussed in chapter 17.

Medications and Herbs

Certain medications and herbs can cause both acute and chronic inflammation of the liver, in addition to other liver damage. This particular type of hepatitis is known as *drug-induced* or *toxin-induced hepatitis.* A substance that is harmful or damaging to the liver is referred to as *hepatotoxic* or as a *hepatotoxin.* In drug- or toxin-induced hepatitis, withdrawal of the hepatotoxic herb or medication combined with subsequent resolution of elevated transaminases (AST and ALT) is often the only means of confirming the diagnosis. Some of these hepatotoxic herbs and medications will be discussed in chapters 21 and chapter 24, respectively.

THE SYMPTOMS AND PHYSICAL SIGNS OF HEPATITIS

Due to the overlapping nature of the different types of hepatitis, it is difficult to determine a specific cause based solely on associated symptoms and signs.

Symptoms and signs of hepatitis may vary greatly; however, most people with hepatitis are asymptomatic, meaning that they have no symptoms. In fact, many cannot remember ever having had an episode of acute hepatitis. This accounts for why many people with hepatitis are surprised when they are first told that something is wrong with their liver. Other people with hepatitis have vague, nonspecific symptoms, such as mild fatigue, which they often attribute to their daily agendas. Others have relentless fatigue, which often is what prompts a visit to the doctor. It is crucial to understand that the severity of symptoms that a person is experiencing bears no correlation to the amount of damage done to the liver. On a physical exam, there may be no clues that a person has hepatitis, and, in fact, the exam may be totally normal. Alternatively, hepatomegaly (an enlarged liver), jaundice, a rash, or even signs suggestive of liver failure may be the initial findings. Often even the physical exam does not bear any correlation to the amount of liver damage.

DIAGNOSING HEPATITIS

The discovery that a person has hepatitis may occur in a number of different ways. Some people are found to have hepatitis during a visit to the doctor for an evaluation of symptoms, others during the course of a routine checkup. Some people first learn that they have hepatitis upon being rejected for a life insurance policy due to a finding of abnormal liver function tests (LFTs). And some people first learn that they have hepatitis upon being rejected as blood donors due to having an elevated ALT level or testing positive for hepatitis B or C. Still others first find out they have hepatitis after developing signs of liver failure.

Symptoms, physical signs, and results from routine blood tests commonly overlap among the different types of hepatitis, and as such they rarely indicate a specific cause. Although imaging studies may suggest liver inflammation, they are generally normal and are not helpful in the diagnosis of hepatitis. However, an abdominal sonogram is usually obtained in order to make sure that other abnormalities, such as gallstones, are not the cause of elevated LFTs. In general, the only way to reliably determine the type of hepatitis, what caused it, and the degree of damage done to the liver is through a combination of serial LFTs, hepatitis-specific blood tests (see the specific chapters pertaining to each type of hepatitis), and a liver biopsy.

TREATMENT OF HEPATITIS

Treatment of hepatitis will normally be based on whether it is chronic, as opposed to acute, as well as the cause of the hepatitis. Specific treatments will be discussed in the chapters corresponding to specific types of hepatitis. This section discusses general treatments of hepatitis.

Treatment of Acute Hepatitis

Treatment of acute hepatitis is mostly supportive. This means that treatment is based upon the symptoms being experienced. If a person feels fatigued, she will likely be advised to take multiple naps during the day and to stay out of work for a few days. However, if the person is not feeling sick, there is no reason for extra bed rest—although it is important not to overdo activities during this time. The key for individuals with acute hepatitis when it comes to activity is to listen to their bodies. Alcohol and recreational drugs should be avoided altogether. As a person may experience a loss of appetite, several small meals instead of a few large meals each day may be advisable. People with acute hepatitis should stick to a healthy, low-fat diet and drink plenty of water. No medications or shots are necessary. Furthermore, people with acute hepatitis should avoid taking unnecessary medications, including vitamins (in excess) and herbs.

Treatment of Chronic Hepatitis

Treatment of chronic hepatitis is somewhat more complicated than treatment for acute hepatitis. Therefore, the treatments pertaining to each type of chronic hepatitis will be discussed in specific chapters later in this book. Beneficial changes that a person can make in respect to diet, exercise, alcohol abstinence, tobacco avoidance, and other lifestyle modifications are covered in chapters 23 and 24.

Treatment of Fulminant Hepatitis

Treatment of fulminant hepatitis typically depends on the cause. In general, anyone suffering from fulminant hepatitis requires close monitoring in an intensive care unit (ICU) of a hospital. If the person does not improve or if her condition worsens, she should be considered for liver transplantation as soon as possible. Liver transplantation will be discussed in chapter 22.

MISCONCEPTIONS ABOUT VIRAL HEPATITIS

Viral hepatitis has a history that dates all the way back to ancient times. However, it was only recently that the different types of viral hepatitis were identified by researchers and that the names for each type of hepatitis, including hepatitis A, hepatitis B, and hepatitis C, were coined. There are many common misconceptions about viral hepatitis that often lead to confusion, needless worry, and unnecessary lifestyle changes. The following six false statements and their explanations will help to dispel some of the most common misconceptions concerning viral hepatitis. See chapters 8 to 13 for a more in-depth look at each of the common types of viral hepatitis.

FALSE: All types of viral hepatitis can cause both acute and chronic hepatitis.

HAV, HEV, and (possibly) HFV cause only acute hepatitis. As such, they totally resolve within six months and do not have a chronic stage. In contrast, HBV, HCV, and HDV can cause both acute and chronic hepatitis. Therefore, these viruses have the potential to lead to cirrhosis and its complications. HGV is not believed to be a cause of significant liver disease.

FALSE: A person who was previously infected with one form of viral hepatitis can never catch another form.

Having had one type of viral hepatitis will not make a person immune to becoming infected with other kinds of viral hepatitis. For example, a person who had hepatitis A at some point in the past is now immune to HAV. This person can never get hepatitis A again and cannot transmit it to others. However, this does not mean that she is immune to other forms of viral hepatitis. She is, therefore, still at risk for becoming infected with other types of hepatitis in the future.

FALSE: One type of hepatitis virus can change into another type of hepatitis virus.

One hepatitis virus cannot change into a different hepatitis virus. For example, HBV cannot transform itself into HCV. However, more than one kind of hepatitis virus can exist in the liver at the same time. Thus, an individual may be co-infected with both HBV and HCV.

FALSE: If symptoms of viral hepatitis resolve, it means that the viral hepatitis is gone. Or, since I feel fine, everything must be okay.

Many people are under the misconception that once the symptoms associated with viral hepatitis resolve, the disease is gone. While, in fact, most people recover totally from many types of viral hepatitis, such as hepatitis A, some viruses such as HCV typically progress to chronic liver disease or even cirrhosis and/or liver cancer without causing any symptoms along the way. Because the liver is so resilient, a person may feel great (often for many years) and not realize that the hepatitis virus is still present, replicating, and continuing to attack and damage the liver.

FALSE: Viral hepatitis and the human immunodeficiency virus (HIV) are the same virus.

The viruses that cause hepatitis are very different from HIV (human immunodeficiency virus), the virus that causes AIDS (acquired immune deficiency syndrome). While some of the hepatitis viruses may be transmitted by routes similar to the transmission routes that apply to HIV, all the hepatitis viruses are very different, both biologically and structurally, from HIV.

FALSE: Viruses can be treated with antibiotics.

Only bacterial infections can be treated with antibiotics. Viruses differ greatly from bacteria. They are smaller and more difficult to treat. They also typically require treatment of much longer duration. Whereas a bacterial infection may require only a week or two of antibiotic therapy, a viral infection may require up to a year, or possibly longer, of antiviral therapy. Viruses are treated with antiviral medications such as interferon, which will be discussed in further detail in later chapters.

HOW HEPATITIS VIRUSES ARE TRANSMITTED

Not all viruses are transmitted by the same route. It is important to understand the different ways that a person may catch a virus and/or spread it to others. Some viruses are introduced into the body by way of the digestive tract, whereas others are transmitted through contaminated blood, during sexual contact, or from mother to child during childbirth. See the chapters on each type of hepatitis later in the book to learn how each is transmitted.

THE IMMUNE SYSTEM AND VIRAL HEPATITIS

Each person has a built-in natural defense system—an army of defenders known as the *immune system*. The immune system fights against foreign substances that enter the body and are perceived as dangerous intruders, such as the hepatitis viruses. A person with a weak immune system who has been exposed to a virus is less likely to be able to eliminate the virus from her body as compared with a person with a well-functioning immune system who is, therefore, less prone to infection.

Two important terms that are frequently used when discussing the immune system are *antigen (Ag)* and *antibody (Ab)*. Think of an antigen as a foreign substance (such as a hepatitis virus) and of an antibody as one of the immune-system soldiers battling the antigen. For example, when an antigen, such as hepatitis B antigen, is present in the body, an antibody—in this case, the hepatitis B antibody—is produced by the immune system. The antibody combines with the antigen with the intent of eliminating it from the body and thereby making the person immune to hepatitis B.

The specific hepatitis antigens and antibodies may be detected from specific blood tests. These tests may indicate that a person currently has or was at one time exposed to viral hepatitis. This blood work is referred to as serologic testing or, more specifically, as hepatitis *serology*. (See table 3.1 in chapter 3.) The hepatitis serology is necessary in order to determine if viral hepatitis is the cause of a patient's liver-related abnormalities and to determine which specific hepatitis virus is the culprit.

CONCLUSION

After reading this chapter, you now know the correct meaning of the medical term *hepatitis*. Most important, this chapter distinguished between viral hepatitis and all other forms of hepatitis. The symptoms and physical signs associated with hepatitis should now be more familiar to you. This chapter also gave you a closer look at viral hepatitis and introduced you to the role that the immune system plays in combating this viral disease. The next chapter discusses hepatitis A in greater detail.

Eight

UNDERSTANDING AND TREATING HEPATITIS A

Marty, a forty-two-year-old lawyer, had never missed a day of work due to illness. After three days of hearing him complain of excessive fatigue and nausea, Marty's wife, Pam, demanded he call in sick to work. When he began to have uncontrollable loose bowel movements almost every hour, he had no choice but to stay home to be near the bathroom. Finally, when Marty noticed that his urine resembled fresh brewed tea and his stools looked like clay, he agreed to see a doctor. He made an appointment for the end of the week, figuring his problem would clear up way before then.

But over the next few days, Marty's symptoms actually worsened. Pam called an ambulance when Marty began to show signs of mental confusion. At the hospital, Marty was immediately taken to the intensive care unit (ICU). Pam, frightened and confused, listened to the doctor as he told her that something was wrong with Marty's liver and that it could be a form of hepatitis. He also told her that they would need to wait for the blood test results to confirm this. And because Marty was jaundiced and encephalopathic (disoriented), he would need to remain in the ICU.

Then the doctor asked Pam if Marty had a history of intravenous drug use or if he ever had a blood transfusion. She replied no to both questions. Next, the doctor asked if Marty had eaten any seafood recently or if anyone else in the family was ill. Pam recalled that about a month earlier, Marty had taken their five-year-old son Jason to the beach. Afterward the pair had stopped at a fish stand for some clams. Jason had developed what appeared to be a mild cold that lasted only a short time. With this added information, the doctor concluded

*that Marty probably had hepatitis A. This diagnosis was subsequently
confirmed by the results of Marty's blood test.*

*Marty's condition seemed touch and go for a while, but after one
month, Marty was discharged from the hospital. By six months, Marty
was totally better and his jaundice totally resolved.*

This chapter discusses the hepatitis A virus (HAV). You will learn the routes
by which HAV is transmitted to others, as well as which people are at particularly high risk of becoming infected. In addition, the symptoms and
physical signs associated with hepatitis A and the manner in which a person is diagnosed are explained in this chapter. The treatment of hepatitis A and the prognosis for those infected are also covered.

WHAT IS HEPATITIS A?

Hepatitis A is inflammation of the liver due to a virus called the hepatitis A virus
(HAV). Prior to its identification in 1973, it was known as *infectious hepatitis,*
due to the fact that HAV is so contagious. HAV only causes acute hepatitis. This
means that within six months time, the inflammation in the liver due to the hepatitis A virus totally subsides, and all of the symptoms, signs, and LFT abnormalities resolve. The liver repairs any short-term damage it may have suffered. No
permanent damage is done, and no long-term consequences are suffered.

In the United States, HAV is the most common cause of acute viral hepatitis.
Each year, approximately 134,000 people in the United States are infected with
HAV. In fact, around 33 percent of all people in the United States have, at some
point, been infected with HAV, and approximately 47 percent of adults over fifty
years old have evidence of exposure to this virus. Almost 100 percent of people
who live in communities in the United States with substandard water and sewage
sanitation systems have been infected during childhood, as have people living in
economically developing countries such as Africa, Asia, and Latin America.

HAV is usually thought of as the least serious of all the hepatitis viruses. This
is due to the fact that—unlike the hepatitis B and C viruses—HAV does not cause
chronic liver disease, and therefore the disease lasts no longer than six months.
Cirrhosis and its complications can never result. Moreover, hepatitis A will not
result in liver cancer. However, each year, hepatitis A causes a substantial number of people to get very ill. Some of these people require hospitalization. Many
others, although not needing hospitalization, lose a significant amount of time
from their jobs.

Though it is typically not fatal, hepatitis A accounts for approximately one
hundred deaths each year in the United States. Although the incidence of hepatitis A declines with advancing age, people greater than fifty years old are at five
to ten times greater risk of having a fatal outcome due to hepatitis A compared
with all ages combined. Furthermore, it has been shown that when a person with
another liver disease, such as chronic hepatitis C or B, becomes infected with HAV,

she may experience a particularly serious and potentially life-threatening form of hepatitis. This is especially applicable to people over fifty years of age. Fortunately, hepatitis A is vaccine preventable. In fact, it is interesting to note that hepatitis A is the most common vaccine-preventable disease in the entire world. See chapter 24 for information on prevention and vaccination.

HOW HAV IS TRANSMITTED

HAV transmission may occur through person-to-person contact, from consumption of contaminated food or water, or by other routes, all of which will be discussed on the following pages. HAV is not spread through pregnancy or through sexual transmission.

Person-to-Person Contact

HAV is most commonly transmitted by person-to-person contact via a fecal-oral route. Fecal-oral transmission, also known as the *enteric route,* occurs when HAV embedded in the feces of an infected person enters the digestive tract of another person. More precisely, the virus enters through the mouth, passes from the stomach into the small intestine, and then gains entry into the liver. The liver is the major site of HAV replication. After the virus is finished multiplying and infecting the liver, it leaves the liver via the bile ducts and is excreted into the bile. As discussed in chapter 1, the bile ducts enter into the small intestine. So HAV goes back into the small intestine, which directly connects with the large intestine, and is mixed in with the stool and eliminated from the body through the rectum. HAV is now ready to infect the next unsuspecting victim.

People living in the same household with an infected person are at increased risk of becoming infected themselves. People who live in communities where sanitation standards are poor, or where living conditions are crowded, are also at increased risk for infection.

A person with hepatitis A is most infectious during the two-week time period preceding and the one-week period following the development of any symptoms or signs of infection and is no longer infectious to others approximately a week or two after symptoms and signs of hepatitis A have begun.

Many people, especially young children infected with HAV, have no symptoms at all. As a group, young children are major transmitters of HAV, as they commonly harbor the virus unknowingly. Furthermore, their hygiene habits tend to be less meticulous than those of adults. Of all age demographics, children are most likely to spread the virus to others, as they tend to play in close contact with other children and are closely handled and cared for by adults. Therefore, a common source of hepatitis A outbreaks has been day-care centers—particularly day-care centers that provide care to children who wear diapers.

Another common source of outbreaks has been institutions for the mentally disabled, since people living in these facilities often have poor personal hygiene and live in crowded conditions. Note, however, that outbreaks have become less frequent as a result of improvements made to conditions within institutions.

Sexual Contact

In some, but not all studies, men who have sex with men, and people who practice anal-oral sex, have been linked with the transmission of HAV. In general, however, there is no evidence that sexual transmission plays a role in spreading HAV.

Contaminated Food and Water

Ingestion of contaminated food and beverages is a common route of HAV transmission. Foods that have been reported to transmit HAV have included milk, strawberries, pastries, hamburger meat, and salads. In these instances, the food was either uncooked (or was undercooked) or was handled after cooking by an HAV-infected person who did not properly wash her hands after defecating.

Shellfish often live in bodies of water that are polluted with HAV. Thus, they appear to have a particularly high incidence of transmitting HAV when eaten raw or incompletely cooked—as is often the case with clams, oysters, and mussels. There have been few incidents of transmission of HAV by water—either by drinking contaminated water or by swimming in HAV-infested water. Don't forget: Bottled water containing non-bottled ice cubes is also a risk.

Other Routes

While there are a few incidents where a blood transfusion was believed to be the source of a hepatitis A infection, the blood supply is considered safe, and transfusions are not considered to pose a risk for HAV transmission. While intravenous drug users (IVDUs) are at a somewhat increased risk of acquiring HAV as compared with the general population, it does not appear that intravenous drug use is a very significant mode of HAV transmission. Other factors, such as poor personal hygiene and unsanitary living conditions, may explain the increased incidence of hepatitis A among IVDUs. In general, it appears that blood-to-blood transmission of HAV occurs infrequently. HAV has occasionally been detected in other body fluids, such as saliva and urine. However, it is believed that these are not routes of HAV transmission.

THOSE AT AN INCREASED RISK FOR HEPATITIS A

Hepatitis A is the most common vaccine-preventable disease in the entire world. Aside from vaccination, there are other measures that a person can take to minimize her chances of acquiring HAV. In addition, many precautions may be taken by a person infected with HAV to reduce the likelihood of transmitting this virus to others. Prevention of hepatitis A will be discussed in chapter 24. The following groups of people are at increased risk for contracting HAV:

- People who travel to developing countries, including tourists, military personnel, Peace Corps workers, and missionaries

- Men who have sex with men

- People who practice oral-anal sex

- Intravenous drug users (both present and former users)

- People who have contact with sewage (this appears to be an insignificant mode of transmission in the United States)

- Employees and children (particularly those in diapers) at day-care centers

- Employees and patients in institutions for the mentally disabled (incidence has greatly decreased since sanitary conditions have improved)

- People who work with primates, such as apes and monkeys, which can also transmit HAV

- People who live in crowded conditions with poor sanitation

THE INCUBATION PERIOD OF HEPATITIS A

After entering the body, HAV incubates. The *incubation period*—the time between the entrance of the virus into the body and the initial appearance of symptoms and signs of the disease—of HAV is about one month, but may be as short as two weeks or as long as almost two months. The length of the incubation period is inversely related to the quantity of HAV that enters the body. This means that if a large amount of HAV enters the body, the incubation period is shorter than if only a small amount is ingested. As noted above, a person is most infectious during the two-week period prior to and the one-week period after exhibiting any symptoms or signs of hepatitis A. This helps explain why hepatitis A is so contagious. People are not aware that they harbor the virus, which prevents them from taking the necessary precautions to ensure that they do not pass it on to others.

THE SYMPTOMS AND SIGNS OF HEPATITIS A

The development of symptoms of hepatitis A is directly related to the age of the person. The younger the person, the more likely the infection will be asymptomatic—without symptoms. In fact, approximately 90 percent of HAV-infected children who are younger than five years old are asymptomatic. Thus, children silently pass the virus in their stools, and it is their parents, exposed unknowingly to HAV, who are the ones most likely to experience symptoms due to infection.

The degree of symptoms among people with hepatitis A varies greatly. Some people have no symptoms at all and are surprised to learn that they were ever exposed to the virus. Others may have nonspecific symptoms such as fatigue or symptoms that may be confused with a very bad cold or flu—chills, loss of appetite (especially for fatty foods), and a headache. Often symptoms include a sudden fever, abdominal pain, diarrhea, nausea, and vomiting. Many adults become jaundiced and seek the attention of a doctor when they notice their urine is dark or tea-colored and/or their stools are light or clay-colored. These people often have pruritus (intense itching). Usually, a week prior to becoming jaundiced, these people experience some nonspecific symptoms such as malaise and weight loss. Some HAV-infected individuals state that cigarettes taste unpleasant to them, and they actually stop smoking during this time. When adults become very ill, studies have shown that approximately one month is typically lost from work. In fact, approximately 15 percent of people with hepatitis A become so ill that they require hospitalization.

On occasion, people develop symptoms that are unrelated to the liver. These are known as *extrahepatic*—outside or unrelated to the liver—manifestations of hepatitis A. These manifestations may include arthritis (inflammation of the joints); *vasculitis* (inflammation of the blood vessels), often associated with a rash; cryoglobulinemia (abnormal proteins in the blood associated with poor circulation); kidney failure; diabetes (elevated blood sugar levels); and gallbladder disease.

Rarely, people develop cholestatic hepatitis A. These people have a prolonged course of disease marked by jaundice. Jaundice may last from two to eight months, and bilirubin levels may exceed 20 mg/dl. Relentless itching is usually the most prominent and annoying symptom in these patients. Although these patients have a severe and protracted course of disease, total resolution occurs in all patients.

In very rare instances, people with hepatitis A develop a particularly severe form of acute hepatitis known as fulminant hepatitis A, which was discussed in chapter 7. These people become extremely ill, developing severe jaundice, encephalopathy (mental disorientation or coma), and coagulopathy (bleeding tendency noted by a prolonged prothrombin time). Liver failure develops abruptly—usually within eight weeks from the onset of symptoms, or within two weeks from the onset of jaundice. All people with fulminant hepatitis A require immediate hospitalization in an intensive care unit (ICU) and prompt referral for a liver transplant. Liver transplantation is discussed in detail in chapter 22.

People with hepatitis A will usually appear to be in good or normal health during a physical exam. Occasionally, the physical exam may reveal an enlarged, tender liver or jaundice. Though not a frequent occurrence, a person may have a rash.

Symptoms and signs usually last a month or two. Once jaundice appears, symptoms often begin to resolve. Jaundice, accompanied by urine and stool discoloration, typically begins to resolve within a few weeks. About 10 to 15 percent of people with hepatitis A may experience a prolonged course known as relapsing hepatitis A. Relapsing hepatitis A is more common in children than adults. During the period of *relapse,* symptoms and signs return after a previous resolution. Blood work again becomes abnormal, and the person is again infectious. In any scenario, by six months all symptoms and signs of hepatitis A will resolve.

DIAGNOSING HEPATITIS A

Neither symptoms, signs, nor LFT abnormalities can definitively confirm that a person has hepatitis A nor can these indicators distinguish hepatitis A from other forms of hepatitis.

The only way of definitively diagnosing that a person is infected with HAV is by obtaining specific blood tests known as the *hepatitis A serology.* The standard hepatitis A serology includes both the immunoglobulin M (IgM) antibody to HAV and the immunoglobulin G (IgG) antibody to HAV. The other liver function tests, which were discussed in chapter 3, are routinely performed when any type of liver disease is suspected.

HAV Antibody Immunoglobulin M (IgM) (HAV Ab IgM)

When a person tests positive for the existence of immunoglobulin M (IgM) antibody to HAV (HAV Ab IgM), it indicates that the person is currently infected with HAV or has been infected recently. HAV Ab IgM becomes positive approximately one week after a person has been exposed to HAV and may remain positive for up to six months thereafter. This antibody then becomes undetectable in the blood; thus HAV Ab IgM will be negative on blood test results after six months.

HAV Antibody Immunoglobulin G (IgG) (HAV Ab IgG)

When a person tests positive for the existence of immunoglobulin G (IgG) antibody to HAV (HAV Ab IgG)—in cases where HAV Ab IgM is no longer detected—it indicates that the person was exposed to HAV at some point in the past, but no longer has an active infection. (Note, however, that in the acute phase, HAV Ab IgG will be positive.) These people can never become infected with HAV again and are no longer infectious to others. Though these people are protected against future HAV infections, they are not protected against other hepatitis infections, such as B and C. The HAV Ab IgG remains positive lifelong and will always be detected in blood tests (HAV Ab IgG positive) when a test for HAV Ab IgG is specifically ordered by a doctor.

AST and ALT (Transaminases)

People with hepatitis A may have very elevated transaminases (ALT and AST) around 500 IU/l to 2,000 IU/l. The degree of elevation of the transaminases does not correlate with the severity of symptoms, nor is it predictive of the outcome of the disease. In most people, transaminases return to normal in about one month. In virtually everyone with hepatitis A, they return to normal by six months. Thus, if transaminases remain abnormal after six months time, another cause for these elevated liver enzymes must be searched for. For example, on rare occasions HAV may trigger the onset of a liver disease known as autoimmune hepatitis, which will be discussed in chapter 14.

Bilirubin

An elevated bilirubin level occurs in approximately 70 percent of adults with hepatitis A. In contrast, only 20 percent of children younger than two years old are jaundiced. The bilirubin level usually does not rise greater than 10 mg/dl and usually returns to normal within eight weeks. In cases where the bilirubin level remains elevated for ten weeks or more, the person is considered to have cholestatic hepatitis. In people with cholestatic hepatitis, the bilirubin can reach levels as high as 20 mg/dl and is often accompanied by pruritus (itching). The bilirubin level typically returns to normal by six months time.

Imaging Studies and Liver Biopsy

Imaging studies are usually normal for people with hepatitis A and will not provide a basis for a diagnosis. However, in jaundiced people, an imaging study—usually a sonogram—is performed in order to eliminate the possibility that another disorder, such as gallstones, is present. A liver biopsy is not needed to establish a diagnosis of hepatitis A. Therefore, liver biopsies are infrequently performed when hepatitis A is suspected.

TREATMENT OF HEPATITIS A

There are no specific medications used to treat hepatitis A. Treatment decisions are usually based on the symptoms experienced by the patient. Bed rest and decreased physical activity are not necessarily required. Each person should, on her own, determine a comfortable level of activity based on how she feels. If a person feels well, she may go to work. If she feels fatigued, a decreased level of activity or a midday nap is in order. It is always recommended that a person with hepatitis A consume plenty of fluids so as to avoid dehydration. This is especially important if diarrhea is one of the symptoms. All alcohol should be avoided during this time, as alcohol may provoke a relapse of the disease. All nonessential medications, both prescription and over the counter, are best avoided.

THE LONG-TERM PROGNOSIS FOR THOSE WITH HEPATITIS A

People with hepatitis A do not suffer any long-term consequences from the infection and are not chronically infectious to others. Within six months of contracting hepatitis A, symptoms, signs, and hepatitis A-related LFT abnormalities totally resolve. Chronic liver disease does not occur. Therefore, contracting HAV does not put one at risk for cirrhosis and/or liver cancer.

Approximately 0.2 percent of people infected with HAV develop fulminant hepatitis A. Each year, approximately one hundred people either die or require a liver transplant as a result of liver failure due to HAV. Older people and people with underlying liver disease are more likely to develop this complication and are more likely to have a poor outcome from fulminant hepatitis A.

CONCLUSION

Increasingly, healthier and cleaner living conditions—such as improved sewage disposal and more sanitary water and food supplies—have contributed to a decline in the incidence of hepatitis A in the United States over the past several decades. However, outbreaks continue to occur. While outbreaks are typically without consequences for most people, a small yet significant percentage of people become severely ill, requiring time out of work, hospitalization, and possibly liver transplantation. People especially at risk for a particularly debilitating course of hepatitis A are elderly individuals and those already suffering from some other chronic liver disease, such as chronic hepatitis C. Infection with HAV is 100 percent preventable. Prevention is discussed in chapter 24. The next chapter will discuss another preventable type of viral hepatitis—hepatitis B. While the acute symptoms and signs of hepatitis B may resemble those of hepatitis A, the major distinguishing point between these two hepatitis viruses is that, unlike hepatitis A, hepatitis B can lead to chronic liver disease, cirrhosis, and liver cancer. Also discussed in the next chapter is hepatitis D, a hepatitis virus that cannot survive without HBV.

Nine

UNDERSTANDING HEPATITIS B AND D

Charlie, a twenty-seven-year-old construction worker, had recently begun a new relationship. His new girlfriend didn't tell him that she had acquired hepatitis B from the prior use of intravenous drugs. A few weeks after an episode of unprotected sex, Charlie felt so fatigued that he could not get out of bed. His joints hurt, he was nauseous, and he had a pain in the location of his liver. When his girlfriend told him that his eyes looked yellow, Charlie immediately went to the emergency room. The doctor suspected gallstones and admitted Charlie as an inpatient. Charlie's sonogram didn't show evidence of gallstones, but his blood work revealed that he had acute hepatitis B.

In this chapter, you'll learn about the hepatitis B virus (HBV) and the hepatitis delta virus (HDV) and how these viruses are transmitted to others. This chapter also covers who is at risk for contracting these viruses and how people typically discover that they are infected. The differences between acute, chronic, and fulminant hepatitis B are addressed. In addition, factors that determine which individuals are most likely to progress from acute to chronic hepatitis B are discussed. This chapter also explains the blood tests used to diagnose hepatitis B, known as the hepatitis B serology. Also covered are the ways in which people with hepatitis B can become infected with HDV. Finally, the long-term prognosis of people infected with HBV or with the combination of HBV and HDV is discussed. See chapter 12 for treatment options for hepatitis B and D and chapter 24 for ways to prevent contracting these viruses.

WHAT IS HEPATITIS B?

Hepatitis B is inflammation of the liver due to a virus called the hepatitis B virus (HBV). Infection with HBV was originally known as *serum hepatitis.* In 1963, the structure of the virus was identified and named the hepatitis B virus. In fact, HBV was actually the very first hepatitis virus to be identified. Approximately 2 billion people worldwide have been infected by hepatitis B, and almost 400 million people worldwide, including 1.25 million people in the United States, are chronic carriers of this virus. Approximately 65 million of those chronically infected will die of the disease. HBV is the single most common cause of cirrhosis and liver cancer worldwide. Hepatitis B is *endemic* (a disease that is extremely widespread in a particular region) in Southeast Asia, China, and Africa. In these areas of the world, more than 50 percent of the population have been exposed to HBV at some point in their lives. Fortunately, the virus has a relatively low prevalence in North America, Western Europe, and Australia, and accounts for only 5 to 10 percent of all chronic liver diseases in these areas.

In most cases, infection with HBV will not prevent a person from leading a normal, productive life. Yet hepatitis B is not entirely harmless. A long-term infection can lead to cirrhosis, liver failure, and liver cancer. As a result, approximately 1 million people die each year from the complications of hepatitis B, making hepatitis B the ninth leading cause of death worldwide. Hepatitis B can present itself in a variety of ways.

HOW HBV IS TRANSMITTED

Approximately one-third of the world's population, or about 2 billion people, have been exposed to or are currently infected with HBV. Approximately 200,000 new HBV infections occur annually in the United States. How did all these people acquire this virus? Well, HBV is an extremely hardy virus. It has been detected in blood, sweat, tears, saliva, semen, vaginal secretions, menstrual blood, and breast milk. However, only blood, semen, and (possibly) saliva have been found to be modes for transmitting the infection. HBV is much harder to catch than the virus that causes a cold or the flu, but a lot easier to catch than HIV (the virus that causes AIDS) or HCV (the virus that causes hepatitis C).

As discussed in chapter 7, HBV is transmitted to others *parenterally* (introduced into the body by any way other than via the intestinal tract). Hepatitis B is not transmitted by the casual contacts that occur in the course of daily life. Thus, a person cannot get hepatitis B from eating food prepared by an infected person, by shaking hands with or hugging an infected person, or by visiting an infected person. Rather, HBV is transmitted in three different ways: through blood or blood products, through sexual contact, or from mother to child during pregnancy and childbirth. In areas of low endemicity, such as the United States, hepatitis B is usually transmitted through sex or intravenous drug use. In areas of high endemicity, such as Africa, Asia, and Alaska, hepatitis B is usually transmitted at childbirth from the infected mother.

Only a small percentage of adults in the United States harbor infectious hepatitis B viral particles that can be transmitted to others. If a person has hepatitis B, it does not mean that they are automatically infectious to others. See table 9.1 on page 100 to find out how a person can determine if she is infectious. The following is a discussion of how HBV is transmitted.

Blood or Blood Products

Prior to 1975, many people developed hepatitis B after having received contaminated blood or blood products, such as fresh frozen plasma (FFP) or platelets, during a transfusion. Since 1975, the blood supply in the United States has been carefully screened for HBV. Consequently, few people nowadays contract hepatitis B through a blood transfusion. Still, there are a lot of other ways a person can come into contact with infected blood, such as through the sharing of toothbrushes, razors, or nail clippers—each of which can carry and transmit infectious hepatitis B viral particles. Therefore, people who have someone with infectious hepatitis B in their household need to take special precautions. People with infectious hepatitis B who have skin conditions that can bleed—such as psoriasis or dermatitis—should take special precaution to cover open lesions or wounds. This is also sound advice for anyone with infectious hepatitis B who has open bleeding cuts or wounds due to any cause.

Needles or instruments used by various professionals can also spread HBV. If not sterilized properly, needles used for tattooing, ear piercing, body piercing, and acupuncture may be tainted with flecks of infected blood. Even barbers and manicurists can transmit the virus if their equipment is contaminated with infected blood. And since being accidentally stuck with a needle or other sharp instrument is an occupational hazard of the medical and dental professions, healthcare workers are particularly at risk for infection with hepatitis B.

By sharing needles, even on one occasion, intravenous drug users can transmit the virus among themselves. Straws, dollar bills, or other instruments shared when "snorting" drugs, such as cocaine, can transmit small amounts of HBV-infected blood from broken blood vessels in the nose from one person to another.

Other people at risk include those with kidney failure undergoing *hemodialysis*—a procedure that helps filter blood—or those receiving a transplanted organ infected with HBV. It should be noted that HBV can remain infectious on a surface for up to one week. Thus, although unlikely, it is theoretically possible to acquire HBV unknowingly from an inanimate object.

Sexual Contact

HBV is one hundred times easier to transmit sexually than HIV (the virus that causes AIDS). HBV has been found in vaginal secretions, saliva, and semen.

Therefore, it doesn't matter if a person's sex partner is of the same or the opposite gender. If one partner has hepatitis B, the other one can get it. Oral sex and especially anal sex (whether it occurs in a heterosexual or homosexual context) are possible ways of transmitting the virus. It is not transmitted by holding hands, hugging, or even dry kissing on the lips. The chance of transmission with deep kissing is unknown, as no infections have been definitively documented after exposure to infected saliva. Yet, since HBV has been found in saliva, the risk of transmission with deep kissing probably exists, and the risk increases if one partner wears orthodontic braces or has open cuts or sores in the mouth. The likelihood of becoming infected with HBV grows with the number of sex partners a person has. Thus, promiscuous individuals are more likely to get HBV. Also, men who have sex with men are ten to fifteen times more likely to catch HBV than the general population.

Childbirth

An infected mother can transmit HBV to her child during childbirth. This mode of transmission is known as *perinatal transmission.* It accounts for the high rates of infection in Asian and African countries, as asymptomatic mothers, unaware that they carry infectious hepatitis B, transmit it to their newborn infants at childbirth.

In the United States, all pregnant women are screened for the presence of HBV, and all babies born to infected mothers immediately receive immunization. In fact, in the United States, it is now common practice to vaccinate infants against hepatitis B, regardless of the mother's HBV status. As a result, there is hope that this infection will, in time, become a disease of the past. For more information on vaccinations, see chapter 24. New mothers are also advised to avoid breast-feeding if they are infectious, even though this mode of transmission has not been considered very significant. Of course, if the mother has bleeding nipples, the risk of transmitting HBV increases.

THOSE AT AN INCREASED RISK FOR HEPATITIS B

Hepatitis B is a disease that is totally preventable through vaccination. Aside from vaccination, there are other measures that a person can take to minimize the chances of acquiring HBV. In addition, there are a number of precautions that may be taken by a person infected with HBV to reduce the likelihood of transmitting this virus to others. Prevention of hepatitis B will be discussed in chapter 24. Meanwhile, take note of the following people who are at increased risk for contracting HBV:

- People who received a blood or a blood-product transfusion prior to 1975

- Hospital and healthcare workers

- Household members of an infected person

- Intravenous drugs users (both present and former users)

- People who have gotten a tattoo or had a body part pierced with an infected needle

- Sex partners of infected people

- Travelers to countries where HBV is endemic

- People who were born to a mother infected with HBV

- Transplant-organ recipients who received an infected organ

And the following groups of people should be screened for HBV:

- People born in areas where HBV is endemic

- Men who have sex with men

- Intravenous drug users (both present and former users)

- Dialysis patients

- HIV-infected people

- Pregnant women

- Family members, household members, and sex partners of HBV-infected people (even if sex occurred on only one occasion)

- Sexually promiscuous individuals (often defined as people with more than one sex partner within a six-month period of time)

WHAT IS ACUTE HEPATITIS B?

Acute hepatitis B is inflammation of the liver due to the hepatitis B virus lasting six months or less. The incidence of acute hepatitis B in the United States has decreased dramatically over the past decade. This is most likely attributable to the widespread utilization of the hepatitis B vaccination among children and health-care workers. However, HBV remains a common cause of acute hepatitis. This section discusses the symptoms and signs associated with acute hepatitis B, how acute hepatitis B is diagnosed, and how it is determined whether acute hepatitis B has resolved or has progressed to chronic hepatitis B.

The Symptoms and Signs of Acute Hepatitis B

The symptoms of acute hepatitis B are usually similar to those of acute hepatitis due to any other cause, which were discussed in chapter 7. Acute hepatitis B can be silent or can be easily mistaken for something else, like a really bad case of the flu. This is one of the reasons why HBV has spread so widely throughout the world. People usually don't know that they have the virus when they pass it on to other people. In fact, the acute phase of hepatitis B is usually detected in only a small percentage of people who are infected. If symptoms do appear, they generally occur after the virus has incubated in the body for about two to three months (a range of 15 to 180 days). The physical exam is usually normal, but it may reveal an enlarged liver, a rash, and/or rarely jaundice.

Symptoms can include decreased appetite, nausea, vomiting, a low fever, abdominal discomfort, and an altered sense of taste and smell. Some smokers with acute HBV claim that cigarettes taste odd. All of these symptoms may last for about a week or two. If jaundice occurs, it usually develops after these symptoms disappear and infrequently lasts more than a month or two. Jaundice may occur in approximately 30 to 50 percent of adults, but is rare in children (as are any signs of acute hepatitis B).

Many people with acute hepatitis B have symptoms and signs related to *extrahepatic* manifestations of hepatitis B. This is partly due to the fact that some body parts other than the liver are caught in the crossfire when the immune system fights back against HBV. The result in many cases is that immune-mediated diseases arise. These include a type of *vasculitis* (inflammation of blood vessels), known as *polyarteritis nodosa (PAN),* and a kidney disease known as *glomerulonephritis* (inflammation of the kidneys). Symptoms of these diseases may include a rash, muscle and joint aches, fever, and excessive protein in the urine. Up to 20 percent of people with acute hepatitis B may suffer from severe joint stiffness and pain. In fact, it is often the rheumatologist, a doctor that specializes in the treatment of diseases of the joints and muscles, who initially discovers that a person is infected with HBV. These extrahepatic manifestations of hepatitis B are discussed further in the section on chronic hepatitis B on page 99.

Diagnosing Acute Hepatitis B

The incubation period of hepatitis B is about two to three months, but may be as short as two weeks or as long as six months. As symptoms may be rather vague, most people never seek evaluation from a doctor during the acute stage of the disease and therefore many people who are infected with the virus never realize it. However, if a person does see a doctor for the evaluation of symptoms or signs of jaundice, acute hepatitis B is usually detected by abnormal results from blood work.

Transaminases (AST and ALT) are often quite elevated initially, and levels in the thousands can occur. As the disease progresses, transaminases typically decrease. The cholestatic liver enzymes (AP and GGTP) are usually only mildly elevated during acute hepatitis B—around two to three times above normal—and bilirubin levels are usually normal. Resolution of acute hepatitis B is usually indicated within six months of the time of infection by the normalization of transaminase levels as revealed by more specific testing called hepatitis B serology tests (see table 9.1 on page 100).

If transaminases remain elevated—usually around two to three times above normal—after six months from the time of infection, this usually indicates progression to chronic hepatitis B. Hepatitis B serology tests will allow the doctor to determine if the LFT abnormalities are in fact due to hepatitis B. Furthermore, the doctor will be able to gather a great deal of information about the status of the HBV infection. This includes determining if a patient is actively infectious to others and determining whether the acute infection has resolved, as opposed to having progressed into a chronic hepatitis B infection. A patient with acute hepatitis B will be positive for hepatitis B core antibody IgM (HBcAb IgM). Please see table 9.1.

Typically, imaging studies are normal. Occasionally, an enlarged liver will be detected. In most cases, imaging studies are performed to eliminate other possible causes of elevated LFTs, such as gallstones. A liver biopsy is usually not performed during the acute stages of a hepatitis B infection.

Determining If Acute Hepatitis B Has Resolved Entirely

After the diagnosis of acute hepatitis B has been made, the doctor will want to see the patient several times over the course of the next few months in order to check on the status of the infection. Six months after the patient has been infected, the doctor will determine if the body has shaken off hepatitis B entirely. Approximately 95 to 99 percent of adults have an immune system strong enough to battle the virus and completely eliminate it from the body. In most cases an adult can eliminate this virus six months from the time of infection, but occasionally (although rarely) it may take up to a year. When elimination of the virus is accomplished, LFT elevations completely normalize, and symptoms, if they were present, totally resolve. Protective antibodies, hepatitis surface antibody (HBsAb), usually will have been formed against HBV. Congratulations are in order. These fortunate people will never have to worry about HBV again, as they are now immune to this virus. (Very rarely, under unusual conditions when one's immune system is severely compromised—as can occur during treatment with immunosuppressive drugs such as steroids—hepatitis B has been known to reactivate.)

Immunity against HBV will protect a person from infection with the hepatitis D virus (HDV); however it won't protect these people against the hepatitis A virus (HAV) or hepatitis C virus (HCV). Also, these people will never again be allowed to donate blood, as they will always have the antibody—hepatitis B core antibody (HBcAb)—for HBV present in their blood, which is a listed contraindication for blood donation.

WHAT IS FULMINANT HEPATITIS B?

Fulminant hepatitis B is a very rare (occurring in less than 1 percent of adults with hepatitis B), but very severe form of acute hepatitis B. It is characterized by sudden liver failure, coagulopathy (a bleeding disorder), jaundice, and severe encephalopathy (coma). Patients with fulminant hepatitis B are severely ill and develop a rapidly progressive downhill course. In the absence of an immediate liver transplant, approximately 85 percent of these patients will die. The treatment of people with fulminant hepatitis B entails immediate hospitalization and contacting a transplant center. Coinfection with other hepatitis viruses such as hepatitis C or D increases the risk of fulminant hepatitis B.

WHAT IS CHRONIC HEPATITIS B?

Chronic hepatitis B is inflammation of the liver due to HBV that continues for more than six months. These people have failed to clear HBV from their bodies. Once a person is chronically infected with this virus, the potential exists for liver damage and cirrhosis along with its complications, including liver cancer.

Determining the Progression from Acute to Chronic Hepatitis B

In the United States, approximately 200,000 people contract HBV each year. However, only 10,000 to 15,000 of these people develop a chronic hepatitis B infection. Why do some people clear the virus from their bodies, while others progress to chronic disease? It appears that the immune system is the most important factor in determining whether a person can rid herself of this virus rather than develop a persistent infection.

The immune system is relatively immature early in life. Therefore, the younger a person is when HBV is contracted, the greater the likelihood that the infected person will become a chronic carrier of the disease. If an adult is infected, her probability of developing chronic disease is very low—approximately 1 to 5 percent. If a person contracts the infection in infancy, there is as much as a 90 to 95 percent chance that her immune system will be unable to eliminate this virus from her body. Children fall somewhere in between, having approximately a 25 to 35 percent chance of going on to chronic disease.

Men are six times more likely than women to become chronic carriers of HBV. The reason for this has not been determined. Also, people with poor immune systems, such as those infected with HIV, organ recipients, and those undergoing chemotherapy, have a much lower success rate of eliminating the virus from their bodies. Patients who are the sickest during their acute illness, especially those who develop jaundice or who survive fulminant hepatitis, have the highest likelihood of totally recovering and thus not progressing to a chronic disease.

The Symptoms and Signs of Chronic Hepatitis B

As is true with liver disease in general, the symptoms of chronic hepatitis B are usually silent or nonspecific. Often people don't know that they have the virus when they pass it on to others. Symptoms may include generalized fatigue and weakness. People who have already progressed to cirrhosis may have symptoms and signs related to the complications of cirrhosis, such as jaundice, encephalopathy, and ascites.

Extrahepatic immune-mediated diseases, such as polyarteritis nodosa (PAN), glomerulonephritis, vasculitis (inflamed blood vessels), or cryoglobulinemia (excess proteins in the blood), may occur. Symptoms of these immune-mediated diseases include pronounced weakness of the muscles, joint aches, rashes, numbness in the arms and legs, high blood pressure (hypertension), abdominal pain, fever, and, infrequently, kidney failure. There is no correlation between the severity of immune-mediated diseases and the severity of the hepatitis. In fact, some people with severe immune-mediated diseases have a very mild hepatitis. These extrahepatic immune-mediated diseases associated with chronic hepatitis B are very uncommon, but may be quite serious. For example, some studies have even reported that as many as 30 to 50 percent of people may die due to complications of hepatitis B–induced vasculitis.

Diagnosing Chronic Hepatitis B

Most people usually find out that they have chronic hepatitis B almost by accident. It is sometimes discovered as part of a routine physical exam, from slight LFT elevations on blood work. Or a person may have been turned down for life insurance because of abnormal LFTs. Or their blood may have been rejected for donation because they tested positive for either the hepatitis B antibody or antigen. Of course, some people find out that they have chronic hepatitis B while under a doctor's care for acute hepatitis B. Others have found out about this condition after complaining of general feelings of fatigue to their doctors. Finally, some people with chronic hepatitis B seek medical help only after having progressed silently to cirrhosis. For these unfortunate people, the first sign of hepatitis B may be a complication of cirrhosis, such as variceal bleeding, ascites, encephalopathy, or liver cancer. (See chapter 6 for more information on cirrhosis.)

Blood Tests

In people with chronic hepatitis B, transaminases (AST and ALT) are usually mildly elevated (two to three times abnormal). AP and GGTP are usually normal or minimally elevated. These tests do not correlate with the severity of liver disease caused by HBV. The bilirubin is generally normal, unless advanced stages of cirrhosis are present. See chapter 3 for more information on the specific tests.

The hepatitis B serology is necessary to obtain an accurate diagnosis of hepatitis B. A lot of crucial information may be gleaned from these specific blood tests, such as the chronicity of HBV, immunity to HBV, and/or infectiousness of HBV to others. The hepatitis B serology is quite complicated. It is detailed in tables 9.1 and 9.2.

Table 9.1. Understanding Hepatitis B Serology

Serological Test	Significance of Serological Test
Hepatitis B Core Antibody IgM (HBcAb IgM) if HBsAg negative	Acute infection with HBV
Hepatitis B Core Antibody IgG (HBcAb IgG) if HBsAg positive	Chronic infection with HBV
Hepatitis B Core Antibody IgG (HBcAb IgG)	A lifelong marker of past infection with HBV that has been successfully cleared from the body (if HBsAg is absent)
Hepatitis B Surface Antibody (HBsAb)	Immunity to HBV or a successful response to the HBV vaccination
Hepatitis B Surface Antigen (HBsAg) if HBcAb IgM positive	Acute hepatitis B infection
Hepatitis B Surface Antigen (HBsAg) if HBcAb IgG positive	Chronic hepatitis B carrier
Hepatitis B "E" Antibody (HBeAb)	Resolved acute hepatitis B infection or inactive (nonreplicating) chronic disease
Hepatitis B "E" Antigen (HBeAg)	Active viral replication—high level of infectivity; seen in both acute hepatitis B and actively replicating chronic hepatitis B
Hepatitis B Viral Deoxyribonucleic Acid (HBV DNA)	Most sensitive marker for HBV replication usually occurs in the presence of HBeAg positivity; when occurs with HBeAg negativity indicates a mutant strain of infectious hepatitis B; disappearance corresponds to resolution of severe infectivity
Hepatitis D Antibody IgM (HDV IgM)	Acute infection with HDV
Hepatitis D Antibody IgG (HDV IgG)	Chronic infection with HDV

Hepatitis B Genotypes

The term "HBV *genotype*" refers to the genetic makeup of the different HBV mutants (variants of HBV) in the hepatitis B viral population of an individual. Seven different HBV genotypes have been identified: genotypes A through G. The HBV genotype can be determined through a blood test. (Note: Not all insurance companies will cover the cost of this test.) HBV genotypes vary in different areas of the world and among different groups of people. For example, in the United States and Europe, genotypes A and D are the predominant HBV variants. And genotypes B and C are most frequent in China and Southeast Asia. Unlike with HCV infection (see chapter 10), in which the genotype correlates with treatment response, the clinical value of HBV viral genotypes is unclear. It has

Table 9.2. Interpreting Hepatitis B Test Results

HBsAg Neg, HBcAb Neg, HBsAb neg	= susceptible to hepatitis B
HBsAg Neg, HBcAb Neg, HBsAb pos	= immune due to vaccination if HBsAb > 10mIU/ml
HBsAg neg, HBcAb Pos, HBsAb pos	= immune due to natural infection
HBsAg Pos, HBcAb pos, HBcAb IgM pos, HBsAb neg	= acute infection (infection within last six months)
HBsAg pos, HBcAb pos, HBcAb IgM neg, HBsAb neg	= chronic infection
HBsAg neg, HBcAb pos, HBsAb neg	= four possibilities:

1. patient is recovering from acute infection
2. testing is not sensitive enough to detect a very low level of HBsAb in the blood; thus, patient is immune
3. testing is not sensitive enough to detect a very low level of HBsAg in the blood; thus, patient is a chronic carrier
4. false positive HBcAb positivity; thus, patient is susceptible to infection

been suggested, however, that HBV genotype C may be associated with more severe liver disease than other genotypes. And genotype B has been associated with the development of liver cancer in young Taiwanese men. Thus, genotypes may have prognostic value. However, more studies on genotypes are needed in order to assess their significance.

Imaging Studies

Usually the doctor will want to obtain at least one imaging study (usually a sonogram) at some point during the diagnostic evaluation of chronic hepatitis B, especially when LFTs are elevated. While an enlarged liver or spleen may be detected on occasion, in general, imaging studies are usually normal—even in advanced stages of the disease. If liver cancer (hepatoma) is present, a mass may be revealed. See chapter 19 for more information on liver tumors. However, just because the liver looks normal on an imaging study does not mean that the liver is normal. That is why a liver biopsy is necessary when more information about the condition of the liver is needed.

Liver Biopsy

As with all liver diseases, even if a person feels fine, that's no guarantee that her liver is fine. The only way to determine the degree to which one's liver is injured is by examining a sample of the liver under a microscope. Therefore, in addition to obtaining a battery of blood tests, including LFTs and the hepatitis B serology, the doctor will need to perform a liver biopsy to determine the full extent of damage done to the liver by the virus and to determine if treatment is necessary. A liver biopsy is the only reliable means of determining the presence or absence of cirrhosis. Some studies have demonstrated that the results of a liver biopsy performed promptly after diagnosis can predict the future course of disease.

The Different Types of Chronic Hepatitis B

People with chronic hepatitis B may be divided into three categories: (1) inactive hepatitis B surface antigen (HBsAg) carrier state; (2) chronic hepatitis B, which is divided into HbeAg positive and HBeAg negative chronic hepatitis B; and (3) resolved chronic hepatitis B. Everyone with chronic hepatitis B is, by definition, both HBsAg and HBcAb positive. (Refer to table 9.1 on page 100 for a discussion of these and some related terms.) This means that both the hepatitis B surface antigen and core antibody are detectable in their blood.

Inactive HBsAg Carrier State

The first type of chronic hepatitis B is found in a person who carries hepatitis B, is HBsAg and HBcAb positive, but who has normal liver enzymes (AST and ALT), a normal physical exam, and is asymptomatic. Such a person is referred to as an inactive carrier of hepatitis B. HBeAg and HBV DNA are negative, and HBeAb is typically positive—indicating that this person is not infectious to others. Inactive carriers of HBV usually have minimal, if any, liver inflammation or damage. They usually live a normal life without any complications due to their liver disease. However, compared with the general population, these people are at a somewhat higher risk for cirrhosis and liver cancer. Therefore, regular observation—in the form of visits to the doctor approximately one to two times per year for a physical exam and blood tests—is necessary to check for early signs of disease progression.

In addition, these people are at risk for reactivation of the virus—return of HBeAg positivity. This occurs approximately 20 to 30 percent of the time. An individual's likelihood of reactivation increases if their immune system becomes suppressed. Such an occurrence may happen during treatment with immunosuppressive drugs, such as steroids (prednisone, for example), or during a severe illness, such as AIDS or cancer. Inactive carriers can also have flares of hepatitis. This may occur with or without the return of HBeAg and is noted by elevations in liver enzymes to approximately five to ten times the upper limit of normal. Repeated flares may lead to disease progression, liver scarring, and even liver failure.

Acute flares of hepatitis B should be distinguished from additional infection with hepatitis A, C, or D. Infection with an additional hepatitis virus is known as *superinfection*. It has been estimated that approximately 20 to 30 percent of such flares are due to superinfection with another hepatitis virus. Superinfection is associated with an increased risk of liver failure.

Chronic Hepatitis B

The second type of chronic hepatitis B is termed chronic hepatitis B and is found in a person who, in addition to carrying the HBsAg, also carries HBV DNA. The presence of detectable levels of HBV DNA indicates that a person is highly contagious or infectious to others. People with chronic hepatitis B may be either positive or negative for HBeAg. In both HBeAg positive and HBeAg negative people, liver enzymes are either persistently or intermittently elevated, and liver biopsy results typically reveal inflammation and damage. People with chronic hepatitis are likely to have a progressive disease leading to cirrhosis.

Chronic Hepatitis B—HBeAg positive

People with HBeAg positive chronic hepatitis B have only an 8 to 15 percent probability each year of becoming negative for HBeAg and HBV DNA. This is known as a spontaneous remission. When this happens, temporary gross elevation in transaminases (AST and ALT) is observed, followed by a rapid return to normal levels. Antibodies to HBeAg (known as HBeAb) are formed. This is known as seroconversion. These people are no longer contagious to others and they experience minimal, if any, liver damage going forward. In fact, any past liver damage often resolves within the next few years. This resolution confirms the transition from chronic hepatitis B into the inactive HBsAg carrier state, as discussed above. Women, older people, and those individuals with genotype B are likeliest to seroconvert. Unfortunately, reactivation to the infectious state can occur in some of these people. Thus, these people must be observed carefully. It is not clear which factors play a role in causing some people to relapse into an infectious state. Certainly excessive alcohol intake may have a harmful effect on people with chronic hepatitis B. And it has been demonstrated that excessive iron intake may promote persistent HBV replication in some people. (Excessive iron in itself can damage the liver and may lead to cirrhosis and liver cancer. This is discussed in more detail in chapters 18 and 23.) Therefore, people with chronic hepatitis B are advised to refrain from alcohol intake and should avoid excess iron supplementation. Seroconverters whose immune systems subsequently become compromised are at risk for a relapse. Immune-system function can become impaired by a number of factors, including infection with the human immunodeficiency virus (HIV), treatment with chemotherapeutic agents for cancer, or use of corticosteroids such as prednisone.

Chronic Hepatitis B—HBeAg negative

People with chronic hepatitis B who are negative for HBeAg have a mutant strain of chronic hepatitis B. A *mutation* is a permanent alteration of the hepatitis B virus's genetic makeup. There are many different types of hepatitis B mutations. In this case, the genetic mutation is characterized by the failure of the virus to make the hepatitis B "e" antigen (HBeAg). This is known as a *precore mutation*. This mutation does not affect the virus's ability to replicate. Therefore, on blood tests, these people are negative for HBeAg, but positive for HBV DNA. Men are more likely than women to have this mutation, and HBeAg negative chronic hepatitis B does not occur with genotype A. Precore mutant hepatitis B has been responsible for several cases of surprised transmission of hepatitis B to others, as these people were unaware that they were infectious. This strain of hepatitis B may be genetically superior to HBeAg positive chronic hepatitis B. Thus, liver disease is usually more active and liver scarring more advanced. These individuals are more likely to develop cirrhosis compared with HBeAg positive people. Furthermore, this strain is usually more resistant to treatment.

Resolved Chronic Hepatitis B

In some instances, a person who is HBsAg positive can become HBsAg negative, which is the last category of chronic hepatitis B, known as resolved chronic hepatitis B. However, it is very uncommon and occurs only at a rate of approximately 0.5 to 2 percent of hepatitis patients each year. Loss of HBsAg is more likely to occur in women than men and is rare in people with the mutant strain.

Most, but not all, people who do resolve will develop the hepatitis B antibody (HbsAb). Liver enzymes (ALT and AST) normalize. Clearance of hepatitis B antigen decreases the risk of progression to liver failure and liver cancer. Most people who have resolved have a benign course of disease. However, approximately half of these people continue to have very low levels of HBV DNA and are considered to be noninfectious to others.

A low level, also considered a noninfectious level of HBV DNA, is defined as less than 10,000 copies/ml. These low HBV DNA levels are only detectable if a very sensitive laboratory assay known as the *polymerase chain reaction (PCR)* is used. The PCR assay has the ability to detect levels as low 200 copies/ml. (These test results are often reported in picograms per milliliters (pg/ml) 1pg/ml = 280,000 copies/ml.) In situations where people with resolved hepatitis B experience severe immune suppression, such as cancer chemotherapy or organ transplantation, chronic hepatitis B can be reactivated. This means that HBsAg will become positive again.

The Long-term Prognosis for Those with Chronic Hepatitis B

The probability each year that a person with chronic hepatitis B will develop cirrhosis is about 2 percent. However, different studies have reported rates varying from 0.1 to 10 percent per year. The cumulative probability of progression to cirrhosis over five years is approximately 15 to 20 percent. After the development of cirrhosis, the probability of developing serious complications, such as decompensated cirrhosis, is about 2 to 10 percent each year. The five-year survival rate after cirrhosis has developed varies from 52 to 80 percent. However, if a person has decompensated cirrhosis, the five-year survival rate decreases to between 14 and 35 percent.

More than 1 million people worldwide die each year from hepatitis B. So, why is it that some people can live a long healthy life with hepatitis B and others experience serious complications? Well, it has been demonstrated that there are many factors that influence the progression from a mild, innocuous illness to a grave outcome. These factors include advanced age, general poor health—for example, depressed immune status such as additionally infection with HIV; the presence of advanced damage found on a liver biopsy sample; and the presence of markers of chronicity and active infectiousness, especially HBV DNA. Similarly, people who do not clear HBeAg (spontaneous remission) tend to have a more aggressive course than those who clear HBeAg. In fact, in some studies it has been shown that people who clear HBeAg rarely progress to cirrhosis. Furthermore, people who clear HBeAg, whether spontaneously or from treatment, have a decreased incidence of liver failure and an improved long-term survival rate. People who are additionally infected with the hepatitis delta virus (HDV) (see page 106) or the hepatitis C virus (see chapter 10) also have poorer prognoses. In addition, it has been shown that the outcome of a person infected with HBV is highly dependent upon the stage at which she first obtained medical attention. Those people who have more advanced disease on liver biopsy samples when initially seen by a specialist have a shorter survival time. It has also been found that people with genotype C have a worse prognosis than those with other genotypes. Lastly, it has been demonstrated that people infected with HBV are more susceptible to the toxic effects of alcohol on the liver than are those without HBV. Therefore, it is important for people with chronic hepatitis B to avoid all intake of alcohol, as alcohol may worsen the course and accelerate the progression of the disease. See chapter 17 for more information on alcohol's effects on the liver.

Chronic Hepatitis B and Long-term Liver Cancer Risk

People with chronic hepatitis B are at increased risk for developing liver cancer. The exact risk is unknown, but in some studies, people with chronic hepatitis B were two hundred times more likely to develop liver cancer compared with people without this disease. Cancer usually occurs in those who have developed cirrhosis. However, cancer can also occur in chronic HBV carriers without cirrhosis. In fact, in some parts of the world where hepatitis B is endemic, such as in Africa, up to 30 percent of people with chronic hepatitis B develop liver cancer without underlying cirrhosis.

From the time a person becomes infected with HBV, liver cancer generally takes about twenty to thirty years to develop. Thus, people who were infected at birth can develop liver cancer as early as the age of twenty. It appears that infection with both HBV and HCV or infection with both HBV and HDV, drinking excessive alcohol, and having a family history of HCC can increase the likelihood that a person will develop liver cancer. It has been noted that men appear to have an increased risk of developing HCC compared to women. Whether this is due to hormonal differences is unclear. See chapter 19 for more information on HBV and liver cancer.

THE HEPATITIS DELTA VIRUS (HDV)

Hepatitis D is inflammation of the liver due to a virus called the hepatitis delta virus (HDV). HDV is a virus that can live only in people with hepatitis B. Approximately 70,000 people in the United States are infected with HDV. Although HDV only accounts for a small percentage of cases of chronic viral hepatitis, it tends to be particularly severe and to have significant long-term consequences. In fact, chronic hepatitis D causes more than one thousand deaths each year in the United States. In the 1970s, hepatitis delta virus infection was endemic throughout Southern Europe. However, by the 1990s the incidence of HDV infection had significantly decreased. In fact, one study done in Italy estimated that the number of cases of HDV within that country decreased by 1.5 percent each year from 1987 to 1997. And, it is anticipated that this trend will continue. Currently, new HDV infections are rare.

HDV infection may be silent or may cause the same kind of fatigue and other symptoms associated with other forms of hepatitis. However, up to 20 percent of hepatitis D patients develop fulminant hepatitis, a particularly serious condition that requires hospitalization. See chapter 7 for a discussion on fulminant hepatitis.

HDV is transmitted through the same blood, sexual, and perinatal routes as HBV, which were discussed on page 92. There are two ways in which a person infected with HBV may become infected with HDV: *coinfection* and *superinfection*. When HBV and HDV are acquired at the same time, it is known as coinfection. In 90 to 95 percent of cases, such people will be able to completely eliminate both viruses from their bodies. This means that only approximately 5 to 10 percent of coinfected individuals go on to develop chronic hepatitis B and D. HDV can also be acquired by someone who already has chronic hepatitis B. This is known as superinfection. In contrast to people infected with both viruses simultaneously, approximately 70 to 95 percent of people who become infected in this two-step fashion progress to chronic hepatitis D.

LONG-TERM PROGNOSIS FOR THOSE WITH CHRONIC HEPATITIS B AND D

Compared with people who have chronic hepatitis B alone, those with chronic infections of both HBV and HDV are more likely to have a poor outcome. These people tend to develop cirrhosis more frequently and more rapidly than those with chronic hepatitis B alone. Approximately 60 to 70 percent of all people with chronic hepatitis D develop cirrhosis, and 15 percent of them develop cirrhosis in two years or less from the time of initial infection. This is much more frequent and rapid than for any other form of chronic viral hepatitis. People with both chronic hepatitis B and chronic hepatitis D are also more likely to develop complications, such as liver failure and liver cancer, and are more likely to require a liver transplant as compared with people suffering from other forms of chronic viral hepatitis.

CONCLUSION

In this chapter, you learned about two hepatitis viruses that can damage the liver: hepatitis B virus (HBV) and hepatitis delta virus (HDV). These viruses lead to the liver diseases hepatitis B and hepatitis D, respectively. The treatment of hepatitis B and D will be discussed in chapter 12, and prevention will be discussed in chapter 24. In cases where treatment fails, a person may be a candidate for liver transplantation. This surgical procedure will be discussed in chapter 22. Meanwhile, the next chapter discusses another viral infection—the hepatitis C virus (HCV). This virus can cause both acute and chronic hepatitis C. Though HCV has some similarities to HBV and HDV, it also has many important differences.

Ten

UNDERSTANDING
HEPATITIS C

*After feeling rundown for about a year, Sue, a thirty-six-year-old of-
fice manager and mother of three, finally went to see her family doctor. After examining her and drawing some blood, the doctor said,
"Sue, you look fine. You probably just need to slow down a little." Sue
went home feeling relieved. She was going to start planning a vaca-
tion for herself. But when the doctor called a week later to inform her
that her blood tests revealed a problem with her liver, she was shocked.
And even more so when subsequent blood tests revealed that she had
chronic hepatitis C. "How could I have contracted hepatitis C?" Sue
wondered. "Could it have been that summer when I experimented a
few times with intravenous drugs? But how could that be? That was
twenty years ago and it only happened a few times!" Sue's doctor advised her to see a specialist.*

This chapter discusses the hepatitis C virus (HCV)—how it is transmitted
and who is at risk for contracting it. It clarifies the difference between the
acute and chronic forms of the disease and the reason why such a high percentage of people who are exposed to HCV become chronically infected. In addition, this chapter covers the various ways that an HCV infection is diagnosed
and what signs and symptoms are common to this virus. Also, the diagnostic
blood tests related to HCV are explained. Toward the end of this chapter, the
probable long-term outcome of chronic hepatitis C and some risk factors that
promote disease progression will be covered. (See chapter 13 for a detailed discussion of the treatment of hepatitis C.)

WHAT IS HEPATITIS C?

Hepatitis C is inflammation of the liver due to a virus called the hepatitis C virus (HCV). After the discovery of the hepatitis A virus in 1973 and the hepatitis B virus in 1963, the remaining hepatitis viruses were lumped into the category of non-A non-B (NANB) hepatitis. Any cases of acute or chronic hepatitis or cirrhosis without identifiable causes were suspected to be a result of the NANB hepatitis viruses. In 1989, a major breakthrough regarding this mysterious and intriguing disease occurred—the hepatitis C virus was identified. Now, HCV is believed to be the virus responsible for more than 90 percent of all cases of NANB hepatitis.

HCV is the most common cause of cirrhosis and liver cancer in the United States. More than 4 million Americans (approximately 2 percent of the United States population) and more than 170 million people worldwide (approximately 3 percent of the world's population) are infected with HCV. (HCV is more prevalent in Africa, the eastern Mediterranean, Southeast Asia, and the western Pacific than in the United States.) The Centers for Disease Control (CDC) estimates that only a small percentage (probably around 5 percent) of infected individuals are even aware that they harbor this virus in their bodies.

People between the ages of forty and fifty-nine are most likely to be diagnosed with HCV. And it is estimated that there will be a fourfold increase in the number of adults diagnosed with HCV by the year 2015. While HCV can infect anyone with risk factors, it has been found to be more common among certain subgroups of people. For example, the prevalence of HCV among prison inmates is between 39 and 54 percent, among intravenous drug users between 70 and 90 percent, and among those attending Veterans Administration outpatient clinics between 18 and 40 percent.

While the incidence of people becoming acutely infected with HCV is decreasing in the United States, approximately 8,000 to 12,000 deaths are attributed to hepatitis C each year. Moreover, it is estimated that in the absence of appropriate therapy, this number will triple within the next two decades. In fact, chronic hepatitis C is the most common reason that a person will need to undergo a liver transplant in the United States.

HOW HCV IS TRANSMITTED

Most people are surprised to learn they have hepatitis C, and many believe they are not at risk for acquiring this virus. Other people have a definable risk factor, such as a history of intravenous drug use, but feel that it occurred such a long time ago that it has no relevance. And some people know exactly how they contracted it.

There are, in fact, many ways that a person can contract HCV. The most efficient mode of transmission is via blood-to-blood contact. This means that blood from an infected person gets into the bloodstream of another person. HCV can only enter the bloodstream by first getting through the protective covering of one's skin. This is known as the *percutaneous route*. Read on for more information about all routes of transmission.

Blood and Blood-Product Transfusions

It has been estimated by the Centers for Disease Control (CDC) that prior to 1990, when screening donated blood and blood products for HCV was begun, almost 300,000 Americans contracted HCV from transfused blood. This occurred as a result of receiving HCV-infected blood—packed red blood cells (PRBC) or blood products, such as platelets, fresh frozen plasma (FFP), or immunoglobulins. In addition, it has been estimated that almost 1 percent of all potential blood donors are infected with HCV. Fortunately, blood banks have been screening all potential donors for HCV since 1990. And since 1992, these screening techniques have been exceptionally accurate.

Today, the incidence of obtaining this virus by receiving a blood transfusion is approximately 1 in 125,000 to 1 in 200,000 per unit of blood transfused (the risk of infection is approximately 0.001 percent per unit of blood transfused). In essence, since 1992, the likelihood of contracting HCV from a blood transfusion has been minuscule. The reason that a small risk still exists is that when a person initially becomes infected with HCV, there is a short period of time, known as the *window period,* in which the HCV antibody (HCV Ab) is not detectable in the blood. If a person donates blood during the window period, her blood will carry HCV, but it will not be detectable. It is recommended that anyone who received a blood transfusion prior to 1992 be tested for HCV. Please note: Once somebody has tested positive for HCV, she should refrain from donating blood or organs.

Intravenous Drug Use

Intravenous drug use (IVDU) is the most common way of transmitting HCV, and it accounts for almost 70 percent of all new HCV infections. HCV has been found in approximately 85 to 100 percent of IV drug users. The longer a person uses IV drugs, the greater the likelihood one has of becoming infected with HCV. HCV is transmitted from one person to another through the sharing of needles and/or other drug paraphernalia. Even a speck of blood so small that it is undetectable to the human eye can carry a great deal of hepatitis C viral particles. Therefore, drug paraphernalia that appears to have been adequately cleaned may still contain HCV.

The decades of the 1960s and 1970s were characterized by considerable experimentation and rebellion. Intravenous drug use was sometimes a part of the culture that prevailed during this era. Though many users were aware that IV drug use was illegal, they were not aware that it had the potential to introduce a serious viral infection (one that had not even been identified) into their livers. For some, IV drug use was a daily occurrence. Others may have tried it only once or twice. But even a one-time occurrence long ago still may have relevance. Remember, HCV can reside in the body for many years, silently doing damage to the liver even though the person feels fine.

Intranasal Drug Use

Intranasal drug use, or "snorting" drugs, is also a potential route of virus transmission. Small blood vessels in the nose may break open and bleed when an instrument such as a straw or a rolled-up dollar bill is used to snort a drug, such as cocaine. Most of the time, the amount of blood on the instrument is so small that it is undetectable. When these instruments are shared, HCV can pass from one person to another. Once again, engaging in this activity even once may be sufficient to infect a person with HCV.

Healthcare and Occupational Exposure

People who work in a hospital or other healthcare facility (e.g., doctor's office, medical labs, blood bank), as well as public-safety and emergency medical workers, are at risk for contracting HCV while on the job, through a needle stick or mucosal exposure (exposure to the mucus-secreting membranes that line a body cavity and communicate with the exterior, such as the inside of the mouth, nose, lips, and vagina) to the blood of an infected person. There is approximately a 2 percent chance of becoming infected with HCV after exposure to the blood of an HCV-positive person. However, the likelihood of contracting HCV ranges between 0 to 10 percent, based on a variety of factors. First, the higher the person's HCV *viral load* (the amount of viral particles per milliliters of blood) at the time of the incident, the higher the risk of acquiring the virus. HCV viral loads (HCV RNA) greater than 500,000 IU/ml increase the likelihood of transmission. Second, the type of body tissue exposure influences the likelihood of transmission. The chance of transmission increases with exposure to mucous membranes, such as an eye splash (blood splashing into someone's eye), and is the highest if there was exposure to breaks in the skin, such as an open wound or sore. HCV-infected blood on someone's intact skin has never been reported as a cause of HCV infection. Third, the longer HCV is outside of the infected person's body, the less chance there is of acquiring the virus. For example, HCV-infected blood from a test tube or lying on a surface is less infectious than HCV-infected blood coming directly from a person's body. This is because the level of HCV infectivity (the level of HCV RNA in blood) declines once it is outside the infected person. Finally, the type of instrument that a person was stuck with is relevant to the likelihood of acquiring HCV. For example, sticking oneself with a solid needle (such as a suture needle) carries a relatively low chance of HCV acquisition since these needles can hold only a small volume of blood. In contrast, sticking oneself with a hollow-bore needle (such as a needle used in drawing blood), which can hold a large volume of HCV-infected blood, carries a higher risk of HCV acquisition.

Even with the potential risk to healthcare workers due to the nature of their profession, the prevalence of HCV infection among this group is actually about the same as that of the general population, which is 1 to 2 percent.

The appropriate testing to obtain after an exposure as well as possible treatment options after exposure are discussed in chapter 13.

Medical Procedures

The World Health Organization (WHO) estimates that approximately 2.3 to 4.7 million cases of HCV occur each year in developing countries as a result of the use of nonsterile, reused needles. The best-known large-scale transmission of HCV from healthcare workers to patients occurred in Egypt, where approximately 7 to 15 million people became infected with HCV due to the reuse of nonsterile needles during a campaign to mass-immunize the population for *schistosomiasis* (a parasite (worm) that may cause severe disease). In the United States, unsterile medical practices, such as reusing needles, have occurred in the past. This may partly explain the presence of chronic hepatitis C in older individuals in the United States who have no other definable risk factor. Many people, particularly those in the military, who received vaccinations prior to the widespread use of disposable needles, acquired the virus by this means. Medical knowledge of appropriate sterility practices has advanced considerably over the past several decades in developed countries such as the United States. As such, transmission of HCV from healthcare workers to patients accounts for less than 0.5 percent of HCV cases. The following is a discussion of the possible ways a healthcare worker or a medical procedure may cause the transmission of HCV to an individual.

People with kidney failure who are undergoing hemodialysis have an increased risk of acquiring HCV. *Hemodialysis* is a medical procedure that involves removing the blood through an artery, cleaning it, and then returning it to the person through a vein. In fact, it is estimated that in the United States, approximately 20 to 30 percent of hemodialysis patients are infected with HCV. This is due to a combination of receiving frequent blood transfusions prior to 1992, possible inadequate sterilization of equipment used during the hemodialysis procedure, and the possible sharing of supplies among patients. Fortunately, the incidence of chronic hepatitis C in this group of people is decreasing due to the use of universal precautions in dialysis units and to improved methods of screening transfused blood.

Another medical procedure that puts one at risk of contracting HCV is undergoing an organ transplant. One may become infected with HCV by receiving an organ (such as a kidney, eye, heart, or even liver) from a person infected with HCV. If an organ donor is infected with HCV, there is approximately a 50 percent chance that she will transmit the virus to the transplant recipient. Since there is a shortage of liver donors, some transplant centers will utilize the liver of a hepatitis C positive organ donor for transplant to a person with hepatitis C in need of a new liver. Unfortunately, prior infection with HCV will not protect the transplant recipient from developing another HCV infection with a different HCV genotype. (See page 131 for a discussion of HCV genotypes.)

The medical practice of sharing multidose vials (vials containing more than one dose of medication) of, for example, local anesthetics, saline, heparin, or other solutions, has been implicated in many small, isolated outbreaks of HCV. Even minimal contamination of a medical product is sufficient to transmit HCV from one patient to the next via this indirect route. Isolated instances of transmission during surgery, from surgeons infected with HCV to their patients, have been noted. Though rare, it occurs primarily during cardiovascular thoracic surgery, as sharp edges of bone are encountered and metallic sutures are used, both of which can penetrate through sterile gloves, thus causing bleeding during surgery. The Centers for Disease Control does not recommend restricting the professional activities of HCV-infected healthcare workers. As a practical matter, any restrictions should be evaluated on a case-by-case basis.

Tattooing and Body Piercing

Tattooing and body piercing, including piercing the ears, are practices that involve breaking the skin with a needle. In the course of these procedures, a small amount of bleeding can occur. If the needles, ink, or other equipment used during these practices are not sterile, HCV may be transmitted as one customer's HCV-infected blood makes its way into the bloodstream of a subsequent customer.

Sexual Contact

Sexual contact, whether it be genital, oral, or anal, appears to be an extremely inefficient means of HCV transmission. In fact, many studies evaluating this mode of transmission have failed to detect the presence of HCV in either the saliva, semen, or urine of HCV-infected people—except when these body fluids have been contaminated by the person's blood. However, it is important to emphasize that HCV has the potential to be transmitted through intimate contact if there is active bleeding such as during menses (if the woman is infected with HCV), or if there are breaks in the skin or in the lining of the mouth, vagina, penis, or anus. Breaks may occur for a variety of reasons including the presence of active, bleeding herpes sores or as a result of traumatic or rough sex, especially anal intercourse. In fact, it has been found that people with sexually transmitted diseases such as trichomoniasis, gonorrhea, and herpes, as well as men who have sex with men, are both factors that have been found to increase the likelihood of sexual transmission. Since HCV can be present in menstrual blood, extra precautions (the use of dental dams and condoms) should be considered during and just after menstruation to decrease the chance of transmission, particularly if the sex partner has open cuts or wounds. Also, sanitary napkins or tampons should be placed in a leak-proof sealed bag and promptly disposed of. Finally, it has been found that people

coinfected with both HIV and HCV may have an increased potential for transmitting HCV through sexual contact. Of interest is that it appears to be easier for
a man to transmit HCV to a woman than vice versa.

Assuming the absence of the above factors, and assuming that blood is not
exchanged during sex, a person who is in a long-term monogamous relationship
with an HCV-infected person is not likely to contract the hepatitis virus from sexual relations with their partner. Therefore, barrier precautions are not routinely
recommended for such people.

Some studies have tested the sex partners of hepatitis C patients to see
whether they, too, were HCV positive. Such studies have produced results ranging from 0 to 6 percent positivity, with approximately 2 percent being the average. However, it is crucial to keep in mind that it is not known whether these sex
partners acquired the hepatitis C virus through sex or by another route.

Household Contact

Transmission of HCV among family members or among other people living together may occur. This can potentially happen through the sharing of razors,
toothbrushes, or any sharp instruments that carry HCV-infected blood. Therefore, it is crucial to keep each person's personal items, such as toothbrushes and
razors, in separate areas of the bathroom, and each item should be clearly labeled.
In this manner, the likelihood of accidentally using a potentially HCV-infected
household item will be decreased. In the United States, the incidence of contracting HCV from accidental household contact is unknown. However, data from
other countries indicate that it is low—approximately 4 percent.

Childbirth

Of great concern to pregnant women infected with HCV and to women with
chronic hepatitis C who are contemplating pregnancy is the likelihood of transmitting the virus to their babies. However, the risk for either of these types of
transmission is very low—occurring only approximately 3 to 7 percent of the
time. Transmission to the newborn has been found to occur only in HCV-infected
women who had high viral loads of at least 2 million IU/ml. It has also been
noted that women who are coinfected with HIV and HCV appear to have
a higher probability of transmitting HCV to their newborns than women who
are not infected with HIV. Please refer to chapter 24 for more information on
this topic.

Breast-feeding is not considered a means of transmitting HCV. Therefore, it
is believed that an HCV-infected mother may safely breast-feed her child, unless
her nipples are cracked and bleeding. Studies comparing the incidence of HCV
in breast-fed versus bottle-fed infants of mothers with HCV showed a fairly
equal incidence of HCV in each group of infants—approximately 4 percent.

Other Routes of Transmission

Though the reasons are not entirely clear, some population groups, such as in certain parts of Africa, some portions of Italy, and some parts of Japan, have been found to have a particularly high incidence of hepatitis C. Some indigenous healing or folk-medicine practices common to these regions, involving skin piercing with unsterilized instruments, are suspected to account for the disproportionately high incidence of the virus. Reuse of nonsterile needles and syringes by health-care workers (as discussed above) is another likely reason for the unusually high incidence in some of these regions.

Another potential, yet unlikely, route of transmission involves insects. Theoretically, transmission by insects can only occur if an insect bites an HCV-infected person and then immediately bites someone else. In this way, the HCV-tainted blood could enter the second person. Viruses other than HCV, such as yellow fever and dengue, have been shown to spread by this route. One study conducted in New Jersey concluded that mosquitoes are unlikely agents of transmission of HCV. Therefore, while not believed to be a significant source of HCV transmission, further investigation into the area of insect transmission is needed.

In some societies, cults and fraternity members mix their blood together as part of a ritual or in order to be inaugurated. Sometimes people will mix their blood with that of a close friend or partner in a process by which they become "blood brothers." This potential mode of HCV transmission also warrants further investigation.

Finally, even a barber or a manicurist may be a risk factor. If the instruments they use are not properly cleaned, they can potentially carry a small amount of HCV. Similarly, people undergoing acupuncture or electrolysis are at risk of becoming infected with HCV if the needles and other equipment being used have not been properly sterilized.

Sporadic Hepatitis C

Some people who have hepatitis C state that they cannot identify a risk factor to account for their HCV infection. This group of people has been classified as having sporadic hepatitis C. Note, however, that some people who have sporadic hepatitis C probably do have an identifiable risk factor but are concealing it for personal reasons. They may fear a lack of confidentiality on the part of their doctors, they may fear being judged as having done something bad (or illegal) in the past, or they may fear being rejected for life or medical insurance. Others do not consider a certain behavior to count as a risk—behaviors such as having a body part pierced or an isolated occurrence of intravenous or intranasal drug use—and therefore deny it when questioned. In fact, in one study, many former IV drug users with hepatitis C who attempted to donate blood denied their IV drug use when screened at the time of blood donation, as they felt that their former habit was such an insignificant event that it would not affect the purity of their blood. Others feel that an episode that happened long ago doesn't count anymore, and therefore they don't disclose it to their doctors. Finally, some people simply do not recall the incident that caused the infection.

THOSE AT INCREASED RISK FOR HEPATITIS C

Unlike hepatitis A and B, hepatitis C is not preventable through vaccination. However, there are measures that a person can take to minimize her chances of acquiring HCV. In addition, many precautions may be taken by an HCV-infected person to reduce the likelihood of transmitting this virus to others. Prevention of HCV will be discussed in chapter 24. Meanwhile, take note of the following categories of individuals who are at increased risk for contracting HCV. All individuals in these categories should be tested for HCV.

- People who have received a blood or blood-product transfusion or an organ transplant prior to 1992 and especially prior to 1990

- Intravenous drug users (past and present)

- Household members of an infected person if toothbrushes, razors, or other objects that may transmit HCV have been shared

- Hospital and other healthcare facility workers after a needle stick or mucosal exposure to the blood of a person with HCV

- Public-safety and emergency medical workers after a needle stick or mucosal exposure to the blood of a person with HCV

- People who have acquired a tattoo or who have had a body part pierced if they suspect unsterile practices

- People who have been born to a mother infected with HCV

- The sex partner of an HCV-positive person, if traumatic sex or bleeding due to mucosal breaks or other reasons (such as prostatitis—an inflammation of the prostate gland with occasional bleeding) may have occurred

- Organ transplant recipients of an HCV-infected organ

- Hemodialysis patients

Note: Anyone with elevated liver enzymes—even those without an identifiable risk factor—should be tested for HCV.

WHAT IS ACUTE HEPATITIS C?

Acute hepatitis C is inflammation of the liver due to HCV lasting six months or less. The number of people who become acutely infected with HCV has been steadily decreasing over the years. For example, in 1984 approximately 180,000 to 230,000 new acute infections each year were estimated to have occurred, compared with 35,000 new acute infections estimated to occur each year as of 2002. The reason for the declining incidence of newly acquired infections is not entirely known, but it has been associated with a decrease in acute hepatitis C among IV drug users. Increased knowledge and publicity about HIV, the virus that causes AIDS, has probably contributed to a decrease in the sharing of drug paraphernalia among IV drug users, thereby resulting in a decreased incidence in HCV transmission. Increased knowledge and awareness about HCV transmission and prevention, as well as improved diagnostic testing for the screening of blood and organ donors, may have contributed to this decline. As knowledge of hepatitis C continues to grow, the number of people who become infected with HCV will likely diminish even further.

The Symptoms and Signs of Acute Hepatitis C

The incubation period—the time between the entrance of the virus into the body and the initial appearance of symptoms and signs of the disease—of acute HCV is about six to eight weeks; however, it may be as short as two weeks or as long as about five months.

When symptoms of acute hepatitis C do occur, they are usually similar to those that characterize acute hepatitis in general (see page 76). However, most people with acute hepatitis C experience no symptoms. Only about 25 to 35 percent of individuals with hepatitis C manifest any symptoms at all. Usually, these symptoms are nonspecific and may easily be mistaken as stemming from something unconnected to hepatitis C, such as the flu. Symptoms, if they do occur, may include fatigue, decreased appetite, and weakness. Occasionally, a person may experience a skin rash and/or muscle and joint aches. People with acute hepatitis C become jaundiced approximately 25 percent of the time. It has been shown that people with another liver disease, such as hepatitis B, who become additionally infected with acute hepatitis C, are particularly likely to experience a severe course of acute hepatitis C. Usually, the physical exam of a person with acute hepatitis C appears normal. Occasionally, a physical exam will reveal an enlarged and tender liver, jaundice, and/or a rash.

Diagnosing Acute Hepatitis C

As mentioned previously, approximately 35,000 new acute hepatitis C infections are estimated to occur each year. However, it is also estimated that only 25 to 30 percent of these newly acquired infections are actually diagnosed. The most likely explanation for this low percentage is that most people with acute hepatitis C are either asymptomatic or have very vague symptoms. Therefore, evaluation by a doctor during the acute stage of this disease is not common. As such, the majority of people with hepatitis C do not discover that they harbor this virus until years or, often, decades later. Therefore, there are probably millions of people who currently have hepatitis C and have no idea that they are infected. However, if a person sees her doctor for an evaluation of symptoms, acute hepatitis C is usually detected from abnormal blood test results.

Transaminases (AST and ALT) are often quite elevated initially. Levels of approximately 200 to 600 IU/l can occur. (The normal range is approximately 0 to 45 IU/l.) Elevations in transaminases usually occur approximately six to eight weeks after infection with HCV (or within a range of two to twenty-six weeks). As the disease progresses, transaminases typically decrease. Transaminase levels often fluctuate between normal (or near normal) and elevated before permanently returning to normal. This fluctuation is a typical characteristic of hepatitis C. Persistent normalization of transaminases by six months usually indicates that acute hepatitis C has resolved. This occurs 15 to 25 percent of the time. If transaminases remain elevated (usually around two to three times normal) after this period or if the ALT levels elevate after a period of normalization, it usually indicates progression to chronic hepatitis C (see page 120), which occurs approximately 60 to 85 percent of the time. Progression to chronic disease is always accompanied by an elevated HCV viral load.

Cholestatic liver enzymes (AP and GGTP) are usually only mildly elevated during acute hepatitis C—around two to three times normal—and bilirubin levels are usually normal. Around one-fourth of all people with acute hepatitis C become jaundiced. Even among these people, bilirubin levels usually normalize rapidly, usually within about one month.

None of these blood test abnormalities is diagnostic of acute hepatitis C. But once the doctor detects abnormal LFTs, additional blood work specific for hepatitis C, known as the hepatitis C serology, will be performed (see page 120 for a detailed discussion of HCV serology). From the results of these tests, which detect antibodies to the hepatitis C virus (HCV Ab) and the hepatitis C viral load (HCV RNA), the doctor will be able to determine if the LFT abnormalities are due to hepatitis C. The hepatitis C antibody (HCV Ab) can be detected in the blood in 90 percent of people within three months, and in almost all people by six months of exposure. The HCV viral load (HCV RNA) can be detected in the blood as early as one to four weeks after exposure. HCV RNA levels vary markedly during this time. As such, a single test for HCV RNA showing an undetectable level does not exclude the possibility of acute infection. Instead, multiple determinations of HCV RNA are needed to confirm acute infection.

Imaging studies are typically normal and are not needed to make a diagnosis of hepatitis C. If performed, imaging studies are generally done in order to eliminate other possible causes of elevated LFTs, such as gallstones. A liver biopsy is usually not performed during the acute stage of a hepatitis C infection.

Determining Whether Acute Hepatitis C Has Resolved

After the diagnosis of acute hepatitis C has been made, the doctor will probably want to see the patient several times over the next few months in order to check on the status of the infection. Six months after the patient has been infected, the doctor will determine whether the patient has shaken off HCV entirely or whether she has progressed to chronic hepatitis C.

Hepatitis C is limited to acute infection in around 15 to 40 percent of people. Typically, those people who suffered from the most symptoms (such as those who were jaundiced) are the ones most likely to clear the virus. These fortunate people have a complete resolution of symptoms, physical signs, and any LFT abnormalities due to infection with HCV. Also, their HCV RNA will permanently return to normal. These people do not develop chronic infection and, therefore, are not at risk for the long-term consequences of hepatitis C. Nor can they transmit HCV to others. However, eradicating one particular "strain" of HCV does not protect a person from becoming infected with other "strains" of HCV, or from other hepatitis viruses such as hepatitis A and B (see page 131 for a discussion of the different strains of HCV, also referred to as genotypes). Also, these people will never be allowed to donate blood, as they will always have the antibody for hepatitis C present in their blood.

WHAT IS FULMINANT HEPATITIS C?

Fulminant hepatitis C is a very rare but severe form of acute hepatitis C. It is characterized by the sudden onset of liver failure, coagulopathy, jaundice, and encephalopathy. Patients become severely ill and develop a rapidly progressive downhill course. Approximately 85 percent of these people are likely to die unless immediate liver transplantation is undertaken. Fortunately, this complication of acute hepatitis C is a very rare occurrence.

WHAT IS CHRONIC HEPATITIS C?

Chronic hepatitis C is defined as the persistence of HCV RNA in the blood for six months or more. In people with chronic hepatitis C, the immune system has failed to clear the virus from the body. Therefore, all individuals with chronic hepatitis C will always have an elevated HCV RNA. Once a person is chronically infected with HCV, the potential exists for liver damage and cirrhosis along with its complications, including liver failure and liver cancer. (The treatment of chronic hepatitis C will be discussed in chapter 13.)

The Reason So Many Cases of Acute Hepatitis C Become Chronic

HCV is a virus that is very difficult to clear from the body. Thus, most people who become infected with HCV (acute hepatitis C) develop chronic disease (chronic hepatitis C). In fact, approximately 60 to 85 percent of infected people develop chronic hepatitis C. This is in stark contrast to the incidence of progression from acute to chronic in other forms of viral hepatitis. For example, hepatitis B progresses to chronic disease only about 5 percent of the time when the infection is acquired as an adult. And hepatitis A never leads to chronic disease. It appears that the immune system is not very efficient in clearing HCV. So, what makes HCV so formidable?

The genes that make up HCV can vary slightly from one strain to another. These different genetic variations of HCV are known as hepatitis C mutants, or *quasispecies*. The entire hepatitis C viral population that is present in a person infected with HCV is made up of a conglomerate of related, yet slightly different, HCV species. This virus population usually consists of one HCV mutant group that is strongest and dominant and numerous other HCV mutants that are weaker. These mutants are all similar in structure but differ slightly from one another. These slight variations in structure account for the fact that some HCV mutants are stronger and thus better equipped to fight the immune system than other HCV mutants. This is analogous to Darwin's theory of evolution: the survival of the fittest.

The fact that HCV is such a resourceful and cunning virus probably accounts for why most people progress to chronic disease. When HCV is being attacked by the immune system during the acute infection, it can mutate into a stronger quasispecies variant. In this manner, HCV is able to outwit the body's immune system and thwart its attempts to eradicate it. Thus, HCV tricks the body's immune surveillance and escapes eradication, allowing for progression to chronic disease. This partly explains why long-term response rates to therapy with interferon (see chapter 13), although getting much better, are still not 100 percent successful. It also may explain why it is so difficult to create a vaccination against HCV (see chapter 24).

Certain factors have been identified as being predictive of which people are most likely to progress to chronic disease (that is, least likely to clear acute HCV). These are listed in the sidebar below.

THE SYMPTOMS AND SIGNS OF CHRONIC HEPATITIS C

Most people with chronic hepatitis C are surprised to find out that they harbor this virus. This is because, even at advanced stages of the disease, symptoms are usually absent. This is true even in some people who have progressed to cirrhosis. And, as with many other liver diseases, if symptoms are present, they are usually nonspecific. Only approximately 25 percent of people with chronic hepatitis C experience symptoms—most commonly fatigue and generalized weakness. Some people complain of vague abdominal discomfort, often in the area over the liver. Others suffer from a decreased appetite, weight loss, and depression. The severity of symptoms is not a good indicator of the amount of liver inflammation and damage (nor even is a lack of symptoms).

Physical findings are often normal in people with chronic hepatitis C. An enlarged, tender liver is rarely detected. Other physical findings, such as an enlarged spleen (splenomegaly) or jaundice, may be indicative of cirrhosis. In general, symptoms and signs of chronic hepatitis C will not provide the basis for its diagnosis.

Risk Factors Predictive of Progression from Acute to Chronic HCV

Gender: Being male increases the chance of progression

Age: Those older than forty at the time of infection have a 60 to 85 percent chronicity rate; children have a chronicity rate of 50 to 60 percent

Ethnicity: African-American men

Route of Transmission: Blood transfusion

Immunosuppressed State: E.g., HIV infection or chronic dialysis

Asymptomatic Acute HCV: Lack of jaundice, fatigue, joint aches, etc., during acute infection

Genetic Predisposition: Certain histocompatibility genes code for disease progression

Disorders Chronic Hepatitis C Can Cause Outside of the Liver (Extrahepatic Manifestations)

Chronic hepatitis C may cause disorders in organs other than the liver, known as *extrahepatic manifestations.* This is partly due to the fact that other parts of the body are often caught in the crossfire when the immune system fights against an HCV infection. Most of these extrahepatic manifestations are due to immune-mediated diseases. However, HCV has also been found in various other parts of the body besides the liver, such as the stomach, lymph glands, bone marrow, and brain. The severity of these extrahepatic manifestations does not correlate with the extent of damage found in the liver, the duration that one has had hepatitis C, or the hepatitis C viral level. Sometimes, these extrahepatic manifestations of HCV are what initially prompted a visit to the doctor. And sometimes these extrahepatic manifestations can cause severe symptoms and may even result in death. Yet, this may occur even when HCV-related liver disease is in an early stage. The following is a discussion of some of the extrahepatic manifestations of chronic hepatitis C.

Skin Diseases

- *Vasculitis*—inflammation of blood vessels—may present as a raised, purplish skin discoloration, known as purpura, which is most commonly located on the legs. The discoloration is due to the leakage of blood under the skin. Vasculitis that occurs in people with HCV is typically associated with cryoglobulinemia—

abnormal proteins in the blood (please see below for full discussion of cryo-globulinemia). The severity of vasculitis usually correlates with the hepatitis C viral level. Thus, treatment of HCV with interferon often results in improvement of vasculitis.

• *Porphyria cutanea tarda (PCT)* is a skin abnormality due to accumulation of porphyrins, substances involved in making blood, under the skin. PCT usually manifests as blisters on the back of the hands and on the forearms, neck, face, and other sun-exposed areas. These blisters bruise and bleed easily, especially when subjected to mild trauma or sun exposure. Other manifestations of PCT include areas of increased or decreased skin pigmentation and increased hair growth, known as *hirsuitism*. Blood tests will indicate an iron overload (please refer to chapter 18 for a discussion of iron overload). Patients with PCT often have high sugar levels, diabetes, or fat deposits in the liver known as a fatty liver (please refer to chapter 16 for a discussion of a fatty liver). In addition to the causative factor of HCV, alcohol consumption, excessive iron intake, and estrogens may precipitate PCT in predisposed people.

Treatment consists of avoidance of all alcohol, estrogens, and iron supplements. If iron overload is present, foods high in iron content (such as red meats and foods fortified with iron, such as some cereals) should be avoided. If symptoms persist after these measures are taken, *phlebotomy* (removal of blood though a vein to reduce iron levels) should be started (please refer to chapter 18 for a discussion of phlebotomy). Drugs such as chloroquine or hydroxiquin, used to treat malaria (a parasite), may also be beneficial for treatment of PCT. Improvement or total remission of PCT will normally occur when treatment of HCV with interferon reduces or eradicates the virus.

• *Lichen planus* is a raised, itchy skin rash that can occur in the mouth, hair, and nails of people with HCV. The inside of the mouth (oral mucosa) will have raised, thin, white streaks surrounded by inflammation and irritation. Lichen planus is typically treated with prednisone (an oral steroid). It should be noted that prednisone also causes the hepatitis C virus to replicate, thereby resulting in raised viral levels.

• Other skin disorders, such as pruritus (excessive itching) and *vitiligo* (a loss of skin pigmentation), may occur in association with chronic hepatitis C.

Hematological (Blood-Related) Diseases

• *Cryoglobulinemia* is the presence of cryoglobulins, abnormal proteins (immuno-globulins), in the blood that become solid in cold temperatures and dissolve at normal body temperature. Thus, when a person with cryoglobulinemia is exposed to cold she may experience poor circulation because cryoglobulins are clogging her small blood vessels. Cryoglobulinemia occurs in approximately 40 percent of all individuals with chronic hepatitis C. It manifests as bleeding into the skin (known as palpable purpura), joint aches, and weakness. However, only approximately 50 percent of people with hepatitis C and cryoglobulinemia experience symptoms. Cryoglobulinemia may also affect the kidneys, brain, and nerves. Rheumatoid factor (RF) is commonly found on the blood tests of those with cryoglobulinemia, although this rarely indicates the presence of rheumatoid arthritis. Some experts believe that cryoglobulinemia is associated with an increased risk of cirrhosis. Cryoglobulinemia improves when hepatitis C viral levels decrease. Thus, treatment of cryoglobulinemia consists of using interferon to treat HCV, which results in improvement or elimination of symptoms in approximately 50 percent of people. Patients with cryoglobulinemia should not be given ribavirin if they also have kidney involvement.

- *Non-Hodgkin's B-cell lymphoma* is a malignant tumor of the lymphoid tissue (cells related to the immune system). In some studies, chronic hepatitis C was found to be present in a significant percentage of people (9 to 37 percent) diagnosed with non-Hodgkin's B-cell lymphoma, suggesting an association between this type of cancer and HCV. In fact, in some instances, lymphoma has been found to shrink as HCV is treated with interferon. The link between non-Hodgkin's B-cell lymphoma and HCV has not been found in all studies; however, there appears to be enough evidence of an association to warrant treatment with interferon as a possible adjunct to therapy for lymphoma in patients with chronic hepatitis C.

- *Idiopathic thrombocytopenic purpura (ITP)* is a disease characterized by an abnormally low platelet count of unclear origin. It is generally manifested in the form of a rash. The disease is believed to be caused by an immune attack on platelets. One consequence of ITP may be a bleeding disorder, as the function of platelets is to facilitate the clotting of blood.

- *Autoimmune hemolytic anemia* may be caused by HCV. Autoimmune hemolytic anemia is a process of *red blood cell (RBC)* destruction, in which the immune system mistakes red blood cells as "foreign invaders," and therefore attempts to destroy them. It is believed that the hepatitis C virus may attach to the surface of red blood cells. The body's immune system wishes to attack the hepatitis C virus but, being unable to distinguish the RBC from HCV, kills the RBC in the process. Autoimmune hemolytic anemia is reversible if treated promptly with the steroid prednisone.

- *Other:* The hepatitis C virus has been found to replicate in the bone marrow. This may cause decreased red blood cell counts (*anemia*), decreased white blood cell counts (*neutropenia*), and decreased platelet counts (*thrombocytopenia*). These counts may worsen further once therapy for hepatitis C (interferon and ribavirin) has begun. (See chapters 11 and 13 for a discussion of how to treat these possible complications.)

Endocrine Disorders

- *Thyroid disease* is the most common autoimmune disorder occurring in people with HCV. An *autoimmune reaction* is a condition in which the body's immune system attacks its own organs because it mistakenly identifies the organ (in this case the thyroid) as being an intruder. Both *hypothyroidism* (an overly slow thyroid) and *hyperthyroidism* (an overly fast thyroid) have been noted to occur. Thyroid disease may worsen once therapy with interferon (see chapter 13) has been initiated, especially if antithyroid antibodies were present prior to treatment.

- *Diabetes* is manifested by elevated sugar (glucose) levels in the blood. Diabetes occurs more commonly among people with chronic hepatitis C than among those with other liver diseases, and studies have suggested a strong association between diabetes and HCV. While interferon therapy has been associated with an increased risk of developing diabetes, there have been some reports of diabetes resolving in patients whose HCV was eradicated with interferon.

Eye Disorders

Although multiple eye disorders have been found in some people with chronic hepatitis C, a direct association has not been proven. However, all of the following have been reported to occur in people with chronic hepatitis C: ulcers in the cornea of the eye, (known as Mooren's corneal ulcers); uveitis, an inflammation of the uvea (the middle layer of the eye); Behçet's syndrome—a syndrome characterized by uveitis as well as ulcers of the mouth and genitalia; retinal vein thrombosis (a blood clot in the eye); and Sjögren's syndrome (dry eyes and dry mouth).

Kidney Disorders

Inflammation of the kidney, known as glomerulonephritis, has been associated with chronic hepatitis C. Approximately 20 percent of patients with both HCV and cryoglobulinemia (see page 123) also have glomerulonephritis. People with glomerulonephritis have either blood (hematuria) or, more commonly, excess protein (proteinurea) in their urine. Treatment of HCV with interferon often results in remission of this type of kidney disease. However, when interferon therapy is stopped, proteinurea typically returns. This often necessitates long-term interferon treatment.

Rheumatologic Disorders

Muscle weakness (*myalgias*) and joint pains (*arthralgias*) have been noted to occur in approximately 30 percent of people with chronic hepatitis C. The areas of the body most typically affected include the ankles, toes, hands, elbows, and wrists. Cryoglobulinemia is often found to be present in these individuals. Blood levels of rheumatoid factor (RF) may be elevated, but this does not indicate that one has rheumatoid arthritis. Treatment with interferon often improves muscle and joint aches once the hepatitis C viral level has been diminished. However, since interferon in itself may causes muscle and joint aches, occasionally these symptoms become worse.

Many other rheumatologic disorders have been found in people with HCV. These include polymyositis (a disease that causes inflammation of the muscles); dermatomyositis (a disease that causes a rash, as well as inflammation of the muscles); fibromyalgia (a disease causing fatigue and muscle pain); and antiphospholipid syndrome, a disorder associated with recurrent blood clots (thrombosis) and low platelet counts (thrombocytopenia).

Psychological Disorders

Many studies have indicated a possible link between HCV and brain dysfunction. People with HCV are often found to have impaired learning abilities, difficulty concentrating, and chronic fatigue. When these symptoms occur, they do not correlate with the severity of liver disease. As such, even people with little or no scarring of the liver (stage 0 or stage 1 disease, respectively) often report these symptoms. Psychiatric disorders, including depression, psychosis, and anxiety are more common among people with HCV than among people without HCV. And, HCV is found to be eleven times more common among people with psychiatric disorders than among those without psychiatric disorders. These findings suggest a strong association between brain dysfunction and HCV, an area that is currently being studied.

Neurological Disorders

Peripheral neuropathy, a disease causing numbness of the legs, occurs in approximately 10 percent of people who have both HCV and cryoglobulinemia. Interferon treatment sometimes worsens peripheral neuropathy.

Other Problems

Other disorders that appear on rare occasions in people with chronic hepatitis C include pulmonary fibrosis (lung scarring); a type of vasculitis known as polyarteritis nodosa (PAN); and cerebral infarction (a stroke). Further studies will need to be conducted in order to confirm that these disorders are in fact associated with chronic hepatitis C.

DIAGNOSING CHRONIC HEPATITIS C

Most people find out that they have chronic hepatitis C purely by accident. Since the majority of people either have vague symptoms or no symptoms at all, an evaluation for hepatitis C is usually prompted by the discovery of abnormal LFTs—most commonly and characteristically ALT (see chapter 3 for more information on LFTs). These abnormalities may be found during a routine annual physical, during a physical for a life insurance application, or during a medical evaluation for an unrelated problem. Others discover that they have chronic hepatitis C in the course of seeing their family doctor for the evaluation of one of the nonspecific symptoms associated with chronic hepatitis C, such as fatigue or loss of appetite.

Sometimes a specialist, rather than the family doctor, will discover that a person has chronic hepatitis C—perhaps during an evaluation of one of the extrahepatic manifestations of hepatitis C. Others seek medical evaluation for ascites or jaundice and, therefore, find out that they have chronic hepatitis C when the disease has already advanced.

Some people learn that they have chronic hepatitis C when they are rejected for blood donation due to testing positive for the hepatitis C antibody. The hepatitis C test that is used for blood-donor screening is known as the *ELISA,* which stands for *enzyme-linked immunosorbent assay* (see page 129). Approximately 40 percent (a range of 30 to 70 percent) of people who test positive for HCV by this blood screening test actually do not have hepatitis C. This is known as a false-positive test. Therefore, if a person tests positive by the ELISA method of HCV detection, it is imperative that she be tested again using a more accurate method known as *RIBA (recombinant immunoblot assay).* The following is a discussion of the tests used to diagnose chronic hepatitis C.

Liver Function Tests (LFTs)

Transaminases (ALT and AST) are elevated in approximately 70 percent of all individuals with chronic hepatitis C. The ALT value is more likely to be elevated, and it is more characteristic of a hepatitis C infection than an AST elevation. In fact, the ALT level is often used as a marker of HCV inflammation. However, it should be stressed that the ALT level, especially a single determination of ALT, is not an accurate indicator of the extent of inflammation in the liver. In people with chronic hepatitis C, ALT and AST levels usually range from approximately 80 to 180 IU/l. This is around two to four times the upper limit of normal (normal value being approximately 0 to 45 IU/l). But a person may have values as high as 450 IU/l or as low as 46 IU/l and still have chronic hepatitis C.

It is important to remember that transaminase levels in people with chronic hepatits C typically fluctuate and that decreased or normalized levels do not indicate that chronic hepatitis C has improved or gone away. By the next day, week, or year, the transaminase levels may be elevated again. Also, the level of elevation of transaminases usually bears little relation to the severity of liver disease caused by HCV, and, furthermore, the level of elevation rarely predicts the outcome of disease. Regardless of the degree of transaminase elevation, the findings on liver biopsy specimens may range anywhere from mild inflammation to advanced cirrhosis.

However, although transaminases levels usually are poor predictors of inflammation and scarring of the liver, some studies have found that elevations persistently greater than ten times the normal value are a predictor of excessive liver scarring. Also, while ALT levels are typically higher than AST levels, a reversal of this finding—AST being higher than ALT—has been found to be indicative of cirrhosis.

Approximately one-third of people with chronic hepatitis C have transaminase levels that are persistently normal. This means that transaminase levels have never been elevated, even after being tested multiple times, preferably over a period of many years. Despite normal transaminase levels, these people have an elevated HCV RNA. Thus, these people are sometimes referred to as "healthy chronic carriers" of HCV (however, further research is needed to confirm the validity of this designation). Most "healthy chronic carriers" will never experience a progressive course of their liver disease and will never experience any significant consequences due to chronic hepatitis C. However, some experts feel that a small percentage of these individuals may progress to cirrhosis. Unfortunately, there do not appear to be any concrete factors that can predict which people with persistently normal ALT levels will experience progressive disease and which ones will continue to remain stable with no long-term consequences due to HCV. It has been observed, however, that approximately 30 percent of people with persistently normal ALT levels will at some point fall out of the category of "healthy chronic carriers," and their ALT levels will become elevated. Elevated ALT levels will now put these individuals at higher risk of progressive liver disease.

In summary, transaminase elevations provide little significant information about the nature of the liver disease caused by chronic hepatitis C. If levels are very elevated, they may predict severe damage of the liver in some people. In general, however, they merely provide a clue that something is wrong with the liver. Finally, transaminase levels do have significance when used to monitor a person's response to therapy (see chapter 13).

In people with chronic hepatitis C, bilirubin levels are usually normal unless the person has advanced liver disease. GGTP is often mildly abnormal. Immunoglobulin G is usually elevated, but has no value in determining a prognosis.

Markers of Liver Scarring

While a liver biopsy is the only way to accurately determine the extent of scarring on the liver, there are many blood tests that may suggest scarring and cirrhosis.

- Iron studies (iron, ferritin, and transferrin saturation), which will be discussed in chapter 18, are often elevated in people with chronic hepatitis C and are generally associated with increased inflammation and damage of the liver.

- A low platelet count as well as a prolonged prothrombin time are typically reliable indicators of cirrhosis.

- An elevated *alpha-fetoprotein (AFP)* level—when elevated to less than 100 nanograms per milliliter (ng/ml) (normal level is less than 20 ng/ml). See chapter 19.

- A hyaluronic acid level of less than 60 micrograms per liter (mcg/l) is usually predictive of the absence of cirrhosis in patients with HCV.

- *FIBROSpect,* which is still considered experimental, is a blood test that can differentiate among degrees of liver scarring in people with hepatitis C. Results are reported as either no to mild liver scarring (stage 0 or 1) or moderate to severe liver scarring (stages 2 to 4). The test is currently not covered by insurance and costs approximately $350.

Hepatitis C Antibody Tests

Blood tests to determine the presence of the hepatitis C antibody (HCV Ab) in the body are necessary in order to make a diagnosis of hepatitis C. These tests determine whether the immune system is producing antibodies against one or more of the hepatitis C antigens (see page 80 for a brief explanation of antigens and antibodies). The presence of the antibody to HCV may indicate that a person was previously exposed to hepatitis C, or, alternatively, it may indicate that a person is currently infected with HCV. It is not possible to determine which scenario applies in a given case from the mere presence of the antibody alone. Therefore, the presence of the HCV Ab does not mean that a person is either immune to or in any way protected against HCV. Nor are these tests capable of distinguishing between acute and chronic hepatitis C. There are currently two blood tests available in the United States that can detect the hepatitis C antibody in the blood. In fact, these tests are currently the only tests approved by the FDA for the diagnosis of hepatitis C. These tests are known as ELISA (enzyme-linked immunosorbent assay) and RIBA (recombinant immunoblot assay).

The ELISA I blood test was the first screening test available to detect the HCV Ab. Made commercially available in May 1990, this test detects the antibody to one of the hepatitis C antigens. ELISA I is capable of detecting HCV Ab approximately sixteen weeks after exposure to HCV. Since 1990, this test has been available to doctors to determine whether the cause of a person's elevated LFTs was in fact due to hepatitis C. This test was supplanted by the ELISA II in May 1992. ELISA II detects the antibody to four of the hepatitis C antigens and is, therefore, significantly more accurate than the ELISA I test. ELISA II is capable of detecting HCV Ab in the blood approximately nine to ten weeks after exposure to HCV. ELISA III is the test used since May 1996 to screen blood products in the United States for HCV. This test detects the antibody to five of the hepatitis C antigens and is, therefore, more accurate than ELISA II. This blood test can detect the HCV Ab approximately six to eight weeks after exposure to HCV. ELISA test results are typically reported as being either "positive" or "negative." ELISA test results may be negative in someone who actually has HCV. This can occur in people with a deficient immune system, such as those with human immunodeficiency virus (HIV) or those on chronic hemodialysis for kidney failure.

RIBA 2.0, made commercially available in June 1993, was formerly used as a supplemental blood test for people at a low risk for infection with HCV who had tested positive for HCV Ab by ELISA II. People considered at low risk for infection include those individuals without an apparent risk factor for HCV such as intravenous drug use. Results of this test are reported as being either positive, negative, or indeterminate. An indeterminate result must be carefully evaluated by a specialist to assess whether the result is really positive or negative. RIBA testing for HCV Ab is currently used by blood banks for screening blood donors (however, blood banks may replace this test with HCV RNA levels in the near future). Given the accuracy of the current ELISA testing, RIBA is otherwise rarely used.

In 1999, the first over-the-counter home test was made available to the public to diagnose hepatitis C. This home test, called the "Hepatitis C Check," allows people to collect a sample of blood on their own at home and mail it to a designated laboratory for hepatitis C antibody testing. The results are available by phone within a week or two and are strictly confidential. One can obtain the "Hepatitis C Check" through various Internet websites.

Hepatitis C Viral RNA (HCV RNA)

There are two types of tests that can detect the amount of the HCV ribonucleic acid (HCV RNA—the genetic material of HCV) in the blood. They are HCV RNA polymerase chain reaction (PCR) and the HCV RNA target mediated amplification (TMA). These tests can detect HCV in the blood approximately one to two weeks after exposure to the virus. Both of these tests are capable of determining the presence—positive or negative (qualitative)—and the actual amount, also known as the *viral load* or viral level (quantitative), of HCV in the blood. These tests are used both to confirm that a person is infected with HCV and to monitor and predict response to antiviral treatment (see chapter 13). A positive result on both tests also confirms that the person is infectious to others.

The HCV RNA quantitative test is measured in international units (IU)/ml. IU/ml represents the amount of HCV RNA in a blood sample. It does not measure the actual number of viral particles in the sample. The former method of measurement—copies/ml, is now obsolete. If you have old test results that reported your HCV RNA level in copies/ml, you should ask your doctor to convert these results into IU/ml, if needed. The current tests have the ability to detect HCV RNA of a much lower level (2 IU/ml to 50 IU/ml) than those used in the past (600 IU/ml to 2,000 IU/ml). The two assays currently available that can detect the lowest levels of HCV RNA are the HeptiMax (Quest Diagnostics), which has the capability of detection of HCV RNA to less than 5 IU/ml, and the HCV RNA UltraQual (NGI), which can detect levels as low as 2 to 3 IU/ml. The use of a blood test with a low level of detection of HCV RNA is crucial for determining response to therapy as well as whether the patient has been cured. In the future it is likely that many other tests will become available that have even lower levels of detection of HCV RNA.

It is important to understand that the viral load does not correlate with the severity of liver disease nor does it affect or predict disease progression. Therefore, a person with a very high viral load (say, 5 million IU/ml) will not necessarily have more liver inflammation and damage or a higher likelihood of disease progression than a person with a lower viral load (say, 500 IU/ml). Furthermore, the viral load typically fluctuates and does not correlate with the degree of elevation of the transaminases (AST and ALT). Thus, people who are not undergoing treatment gain no useful information by having viral loads repeated. However, people who are planning to start therapy should have their viral loads determined. A low viral load (under 1 million IU/ml) prior to starting therapy may be an indicator of possible treatment success.

It appears that the level of HCV RNA in the blood and in the liver is very similar. Therefore, measuring HCV RNA directly from a liver sample adds no significant additional information.

Hepatitis C Antigen

Hepatitis C core antigen (HCV core Ag) is currently not available outside of research studies. Preliminary test results have shown that the HCV core Ag appears to correlate closely with the level of HCV RNA. However, the current version of this test has a lower limit of detectability equivalent to an HCV RNA level of 20,000 IU/ml. As such, the HCV core Ag test adds little information to currently available testing. Further research is being conducted to improve its level of detectability.

HCV Genotypes

The term *HCV genotype* refers to the genetic makeup of the different HCV mutants in the hepatitis C viral population of a single person. There have been six different HCV genotypes clearly identified: genotypes 1 through 6. The HCV genotype is determined through a blood test. The HCV genotype need only be determined once, as the genotype will not change during the entire course of infection.

One HCV genotype may differ genetically from another by as much as 35 percent. To further complicate matters, within each genotype there are at least two or three subtypes, each of which may differ genetically from one another by about 15 percent. These subtypes are classified alphabetically as "a, b, and c." Different HCV genotypes are common to different areas of the world and different groups of people. For example, genotype 1a and 1b accounts for 70 to 75 percent of all HCV infections in the United States; genotype 2 is most commonly found in people with HCV in Italy, North Africa, and Spain; genotype 3a is believed to be the predominant HCV genotype among intravenous drug users in Europe; and genotype 4 is commonly found among people with HCV in Egypt and the Middle East. Genotypes 5 and 6 are very uncommon.

Genotypes are not predictive of disease progression. However, genotypes do have predictive value as to the outcome of interferon therapy, as certain genotypes respond less favorably than others. Furthermore, certain genotypes require a shorter duration of therapy and respond well to lower doses of ribavirin. Therefore it is important to determine the genotype, as it can be useful in making certain treatment decisions. Studies have found that people with genotypes 1 and 4 have a poorer response to interferon treatment and require higher dosages of the medication ribavirin than people who have genotypes 2 and 3. The former group—genotypes 1 and 4—typically requires at least forty-eight weeks of therapy, whereas the latter group—genotypes 2 and 3—typically require twenty-four weeks of therapy (please refer to chapter 13 for a full discussion of genotypes and treatment). Genotypes do not correlate with the amount of inflammation and scarring of the liver. Genotype 3a has been shown to correlate with the degree of fat (*steatosis*) on liver biopsy specimens.

Imaging Studies

Usually the doctor will want to obtain at least one imaging study—typically a sonogram—as part of the diagnostic evaluation of chronic hepatitis C, especially when transaminases are elevated. Imaging studies are usually normal, even in advanced stages of the disease. While an enlarged liver may occasionally be detected, it is not indicative of the degree of scarring of the liver. An enlarged spleen, small nodular liver, ascites, and varices can sometimes be detected with an MRI or CT scan. These findings are usually diagnostic of advanced cirrhosis. If liver cancer (hepatoma) is present, a mass may show up on the sonogram, CT scan, or MRI (see chapter 19).

Note, however, that just because the liver looks normal on an imaging study doesn't mean it actually is normal. In order to provide maximum information about the condition of the liver, a liver biopsy is necessary.

Liver Biopsy

As with all liver diseases, even if a person feels fine, that's no guarantee that her liver is fine. Furthermore, physical findings, LFT abnormalities, HCV RNA viral load, HCV genotype, and imaging studies typically cannot accurately determine the extent of liver inflammation and damage caused by HCV.

The only way to determine the degree to which a liver is inflamed and injured is by examining a sample of the liver under the microscope. A liver biopsy is the only reliable means of determining the presence or absence of cirrhosis. Thus, a liver biopsy is necessary in order to assess the amount of liver inflammation due to the virus—known as the grade of hepatitis C. A liver biopsy is needed to determine the amount of scarring or fibrosis on the liver—known as the stage of disease. The results obtained from a liver biopsy provide crucial information that is used to guide treatment decisions and assess a person's long-term prognosis. See chapter 5 for more information on liver biopsies.

THE LONG-TERM PROGNOSIS FOR THOSE WITH CHRONIC HEPATITIS C

Chronic hepatitis C typically progresses at a very slow pace. That means that most people will not develop significant liver inflammation or damage until at least twenty years after becoming infected with the virus. Some may even take as long as forty to fifty years. And others may never develop serious liver disease.

It appears that cirrhosis develops in about 20 percent of all individuals with chronic hepatitis C within approximately twenty years after they are infected; however, percentages as high as 50 and as low as 5 have been cited. Moreover, because HCV was only identified in 1989, long-term studies of disease progression have not been able to be conducted. Nevertheless, some experts estimate that more than 50 percent of people will develop cirrhosis approximately thirty to forty years after they have been infected. Even after cirrhosis has developed, most people live long, healthy lives with chronic hepatitis C. However, once a person has developed one of the complications of cirrhosis, such as variceal bleeding, encephalopathy, or ascites (which is known as decompensated cirrhosis), without appropriate treatment she has a 50 percent chance of dying within the next five years. In a given year, decompensated cirrhosis occurs in approximately 6 percent of people with compensated cirrhosis due to HCV. And in a given year, liver cancer develops in approximately 4 percent of people with cirrhosis.

From these statistics, it is apparent that some people with chronic hepatitis C have a relatively innocuous course of disease, whereas others have a more progressive and serious, possibly even fatal, course of disease. So the question is, why do some people with chronic hepatitis C fare so much better than others? Unfortunately, no one knows the complete answer to this question, but there are many contributing factors that can accelerate the rate of disease progression. Read on for a discussion of some of these factors.

Prognosis Based on Viral Characteristics

Viral characteristics are believed by some researchers to play a role in determining disease progression. However, results from studies on some of these parameters, such as viral load and transaminase elevation, have been inconsistent, and therefore no definitive conclusion can be drawn as to the utility of these parameters in predicting the course of disease. On the other hand, liver biopsy results tend to be quite useful in predicting the future course of disease.

Viral Load

The viral load bears no correlation with inflammation and scarring of the liver. Nor does it affect disease progression. Viral loads are important to follow while on interferon therapy to assess efficacy of treatment. However, for patients who are not undergoing treatment, there is no additional information to be gained by following viral loads.

Viral Genotype

While some studies have found that people with genotype 1b have a particularly progressive disease course compared to those with other HCV genotypes, other studies have been unable to document any correlation between genotype and disease outcome. Therefore, the viral genotype, while important for treatment decisions, is not a predictor of disease progression for people with HCV.

Viral Diversity

Some researchers have found that the more diverse the population of HCV quasispecies is in a given person, the more likely it is that the person will progress to advanced disease. Further studies need to be conducted on HCV quasispecies before definitive conclusions can be drawn.

Transaminase Levels (ALT and AST)

As noted previously, the level of transaminase elevation neither correlates with hepatitis C disease progression nor with the development of advanced liver disease. However, it has been noted that people with persistently normal transaminase levels tend to have neither an aggressive course nor a poor outcome of disease. One study demonstrated that liver disease progression in people with persistently normal ALT levels is at least twice as slow as in people with elevated ALT levels. And another study suggested that in people with persistently normal ALT levels, it may take about eighty years for cirrhosis to develop, especially if they refrain from drinking alcohol. By contrast, a few studies have pointed to instances of significant liver damage in people with chronic hepatitis C and persistently normal ALT levels. However, consensus is that people with HCV and persistently normal transaminase levels typically have a benign course of disease.

Liver Biopsy Results

As discussed in chapter 5, the way to effectively determine the extent of inflammation and damage in the liver is by sampling a piece of liver tissue. It has been shown that the amount of inflammation and scarring found in liver biopsy samples may be used to predict the likelihood of a person's progression to cirrhosis, as well as the rate of progression thereto. For example, people whose liver biopsy specimens indicate severe inflammation and scarring have been shown to progress to cirrhosis rapidly—in approximately ten years. Those whose biopsy specimens indicate mild inflammation and no scarring can expect their disease to progress very slowly. It is estimated that these individuals will not advance to cirrhosis for many decades.

Prognosis Based on a Patient's Characteristics

Certain individual patient characteristics have been noted to have an impact on the course of chronic hepatitis C. These include age, gender, race, duration of infection, genetic predilection, route of transmission, and immune status.

Age

Studies have consistently found that people who become infected with HCV after the age of forty have a more progressive course of disease compared with those who became infected under the age of forty, and 20 percent of these people develop cirrhosis within twenty years after becoming infected. The younger a person is at the time of infection, the slower the disease progresses. It has been observed that people who contract HCV below the age of forty will develop cirrhosis within twenty years of infection only 2 to 8 percent of the time. The reason for this association with age is unclear but is believed to be related to the immune system. It has been suggested that as a person who was infected at an early age gets older, the rate of progression of HCV-related liver disease accelerates. This may be due to the inability of the aging immune system to control the effects of HCV.

Gender

Gender differences in HCV may be related to the effects of sex hormones on the liver. Women, especially if they were young at the time they acquired the virus, appear to progress to cirrhosis less often than men. In fact, studies have shown that women have a 5 percent likelihood of progressing to cirrhosis, compared with 20 to 30 percent likelihood for men. Also, some studies have found that men are as much as four times more likely than women to develop liver cancer from HCV.

It appears that sex hormones, particularly estrogens, may play a significant role in delaying progression of HCV to cirrhosis and in enhancing the response of HCV to therapy. Therefore, it is possible that hormone replacement therapy (HRT) may have a beneficial effect in postmenopausal women with HCV. However, this issue has not been studied. Clearly, the role of sex hormones in people with HCV needs further investigation.

Race

African Americans with HCV appear to have poorer prognostic factors than Caucasians. They have a higher prevalence of hepatitis C than Caucasians. In fact, the prevalence among African Americans is almost three times as great as that of Caucasians. African Americans, especially males, are more likely to progress to chronic disease than are Caucasians. Approximately 90 percent of African Americans are infected with genotype 1 (which does not respond as well to therapy) as compared with 70 to 75 percent of Caucasians. While African Americans appear to have a slower rate of progression of HCV, once cirrhosis develops they are more likely to suffer from complications such as liver cancer and death. Finally, the response rate to treatment is poorer for African Americans than for Caucasians.

Duration of Infection

Some experts believe that since hepatitis C is a progressive disease, the longer a person is infected with the virus, the greater the likelihood is of developing the possible complications of chronic hepatitis C, including cirrhosis, liver failure, and liver cancer.

Genetic Predilection

Some studies have suggested that some people infected with chronic hepatitis C may possess a genetic predilection that protects them from developing the potential complications of the disease. Similarly, it is possible that some people possess genetic characteristics that promote progression of HCV. Further studies need to be conducted to confirm these theories.

Route of Transmission

In people with chronic hepatitis C, the route by which the person became infected with HCV probably influences the course of the disease. Several studies have demonstrated that people who acquire HCV by a blood transfusion have a greater chance of developing significant liver disease than those who acquired HCV through other routes. This could be due to the fact that a large amount of hepatitis C viral particles may potentially be transmitted to a person in the course of a blood transfusion, whereas the sharing of a needle through illicit drug use, for example, provides the opportunity for a comparatively small amount of HCV to be transmitted. Fortunately, the application of accurate screening tests for HCV to all potential blood donors has made the transmission of HCV via blood transfusion an event of the past.

Immune Status

The immune status of a person with chronic hepatitis C may influence the rate of progression to liver disease. People with poor immune systems are known as being *immunocompromised* or *immunosuppressed*. Examples include those with AIDS, those who are on immunosuppressive medications (such as tacrolimus or prednisone) in the aftermath of an organ transplant, and those undergoing cancer chemotherapy. These people often have a severe and aggressive course of liver disease due to chronic hepatitis C, as compared with people who have chronic hepatitis C and have well-functioning immune systems. However, this finding is not universal and is subject to a number of variables. Some immunosuppressed people, including some with chronic kidney disease, have experienced a particularly mild course of HCV. And in cases where a person has reinfected her newly transplanted liver, the course of HCV is quite variable. Some recent studies have noted an aggressive course of disease, with cirrhosis developing in the new (but now infected) liver within a year. Other studies have noted the development of cirrhosis in 30 percent of these people within five years. Some older studies on this subject have shown that infection with HCV caused virtually no damage to the new liver. It is clear that many factors come into play in the case of one's immune system and how it affects the rate of progression of chronic hepatitis C. For a further discussion of liver transplantation in patients with hepatitis C, see chapter 22.

By reducing the body's immune defenses, immunosuppressive medications (such as the steroid prednisone and the antirejection drug cyclosporine) promote a surge of viral replication manifested by an increased HCV RNA viral load. Therefore, immunosuppressive medications may have the effect of accelerating the progression of chronic hepatitis C. Thus, people with chronic hepatitis C are advised to avoid the use of such medications, unless these medications are absolutely warranted.

Prognosis Based on Other Characteristics

Other factors that may independently cause liver disease may coexist in people with chronic hepatitis C. When combined together, a particularly aggressive course of liver disease with a poor outcome often results. These factors are now discussed.

HCV and Alcohol

Alcohol is a strong toxin to the liver and can lead to cirrhosis and liver cancer. People with chronic hepatitis C who drink excessive amounts of alcohol are at an especially high risk for a particularly accelerated course of liver disease to advanced stages. This has been found to apply even to former excessive alcohol users who currently abstain and even to some people who consider themselves to be social drinkers. Alcohol may cause liver damage in people with HCV at small dosages that would not otherwise be dangerous to the liver in a person without HCV. It appears that alcohol actually promotes replication of HCV. You may accurately visualize alcohol as a potent fuel that HCV utilizes to multiply and prosper in the body. People with chronic hepatitis C who drink alcohol are more frequently found to have cirrhosis and liver cancer and are more likely to die at an earlier age than people who do not subject their livers to this additional insult. Finally, alcohol use has been shown to decrease the efficacy of interferon, as well as the response to interferon treatment. Unfortunately, studies have not been done to determine the effects of moderate alcohol use on the course of HCV. In any case, it would be prudent for all people with chronic hepatitis C to minimize their alcohol intake. In fact, the best advice for these people is to totally abstain from all alcohol. See chapter 17 for more information on alcohol and the liver.

HCV and Cigarette Smoking

Cigarette smoking has been cited as a possible factor in promoting disease progression in people with chronic hepatitis C. In fact, it has been found that people with HCV who smoke cigarettes are more likely to have scarring and inflammation on liver biopsy specimens. Furthermore, people with HCV who smoke cigarettes develop liver cancer more frequently than people with HCV who do not smoke. It is believed that cigarette smoke may contain liver-toxic substances that may cause scarring and liver cancer in people with HCV. Further study is needed to confirm this possible association. Other forms of tobacco, such as from a pipe or cigar, have not been linked to the progression of hepatitis C, but this may be due to the fact that these forms of tobacco have never been specifically evaluated in this context. However, it can most likely be concluded that all forms of tobacco are not healthy for the liver.

HCV and Hepatitis Viruses

It is not infrequent for people with chronic hepatitis C to be additionally infected with another hepatitis virus. It has been noted by some researchers that fulminant hepatitis—a severe form of hepatitis (see chapter 7)—or even death can occur in people with chronic hepatitis C who become additionally infected with the hepatitis A virus (HAV). Some studies have found that people infected with both HCV and HBV have a very aggressive course of disease and are at increased risk of developing cirrhosis and decompensated liver disease. Therefore, everyone with chronic hepatitis C who has not been exposed to HAV or HBV is urged to obtain the vaccinations against these other hepatitis viruses. Vaccinations will be discussed in chapter 24. Coinfection of HCV with the hepatitis G virus (HGV) is not believed to influence the outcome of liver disease due to HCV.

HCV and Human Immunodeficiency Virus (HIV)

Coinfection of HCV and HIV is common among intravenous drug users and people such as hemophiliacs, who have had numerous blood transfusions. Approximately 200,000 people in the United States are infected with both viruses. Progression to chronic infection occurs at a greater rate in people with both HIV and HCV than in those with HCV alone. Approximately 90 to 95 percent of people with HCV who are also infected with HIV progress to chronic disease, compared to 60 to 85 percent of people with HCV alone. Women with both HCV and HIV are less likely to progress to chronic infection than men with HCV and HIV. People with HCV who are also infected with HIV have a particularly rapid progression to cirrhosis, liver failure, and liver cancer.

HCV and Autoimmune Hepatitis (AIH)

A form of autoimmune hepatitis (AIH) may occur in people with chronic hepatitis C. It has been shown that the coexistence of these two liver disorders does not lead to a poorer outcome of disease in a person with chronic hepatitis C. However, the coexistence of these two liver disorders may cause some treatment dilemmas. This is discussed in more detail in chapters 13 and 14.

HCV and Nonalcoholic Fatty Liver Disease (NAFLD)

NAFLD, a very common liver disease, can lead to cirrhosis. This disease, characterized by fat deposits in the liver, is often associated with obesity and diabetes.

NAFLD, obesity, and diabetes are factors that by themselves may contribute to the progression of scarring in people with HCV. Therefore, people with HCV who are overweight are strongly advised to lose weight through a combination of a low-fat, low-sugar diet and exercise. (Please refer to chapter 16 for a full discussion of NAFLD.)

HCV and Iron Overload

Excessive iron can be harmful to the liver and can lead to liver damage and cirrhosis. Chapter 18 is devoted to this topic. Many people with chronic hepatitis C (especially men) have increased iron levels (iron, ferritin, and transferrin saturation) in their blood. This may be due to iron being released into the bloodstream by dying liver cells. Some of these people may carry a gene for hereditary iron overload (hemochromatosis). These people are typically found to have more advanced liver disease and a higher incidence of cirrhosis. It is possible that iron may promote the replication of HCV. Some studies have noted that people with chronic hepatitis C who have high iron levels respond poorly to treatment with interferon (see chapter 13). This is why iron reduction therapy in the form of phlebotomy has been proposed by some researchers as a possible adjunctive treatment option for people with chronic hepatitis C who have high iron levels, especially if they carry a gene for hemochromatosis. In any case, it is probably wise for people with chronic hepatitis C, especially those with high iron studies and those with cirrhosis, to avoid iron supplementation or foods fortified with iron. Nutrition for people with chronic hepatitis C will be discussed in chapter 23.

HCV and Schistosomiasis

Schistosomiasis is a parasitic worm that is common in Egypt. People infected with both schistosomiasis and HCV have a particularly high frequency of cirrhosis, liver cancer, and death. It is unclear why these coinfected individuals have such a poor prognosis. However, an impaired immune system due to schistosomiasis has been postulated as an explanation.

HCV and Herbs

There has been a boom of interest in the use of herbal remedies for the treatment of chronic hepatitis C. However, many herbs are in and of themselves toxic to the liver. Due to the lack of FDA regulation regarding marketing and labeling, it is quite possible that many people are unknowingly ingesting herbs that are actually toxic to their livers in the mistaken belief that what they are ingesting will improve the health of their livers. Herbal remedies and how they may affect the progression of chronic hepatitis C is a subject that warrants further investigation. See chapter 21 for information on herbs.

HCV and Environmental Factors

Environmental toxins—such as toxic fumes and pollutants from work sites, polluted air, waste, paints, and pesticides—may potentially promote acceleration of disease in people with chronic hepatitis C. This association remains largely unexplored. However, since everything that we are exposed to, including what we breathe and absorb through the skin, is filtered through the liver to be detoxified, it makes sense that certain environmental toxins may contribute to a worsening course of liver disease.

Chronic Hepatitis C and Liver Cancer Risk

People with HCV are twenty-five times more likely to develop liver cancer (also known as hepatocellular carcinoma [HCC] or hepatoma) than people without HCV. With rare exception, liver cancer develops only after people with HCV have progressed to cirrhosis. Among people who have cirrhosis, liver cancer occurs at a yearly rate of approximately 4 percent. Approximately 15 percent of people with cirrhosis due to HCV develop liver cancer within ten years from the time cirrhosis occurred. And it usually takes approximately thirty years for liver cancer to develop from the time of initial infection with HCV. In the United States, the incidence of HCV-related liver cancer is rising. This is due to the fact that there are increasing numbers of people who have had HCV for almost thirty years.

In people with chronic hepatitis C, excessive alcohol consumption appears to increase the risk of developing liver cancer, thereby underscoring the importance of abstinence for people with hepatitis C. As stated above, it appears that coinfection with HBV and HCV greatly increases a person's chances of developing liver cancer. As such, it is important for people with chronic hepatitis C who are not already infected with hepatitis B to obtain the hepatitis B vaccination. (See chapter 24 for more information on vaccinations.) Coinfection with HCV and HIV may increase the likelihood of developing liver cancer, although this association needs to be confirmed. Diabetes and obesity have each been linked to the development of liver cancer in people with HCV. However, further study needs to be conducted to prove this association.

Males, people above the age of fifty-five, and people with advanced cirrhosis appear to develop liver cancer more frequently. It has been demonstrated that treatment with the antiviral drug interferon prior to the development of liver cancer may lower the incidence of liver cancer in some people with chronic hepatitis C (see chapters 13 and 19). This underscores the importance of early detection of hepatitis C as well as the need for aggressive treatment of chronic hepatitis C prior to the development of advanced liver disease, so as to slow, or hopefully reverse, its development.

CONCLUSION

Perhaps the most frightening aspect of chronic hepatitis C is its silent and progressive nature. Most people harbor the virus for ten, twenty, or even thirty years, not knowing it's in their bodies and oblivious to the liver damage it has caused. However, there are some encouraging aspects to this disease. The number of new acute HCV infections has declined significantly in recent years. And there is greater awareness and knowledge about HCV transmission and prevention. Currently available diagnostic blood tests to screen prospective blood donors have succeeded in making acquisition of HCV by blood transfusion virtually impossible. This is of tremendous significance, as studies have shown that those people who acquired HCV via this route are the ones most likely to develop progressive disease. Some controllable risk factors that can accelerate progression of disease, such as alcohol consumption, cigarette smoking, obesity, and coinfection with other hepatitis viruses, have been pinpointed. Thus, a person on her own initiative can take measures that will help diminish her risk of disease progression. As the knowledge of HCV continues to grow, the number of people becoming infected with HCV and the number of people having a poor outcome due to HCV will surely diminish even further.

The next chapter is an overview of the treatment of chronic viral hepatitis. As such, interferon, the most effective treatment for both chronic hepatitis B and C, will be discussed in detail.

Eleven

TREATING CHRONIC VIRAL HEPATITIS—AN OVERVIEW OF INTERFERON AND ITS POTENTIAL SIDE EFFECTS, AND HOW TO MANAGE THEM

When diagnosed with an illness, one of the first questions that a person typically asks her doctor is "How is this disease treated?" Prior to 1991, when it came to chronic hepatitis B or C, the answer to this question would have been, "There is presently no effective treatment." Fortunately, this is not the answer that a person asking this question today would receive. While current therapies do not work for everyone, people with chronic hepatitis B and C should consider themselves fortunate. Not only are effective medications available to treat these diseases, but there are a variety of treatment regimens from which a person can choose. Even those people who have carried the virus for several decades can often be successfully treated—and yes, even cured.

This chapter discusses important issues that a person with chronic hepatitis B or C should consider as she decides which treatment option will be best for her. These issues include the difference between FDA-approved and experimental drug therapy; the advantages versus the disadvantages of participating in a clinical research trial of a promising new drug; and what to look for when evaluating a clinical research study. Also included is a general overview of interferon—the first therapy to be proven effective for treating chronic viral hepatitis B and C. This overview includes the history of interferon, its potential side effects, and how best to deal with side effects that do occur. Also, some financial issues regarding interferon are addressed. (More specific information on interferon therapy is covered in chapters 12 and 13.)

WHAT IS ANTIVIRAL THERAPY?

Antiviral therapy is the use of any drug or other agent acting or directed against a virus. The immediate goal of antiviral therapy is to interfere with the replication of the virus. The ultimate goal of antiviral therapy is to totally eradicate the virus from the body. Viruses are much more difficult to treat than bacteria. Bacteria are treated with agents called antibacterials, otherwise commonly known as antibiotics. Antibiotics have no action against viruses. Many different antivirals have been used to treat hepatitis B and C. Chapters 12 and 13 detail these treatments. The remainder of this chapter discusses interferon—the first antiviral therapy proven to be effective for some people with hepatitis B and C.

WHAT ARE INTERFERONS?

Interferons (IFNs) are a family of proteins made naturally by the body. In 1957, it was discovered that when a virus attacks the body, interferon is produced by special cells in the body in an effort to *interfere* with further viral replication and damage and to protect noninfected cells in the body from becoming infected. Thus, interferons were found to have the ability to fight viruses, which is known as *antiviral activity.* It was also discovered that interferons play an important role in fighting cancers, which is known as *antitumor activity,* and in regulating the immune system, which is known as *immunomodulatory activity.* There is even evidence that interferon may be able to reverse scarring that has already occurred to the liver due to the hepatitis B or C virus. This makes interferon an anti-scarring, or *antifibrotic,* medication.

Sometimes the body does not produce enough natural interferon to fight infections, cancers, and immune disorders. It has been shown that supplementing the interferon made in the body with synthetically manufactured interferon given by injection provides benefits to many people. In addition to being used to treat the viruses that cause chronic hepatitis—HBV and HCV—interferons have been used to treat a variety of diseases, including hairy cell leukemia (a rare blood disorder); melanoma (a type of skin cancer); Kaposi's sarcoma (a type of skin cancer that occurs in elderly people and people with AIDS); and condyloma acuminatum (a wartlike growth on the genitals).

Interferon, regardless of the type, is administered by injection only. It is most commonly injected by what is known as the *subcutaneous (SQ)* route (beneath the skin), but can also be injected *intramuscularly (IM)* (into the muscle). Patients can be injected by a doctor or nurse, but typically are taught to inject themselves so that they may administer their own medication at home. Patients are often given an instructional video or pamphlet to supplement any lessons given on self-injection. Unfortunately, interferon is not effective if taken orally and, as such, is not available in pill form. Intranasal sprays are currently being tested, but thus far have not proven to be effective. Devices that can be implanted under the skin to enable a controlled, timed release of interferon are also being studied.

The Classes of Interferon

There are three different classes of interferon: alfa (also spelled alpha), beta, and gamma. Alfa and beta interferons are known as type I interferons, whereas gamma interferon is known as type II interferon. While there is only one form of beta and gamma interferon, there are numerous forms of alfa interferon. The different types of alfa interferon are closely related in structure but differ slightly from one another, and therefore each variant is classified as a different subtype. The slight variations among the subtypes of alfa interferon account for the differences in the three FDA-approved synthetically manufactured alfa interferons currently available.

Interferon and FDA Approval

In 1991, interferon was first approved by the FDA for the treatment of chronic hepatitis C. Known as Intron A (interferon alfa-2b), this form of interferon is manufactured by Schering-Plough Corporation. In 1992, Intron A was FDA approved for the treatment of chronic hepatitis B. Intron A is currently the only type of interferon approved for the treatment of hepatitis B. In 1996, interferon alfa-2a (commercially marketed as Roferon A and manufactured by Roche Pharmaceuticals) was FDA approved for the treatment of chronic hepatitis C. Both Intron A and Roferon are identical to the corresponding natural alfa interferon that occurs in humans.

In 1997, the first bioengineered (i.e., non-naturally occurring) interferon for the treatment of chronic hepatitis C was approved by the FDA. Initially manufactured by Amgen (who sold the rights to this product to the pharmaceutical company Intermune in June 2001), it is marketed under the name Infergen (also known as interferon alfacon-1 or consensus interferon). Infergen represents an effort to create a type of interferon that is superior to those produced naturally by the body.

More recently, pegylated (PEG) interferon—an interferon requiring only a once-a-week administration (as opposed to the previous requirement of three times a week), was FDA approved for the treatment of chronic hepatitis C. FDA approval was granted in January 2001 to PEG-Intron (manufactured by Schering-Plough), and then in June 2002 to PEGASYS (manufactured by Roche Pharmaceuticals). Both forms of pegylated interferons are currently undergoing clinical trial studies for their use in the treatment of chronic hepatitis B. (A full discussion on the rationale behind the pegylation of interferon is discussed in chapter 13.)

Many other interferons are being tested by pharmaceutical companies for their use in the treatment of chronic hepatitis B and C. Examples include alfa interferons such as Wellferon (interferon alfa-n1—manufactured by Glaxo-Wellcome), an interferon that is approved in Canada for treatment of hepatitis C, and Alferon N (interferon alfa-n3—manufactured by Interferon Sciences); long-acting interferons such as Albuferon (manufactured by Human Genome Sciences) and Multiferon (manufactured by Viragen); beta interferons such as Rebif (manufactured by Ares Serono); interferons proposed to target the liver with the hope of diminishing side effects of interferon, such as Omega interferon (manufactured by BioMedicine); oral interferons such as oral interferon alpha (manufactured by Amarillo Biosciences); and interferons specifically aimed to reverse liver scarring, such as Interferon Gamma-1B (manufactured by Intermune).

POTENTIAL SIDE EFFECTS OF INTERFERON THERAPY AND HOW TO MANAGE THEM

All drugs have potential side effects. To realize this, you need only read the informational insert or label that accompanies any medicine—whether prescribed or over the counter. (By the way, if such information is not included, you can ask the pharmacist to provide it to you.) Accompanying any given medication is a list (typically quite lengthy) of potential side effects that may occur as a consequence of taking the drug. This is true even for the most commonly used over-the-counter medications, such as an aspirin or an antacid.

What accounts for such an extensive list of potential adverse reactions? The reason is that when a drug is being evaluated for FDA approval, every symptom that a person experiences while taking that drug must be reported. All of these side effects get listed on the informational insert that accompanies the medicine. Some of the listed side effects may have occurred in only a very small percentage of people, and some of the listed side effects may not even have been due to the drug at all.

There are some important points to keep in mind when evaluating the risks versus benefits of taking a medication such as interferon. Side effects associated with any drug, including interferon, vary from person to person. This means that not everyone will experience a particular side effect. While some people feel quite ill while undergoing interferon therapy, others experience few, if any, side effects. And there are some people who actually feel better while on interferon. That's right! This point bears repeating. It is possible that a person will have minimal to no side effects or will even feel better than usual while on interferon. And those who do experience adverse side effects usually do not experience them all the time. In fact, studies have shown that only approximately 2 to 5 percent of people find the side effects of interferon so debilitating that discontinuation of therapy is necessary.

Side effects are usually the worst during the first few weeks of therapy, so it is important to try to stick with therapy for at least a month or two. Some people schedule time off from work for when they plan to start interferon therapy. Others plan to begin therapy when their work schedule or personal responsibilities are light, thereby making it easier to get through the initial period. Side effects associated with interferon are usually dose related, meaning that the higher the dose of interferon, the greater the side effects. Sometimes a reduction in dosage may satisfactorily mitigate the side effects. However, studies have shown that adherence to the recommended dose and duration of therapy is directly correlated with success of treatment, that is, eradication of the virus and regression of liver scarring.

Most side effects can be successfully managed by a knowledgeable doctor in conjunction with a motivated patient. Thus, it is not advisable to decrease the dosage of medication or interrupt therapy unless the side effects are so severe that they outweigh the benefits of curing the disease: in other words, if the treatment of the disease is worse than the disease itself. If an adverse reaction occurs due to interferon and does not respond to side-effect management or dose reduction, then discontinuation of interferon is necessary.

It has been demonstrated that people with advanced liver disease and cirrhosis are the ones most likely to experience side effects. However, people with cirrhosis may have less side effects if they commence treatment with a relatively low dose of interferon. The importance of treatment in the early stages of the disease, when people are strongest and healthiest and best able to tolerate interferon, cannot be overstated. Finally, the side effects due to interferon will totally abate after interferon therapy has been discontinued.

If people can adopt strategies to cope with the side effects, then interferon therapy need not interfere with their daily lives. Plus, if side effects are managed promptly and aggressively, the dosage of interferon will not need to be lowered. This will allow a person to get the therapeutic dose of interferon that results in optimal effectiveness of the drug. This was mentioned before, but it is a crucial point that bears repeating. Once the dose of interferon is lowered, the chances of eradicating the virus and reversing inflammation and scarring of the liver diminish. Therefore, it is recommended to attempt to continue with the prescribed dosage and duration of therapy, without reduction, while at the same time treating accompanying side effects. Studies have shown that adherence to therapy is directly related to successful outcome.

One positive aspect to interferon therapy is that, unlike insulin injections for diabetes, which continue throughout the patient's life, interferon shots for chronic hepatitis B and C do not last forever. This is important to keep in mind for people who are experiencing difficulty dealing with the side effects of interferon: It's just for a limited amount of time. Try to stick it out!

The following is a discussion of the potential side effects associated with interferon therapy and some tips on how best to manage them. Since many of the side effects of interferon therapy are similar to the symptoms of liver disease in general, the reader is referred to chapter 20 for more helpful hints on managing these symptoms. Cough, skin rashes, dryness and itching, nausea, and anemia are the side effects more commonly associated with ribavirin, a drug used in combination with interferon for the treatment of hepatitis C. Those particular side effects are discussed in chapter 13.

Flu-like Symptoms

Flu-like symptoms are the most common side effects experienced while taking interferon. Flu-like symptoms typically include a low-grade fever, chills, headache, muscle and joint aches, fatigue, and weakness. These side effects may occur throughout treatment, but tend to be most pronounced during the first month of treatment and to diminish as treatment progresses. They are best managed by taking one to two tablets of acetaminophen (Tylenol) about thirty minutes prior to the interferon injection and about four to six hours after the injection. As will be discussed in chapter 24, aspirin and other nonsteroidal anti-inflammatories (NSAIDs), such as Motrin and Naprosyn, are worse for the liver than acetaminophen and should be avoided.

For some, injecting fifteen to thirty minutes prior to going to bed is helpful, since this will limit the side effects primarily to the sleeping hours. However, if the side effects from interferon either cause or contribute to insomnia, then changing the injection time to the morning is advisable. Some people find that it is easiest to handle the side effects of interferon if they are busy working, as this diverts their attention from their symptoms. Taking a lukewarm bath may also help relieve some flu-like symptoms. Never take an alcohol sponge bath, as the fumes from the alcohol are not good for the liver. Cooling packs applied to the body may also be helpful. Muscle and joints aches may be alleviated in some cases by massages and moderate exercise. In clinical trials, the supplement glucosamine chondroitin has been shown to build, and possibly repair, joint cartilage. Thus, some people who have taken this supplement have experienced relief from joint aches.

Amantadine (Symmetrel) is an antiviral medication used to treat people with influenza A (the flu) as well as people with Parkinson's disease, a neurological disorder. Although some studies have demonstrated that amantadine may be an effective treatment for individuals with chronic hepatitis C, this finding has not been confirmed by most of the studies done with this drug. However, amantadine, which is easy to take and has few side effects of its own, may be helpful in combating some of the flu-like symptoms that are associated with interferon therapy. Therefore, amantadine may be a useful adjunctive therapy to control some interferon-associated side effects. Further study needs to be conducted before amantadine becomes routinely prescribed to treat the side effects of interferon.

Hydration, hydration, hydration! Staying hydrated is probably the most important strategy for diminishing flu-like symptoms. Drinking approximately one gallon of water each day is recommended. That's right—one gallon! Several bottles of cold water should be a constant companion. Clear juices such as apple juice can also be consumed. Try to stay away from caffeinated drinks. Hot, humid weather may exacerbate flu-like symptoms. When confronted with this type of weather, staying in an air-conditioned environment, especially during daylight hours, is important. If you must go out in the daytime heat, be sure to wear a hat and apply sunscreen liberally to the entire body and especially to any exposed areas.

Fatigue

Approximately 25 percent of all Americans suffer from fatigue. Hepatitis and interferon both cause fatigue in their own right. The upshot of this is that more than 50 percent of people with hepatitis who are undergoing interferon treatment will suffer from this symptom. Unfortunately, there is no pill or quick fix one can take to eliminate fatigue. However, there are strategies you can employ to boost your energy level.

Poor eating habits intensify fatigue. As such, a healthy, well-rounded diet low in fat and high in complex carbohydrates is important. This should be accompanied by lots of water—at least ten to twelve glasses (one glass = 8 ounces) per day; a gallon is even better. After consuming a large meal, it is common to become tired. Therefore, multiple (at least five to six) small meals throughout the day should become a habit. And avoid grabbing a candy bar as a quick pick-me-up. After a fleeting sugar rush, sugar levels will quickly plummet, thereby worsening fatigue. A baked potato or a small bowl of rice or pasta (complex carbohydrates) will sustain energy levels longer. (Please refer to chapter 23 for more information about diet and nutrition.)

If at all possible, a fifteen- to twenty-minute nap once or twice a day will provide a quick pick-me-up. People with chronic hepatitis, especially those on treatment, should get as much rest as their body requires.

Exercise is crucial. It may seem like a catch-22—a person is too tired to exercise, yet exercise will provide her with a boost of energy. The solution is to start gradually. Even if only ten minutes a day is all a person can manage, by the end of the week she will have exercised an entire hour, which, of course, is better than nothing. With time, most people are able to build up their stamina to the point where they can exercise for at least twenty to thirty minutes each day. (See chapter 23 for more tips on exercise.)

Ondansetron (Zofran) is a medication used in the treatment of nausea and vomiting associated with cancer chemotherapy. Some anecdotal reports have noted the effectiveness of Zofran (4 mg twice a day) in the management of fatigue associated with liver disease. Further studies need to be conducted before this medication can be recommended, but since some people on interferon suffer from nausea and fatigue, Zofran, if its effectiveness can be proven, would be a helpful tool for battling these symptoms. There are medications used to treat fatigue in people with HIV and chronic fatigue syndrome. These include the SSRI bupropion (Wellbutrin), methylphenidate (Ritalin), and modafinil (Provigil). Ritalin has been found to reduce interferon-induced fatigue during melanoma treatment. Also, a preliminary study conducted on a small group of patients with hepatitis C showed that Ritalin significantly improved interferon-induced fatigue. Provigil is a medication approved for the treatment of narcolepsy, a neurological disorder marked by uncontrollable attacks of daytime sleepiness. Anecdotal evidence suggests that Provigil at a dose of 200 mg a day may be a useful adjunct in the treatment of fatigue associated with interferon. More studies need to be conducted on patients with hepatitis before any of these medications can be used routinely in the management of fatigue.

It goes without saying, but bears repeating anyway—alcoholic beverages should be totally avoided. In addition to being bad for the liver, alcohol is also a sedative, and furthermore it induces the hepatitis B and C viruses to replicate. Also, many people have reported that they feel more energetic as a result of totally eliminating caffeine intake. Finally, cannabis (marijuana) has been shown to decrease the effectiveness of interferon. Since smoking marijuana may also contribute to fatigue, it is advised to avoid this activity totally. (See chapter 20 for more tips on treating fatigue.)

Psychiatric/Psychological Side Effects

Interferon may cause depression, fatigue, irritability, confusion, emotional instability, insomnia, lack of concentration, diminished appetite, and weight loss. Approximately 57 percent of people may experience one or more of these symptoms at some point while taking interferon. And between 35 and 57 percent of people with chronic viral hepatitis suffer from these symptoms prior to even starting therapy, due either to a pre-existing condition or to the effects of the hepatitis C virus. In fact, researchers from Canada have recently linked brain dysfunction and hepatitis C independent of the severity or the duration of the disease. Fortunately, psychiatric symptoms, whether pre-existing due to the hepatitis C virus or due to interferon therapy, are controllable and treatable in most patients so as to allow for successful completion of therapy.

All drugs are metabolized, at least to some extent, through the liver. While people with a chronic liver disease should avoid any nonessential medications so as not to subject their livers to additional stress, this directive is outweighed by the great benefit to be obtained by treatment with an antidepressant or an antianxiety medication while on interferon therapy. People who are prone to depression, emotional instability, or other related symptoms will benefit from beginning an antidepressant or antianxiety medication prior to commencing interferon therapy. In fact, it is advisable for most people (including those with no prior psychological problems) to begin one of these medications prior to beginning therapy in order to prevent or diminish potential psychiatric symptoms from occurring. In this manner, treatment is most likely to continue uninterrupted, and the recommended dosage and duration of therapy are more likely to be adhered to.

Patients who take antidepressants during interferon therapy are less likely to have their relationships with family, friends, caretakers, coworkers, doctors, and their staff adversely affected while on therapy. This is an important point, as it is typically these "other" people who bear the brunt of any irrational and aggressive behavior caused, or worsened by, interferon therapy. Most important, a person should never feel reluctant or embarrassed to seek support from a psychological counselor or psychiatric doctor. Obtaining as much additional help as possible is strongly recommended. Those people who have a psychiatric condition or who experience severe psychiatric side effects while on interferon should be managed jointly by a liver specialist and a psychiatrist. People who suffer from severe depression along with suicidal thoughts, who have made suicide attempts, or who suffer from psychosis (delusions and hallucinations) should avoid interferon therapy until their underlying psychiatric problems have stabilized and any suicidal thoughts have abated.

Probably the safest antidepressants are the selective serotonin reuptake inhibitors (SSRIs) such as Paxil, Zoloft, Prozac, Celexa, and Lexapro. Although all SSRIs appear to be equally effective in the treatment of depression and anxiety, comparative studies on the different SSRIs in people with hepatitis on interferon therapy have not been done. In general, it takes approximately two to eight weeks for antidepressant medication to take full effect. (Lexapro's antidepressant/antianxiety action takes effect more quickly than the other SSRIs'.) Therefore, it is recommended to start an SSRI approximately one month before starting interferon therapy. Side effects of SSRIs are infrequent but may include anxiety, gastrointestinal problems, sexual problems, headaches, and weight gain. Wellbutrin may have less sexual side effects than other SSRIs. In addition, Wellbutrin is used for cigarette-smoking cessation. Thus, Wellbutrin may have a doubly beneficial effect for patients who are on interferon and want to stop cigarette smoking.

All SSRIs typically decrease anxiety levels, but additional antianxiety medications are sometimes needed, such as buspirone (Buspar) or alprazolam (Xanax). Xanax use should be limited due to its potential for addiction and liver toxicity. Studies have not shown any benefit to the herb St. John's wort *(Hypericum perforatum)*—an herb some use to treat depression—in the treatment of moderate to severe depression. Furthermore, herbs are not regulated by the FDA and thus are not subjected to purity and standardization control. (See chapter 21 for more information on herbs.) If depression continues, or if suicidal thoughts, delusions, or hallucinations occur, interferon therapy should be stopped and the patient should seek immediate psychiatric evaluation.

Interferon may also cause thyroid abnormalities, symptoms of which may mimic psychiatric disorders. Those on interferon must have their thyroid profile periodically checked via blood tests, especially when any of the above symptoms develop during therapy. Thyroid abnormalities are discussed below.

Thyroid Abnormalities

Thyroid abnormalities occur while on interferon therapy in approximately 8 percent of people. People who are prone to autoimmune disorders are more likely to develop a thyroid disorder than people without this predisposition. A person may develop either a slow-functioning thyroid (hypothyroidism) or a fast-functioning thyroid (hyperthyroidism). Symptoms associated with hypothyroidism include fatigue, weakness, hair loss, dry skin, memory impairment, and psychosis. Symptoms associated with hyperthyroidism include nervousness, heat intolerance, palpitations, weight loss, weakness, shortness of breath, poor concentration, emotional instability, and depression.

As noted above, symptoms of thyroid disorders are similar to those of psychiatric disorders. Thyroid disorders are readily diagnosed by obtaining a thyroid profile from blood tests. Both hypothyroidism and hyperthyroidism are easily treatable with thyroid medication. Occasionally, referral to an endocrinologist is necessary. Thyroid abnormalities that develop while a person is on interferon usually resolve after interferon is discontinued.

Injection-Related Symptoms

Expect to experience mild pain, redness, itching, and swelling at the interferon injection site. This is known as an *injection-site reaction.* It appears to be more common with the newer once-a-week pegylated interferons than with the older three-times-a-week interferons. (See chapter 13 for a full discussion of pegylated interferon.) Redness and swelling around the injection site may encompass an area as large as a half-dollar. While it may look alarming, most of the time it is normal and should be expected. This type of skin reaction typically occurs within a day or two of the injection and may not resolve for up to a month after the injection. If pain, swelling, and redness become severe, it should immediately be reported to the doctor or nurse, as it may be a sign of infection. If an infection is discovered to be present at the injection site, antibiotics need to be started immediately. The infected site should not be used again until it has totally healed.

In order to avoid infection, it is of crucial importance that the injection site is clean. A person should always clean the site with alcohol or an antiseptic, such as Betadine, prior to injecting. Also, it is essential to rotate the site of the injection. For example, the right thigh, the left thigh, and two sites on the stomach should each be used in rotation as injection sites. In this manner, the inflamed site will not be returned to for one month's time, allowing the redness and swelling to totally abate. If redness persists, a local over-the-counter topical steroid preparation such as hydrocortisone cream or Benadryl lotion may be applied to the area. Also icing the area prior to the injection may numb this region, thereby decreasing side effects. Be sure to allow for total drying of the alcohol after cleaning the area prior to the injection, and do not excessively rub or touch the injection site.

The patient can also request that the needle size be changed to a thinner gauge. Thinner needles, such as an insulin-type needle (a 28- or 29-gauge needle), are virtually painless. In patients with particularly sensitive or thin skin, lidocaine, a local anesthetic, may be mixed with the interferon injection to numb the area and decrease pain at the injection site. Lidocaine gel may be used topically to relieve injection-site soreness.

Make sure that the interferon solution is at room temperature. Finally, it is important not to expose the injection site to direct sunlight, as sunlight may exacerbate redness and irritation. So, it's knee-length shorts in the summer! Also, try to avoid tanning salons, as tanning may worsen any rashes that occur while on treatment.

Hair Loss

Interferon can cause hair thinning, hair loss, hair breakage, and can change the texture of hair. However, some people are under the impression that interferon therapy will cause them to lose all their hair. (Isn't that what Pamela Anderson stated as one of her main reasons for not starting therapy?) This is a total misconception. In fact, hair loss while on interferon therapy is infrequent. If it occurs at all, the amount of hair lost is often minimal and usually unnoticeable to others.

People on interferon do not experience hair loss in the way that a cancer patient on chemotherapy does. Hair loss from interferon appears to be most frequent in Caucasians with black hair and Asians. It typically occurs around the third or fourth month of therapy. Hair loss may continue for up to three months after treatment is discontinued.

If hair loss does occur, there are many steps a person can take to minimize this side effect. People should refrain from dying or bleaching their hair while on interferon therapy, since this may exacerbate hair loss. A mild hair rinse may be used as an alternative to coloring. Avoid permanents and hair-straightening procedures while on therapy. Many people have found the vitamin biotin (a B vitamin) to be helpful. It is advisable to take this vitamin daily upon the commencement of therapy. A mild shampoo and a detangling conditioner are advisable. Nioxin shampoo, Nioxin conditioner, and Nioxin hair-growth promoter can help keep hair loss to a minimum while on therapy. Nioxin hair-loss treatment should be started about a month prior to starting interferon. It may be purchased without a prescription, but if you have trouble finding it, you may be able to purchase it via their Internet website, www.nioxin.com. Other recommended shampoos include Tricomin, Revivogen, and Nizoral. Minoxidil (Rogaine) liquid topical medication may be of some benefit. It should be applied only to the scalp and not ingested. It may stop the hair loss and thicken the remaining hair, but continued use twice daily for at least four months is typically required before obvious results are noted.

Other tips for diminishing hair loss include the use of a wide-tooth comb, avoidance of curling irons and rollers, and avoidance of daily shampooing. Avoid cornrowing, tight braids, and pulling hair back in a ponytail with tight rubberbands. A short haircut may be in order. If hair loss becomes a major problem, medical insurances will typically cover the cost of a wig or hairpiece. Often a doctor's note or prescription along with a receipt of purchase is all that is required for insurance reimbursement.

Fortunately, any hair loss induced by interferon therapy is temporary, and regrowth typically occurs within three to six months from the drug's discontinuation. The color and texture of hair may differ from the person's original hair type. In fact, many people have noted that their hair grows back thicker, straighter, and shinier than before!

Nail Irregularities

A person's nails may become brittle while they are on interferon resulting in frequent breaking, cracking, and splitting of nails. Anemia, thyroid abnormalities, dehydration, weight loss, and poor nutrition, all of which can occur on interferon therapy, are possible contributing factors to nail brittleness. Constant nail-biting may be attributable to interferon-induced anxiety. An SSRI may be helpful under these circumstances. To help minimize nail brittleness, gloves should be worn when doing dishes, nails should be cut short, and nail salons and nail polish remover should be avoided. Petroleum jelly (Vaseline) or olive oil may help keep the nails lubricated and moisturized, thereby decreasing breakage. Biotin, zinc, and glucosamine chondroitin may act to decrease breakage; however the effectiveness of these products at reducing nail breakage has not been proven.

Headaches

Headaches are a common side effect of interferon treatment, occurring intermittently in approximately 50 percent of people on treatment. Management of headaches requires both dietary and lifestyle changes, such as reduction of caffeine intake and stress reduction, in addition to pharmacologic treatment. For a full discussion of the treatment of headaches, see chapter 20.

Insomnia

Insomnia occurs in approximately 30 to 40 percent of people while on interferon treatment. Insomnia may cause or worsen anxiety, depression, decreased concentration, poor coordination, and excessive fatigue. Therefore, prompt and aggressive management of insomnia is important in order to facilitate the tolerability of interferon treatment. The management of insomnia is discussed in detail in chapter 20.

Eye Problems

Rarely, interferon may cause eye problems. Symptoms may include dry, itchy eyes, burning eyes, decreased vision, blurry vision, poor night vision, and blind spots. All people with high blood pressure or diabetes need to undergo an eye exam prior to beginning interferon therapy. Anyone who develops any visual disturbances while on interferon should report the symptoms immediately to their doctor. Dry, itchy eyes may be treated with over-the-counter saline eye drops or Natural Tears. If eye problems are accompanied by decreased vision, evaluation by an ophthalmologist is necessary. In these circumstances, interferon may need to be discontinued, depending upon the severity of symptoms. Typically, eye problems resolve once interferon use is stopped.

Weight Loss

Interferon may cause loss of appetite, altered taste sensation, nausea, mouth sores, mouth dryness, abdominal discomfort, flatulence, and diarrhea. Weight loss in the range of ten to twenty-five pounds may occur while a person is on interferon therapy due to these side effects. This should not be a cause for alarm, as weight typically returns to normal soon after therapy is discontinued. However, when weight loss is due to poor eating habits, the patient may experience vitamin and other nutritional deficiencies. This may cause or contribute to hair loss; dry, thin skin; and brittle nails.

Eating multiple—approximately five or six—small meals throughout the day and consuming plenty of water will help maintain a steady weight while on interferon. Large meals should always be avoided. Furthermore, the food consumed should be healthy and low in fat. Using plastic utensils instead of metallic flatware may decrease the peculiar taste often experienced by people on interferon and may make food more appetizing. Mouth sores may be due to excessive oral dryness or infections. Mouth sores are a common cause of decreased interest in food and subsequent weight loss. The management of mouth disorders is discussed on page 157 of this chapter. Nausea, more commonly a side effect of ribavirin therapy, is discussed in chapter 13.

Flatulence (increased gas production) and diarrhea may be lessened by adhering to a lactose-free (dairy-free) diet and by avoiding raw vegetables and fruits. Vegetables may be eaten if well cooked, and fruits may be eaten provided they are peeled first. Fiber supplements that act as bulking agents, such as Metamucil or Citrucel, may help decrease the incidence of loose stools. It is important to avoid fiber supplements containing senna, as there have been reports that some cases of toxic hepatitis have been caused by senna. Over-the-counter antidiarrheals, such as Imodium AD, may be used, but it is important to discuss any medications with your doctor prior to taking them. (See chapter 23 for more information on nutrition.)

Exercise, especially weight-bearing exercise—which increases muscle and bone mass—is important for people on interferon therapy. Furthermore, exercise in general, whether it be swimming, playing tennis, or walking, helps stimulate one's appetite.

Appetite stimulants may be taken if weight loss becomes severe. The safest appetite stimulant is probably Reglan (metoclopramide), a medication typically used in the treatment of nausea. Reglan taken half an hour prior to meals may help increase the desire for food. Megace (megestrol acetate), an appetite stimulant used to treat excessive weight loss in patients being treated with chemotherapy for cancer as well as in patients with HIV, may cause nonalcoholic fatty liver disease and diminish response to interferon treatment. Further studies need to be conducted on Megace before it can be recommended. Marinol (dronabinol), also referred to as medical marijuana, has been used to stimulate appetite and reduce the nausea and vomiting associated with chemotherapy, as well as to increase weight in people with HIV. Studies have not been conducted on people with hepatitis who are on interferon therapy; thus, Marinol use cannot be recommended at this time. Many antidepressant/antianxiety medications such as the SSRIs (Paxil, Celexa, and Zoloft), as well as Ritalin, have been associated with weight gain. The medications may provide a dual benefit to those on interferon who suffer from both depression and weight loss.

Decreased Blood Counts

The bone marrow is responsible for the production of red blood cells, white blood cells, and platelets. Interferon can inhibit the bone marrow from performing this function. This is known as bone marrow suppression. Thus, people on interferon may develop decreased red blood cell counts (anemia), decreased white blood cell counts (neutropenia), and decreased platelet counts (thrombocytopenia). These side effects are most common, but not exclusive to, people who have cirrhosis. These side effects are also more common with the newer, once-a-week pegylated interferons than with the formerly standard three-times-a-week interferon. Bone marrow suppression can also be caused by the hepatitis C virus itself, even in the absence of interferon therapy. This is based on the finding that the hepatitis C virus can replicate in the bone marrow, causing damage and destruction of blood cells. Hepatitis C has also been associated with autoimmune hemolytic anemia (see page 124), which results in the destruction of red blood cells (RBCs), thereby causing anemia. In general, decreased blood counts may be reversed by reducing the dose of interferon or by discontinuing therapy. However, this typically leads to diminished efficacy of treatment and a lower response rate. Thus, maintaining the optimal dose of medication while effectively managing bone marrow side effects is a key element in achieving the best long-term results of therapy. As noted above, interferon causes anemia by suppressing the production of RBCs by the bone marrow. While interferon may cause anemia, anemia is more common (as well as more severe) when given in combination with ribavirin, a medication used in combination with interferon for the treatment of chronic hepatitis C. Anemia is discussed in detail on page 192.

Neutropenia

Neutrophils are special WBCs that are the body's first line of defense against infectious invaders such as bacteria, viruses, and fungal infections. When the number of WBCs or neutrophils go below a certain level (less than 1,500/mm^3 or 750/mm^3, respectively) in the body it is known as *neutropenia*. Pegylated interferon is much more likely to cause neutropenia than three-times-a-week interferon. While complications such as severe bacterial infections are uncommon, it is nevertheless important to take steps to prevent neutropenia, as well as to reverse it when it does occur. Neutropenia is more common among African Americans than Caucasians.

The goal is to prevent and/or reverse neutropenia without unduly compromising interferon therapy. One way neutropenia can be reversed is by decreasing the dose of interferon. However, this will result in subtherapeutic dosages and will compromise viral eradication rates. Granulocyte-colony stimulating factor (G-CSF), marketed by Amgen as Filgrastim (Neupogen), increases the white blood cell and neutrophil counts. Anecdotal evidence suggests that Neupogen at a dose of 300 micrograms administered subcutaneously between one to three times a week will correct most PEG-interferon-related neutropenia without requiring a dose reduction. The most common side effects of Neupogen include nausea and bone pain. Further study on the use of Neupogen to manage interferon-related neutropenia is currently ongoing. Pegfilgrastim (Neulasta) is the pegylated or long-lasting form of Neupogen. It does not need to be administered as frequently. There are currently no published studies on the use of Neulasta for interferon-induced neutropenia in patients with hepatitis, but the infrequent dosing regimen of one injection every other week is a welcome advance.

Thrombocytopenia and Thrombocytosis

Interferon may cause *thrombocytopenia,* which is defined as a low platelet count—less than 80,000cells/mm^3.Thrombocytopenia most commonly occurs in people who have cirrhosis, as these individuals often already have low platelet counts, and in people taking interferon alone without ribavirin, such as those with hepatitis B or those with hepatitis C who cannot tolerate ribavirin.

Ribavirin typically causes *thrombocytosis*—elevated platelet counts. This is why people who take the combination therapy of interferon and ribavirin rarely have significant thrombocytopenia. In fact, this complication occurs in less than 3 percent of people on combination therapy. In cases where people have a platelet count less than 50,000 to 80,000cells/mm^3, it is recommended that the dose of interferon be lowered. Low platelet counts may put one at increased risk for bleeding. However, bleeding is rare if the platelet count remains above 25,000cells/mm^3. Interleukin-11(IL-II) Obrelvekin, marketed under the brand name Neumega, is used to treat thrombocytopenia in patients undergoing cancer chemotherapy. In people with interferon-induced thrombocytopenia, IL-II has been shown to increase platelet counts to over 100,000cells/mm^3. IL-II is given as a daily SQ injection of 25 to 50 micrograms. Platelet count elevations are usually seen about a week or two after the initial injection. Typically, the only significant side effect noted is fluid retention. This is particularly a problem for people with cirrhosis, as some of these people already suffer from this complication. Fluid retention can be treated with water pills. Further study on IL-II is needed before it can be routinely recommended for people with HCV with interferon-induced thrombocytopenia.

Mouth

The mucosal cells of the mouth are sensitive to many types of medication, including interferon. Thus, one may experience a painful, burning, excessively dry or ulcerated mouth while on interferon therapy. This is known as *mucositis* and may lead to a decreased appetite, resulting in weight loss. Cigarette smoking worsens mucositis, another reason to get rid of this bad habit. Good oral hygiene while on interferon is especially important. Meticulous, but not excessive, toothbrushing (three to four times per day) and gentle flossing are essential. If one's gums are already injured, flossing should be avoided. The mouth should be rinsed with baking soda rather than a commercial mouthwash, as many of these contain alcohol. Any necessary dental or periodontal procedures (such as implants or dentures) should be performed at least three to six months prior to commencement of therapy, or one to three months after completion of therapy. Mucositis may be diminished by regularly lubricating the lips and the corners of the mouth with petroleum jelly, especially prior to going to sleep. A topical corticosteroid, such as fluocinomide (Lidex) 0.05%, or clobetasol (Temovate) 0.05% may enhance the healing process. A corticosteroid mouth rinse such as dexamethasone elixir may also be helpful. Xylocaine, a local anesthetic that numbs the mouth, may afford some relief. Other over-the-counter topical anesthetic solutions such as Orabase B may be useful. Medications that coat an ulcer, such as sucralfate (Carafate), Orabase (an adhesive paste with a topical anesthetic), or even Kaopectate may be applied directly to the sore. This may significantly diminish the pain caused by an oral ulcer.

Mouth infections (including those attributable to the herpes virus) and fungal infections (such as thrush) may occur in the mouth due to neutropenia. Oral herpes, also known as herpes simplex 1, causes fever blisters or cold sores. Oral herpes may be treated with acyclovir taken orally (Zovirex) or topically (Denavir). An anesthetic mouthwash or spray, such as Hurricane liquid, may help alleviate the pain associated with oral herpes. Oral thrush requires Mycostatin (nystatin), usually taken as a swish-and-swallow preparation. If this does not eradicate the fungus, Diflucan (fluconazole) tablets taken orally may be necessary.

Interferon therapy may increase the likelihood of tooth decay and dental cavities due to decreased saliva production. Saliva contains antibacterial agents that kill the bacteria that cause tooth decay. It is therefore important to take steps to increase the flow of saliva in the mouth. This can be achieved by chewing sugarless gum and by drinking fluids consistently throughout the day.

Decreased Libido

The female sex drive (*libido*) is a complicated combination of physical and psychological factors. Interferon therapy may make women feel tired, depressed, and irritable. As a result, for many women on interferon, sex is the last thing on their minds. Furthermore, vaginal dryness, which can lead to itching, sensitivity, irritation, and discomfort, can occur while on interferon. Continued dryness leads to yeast infections and vaginitis, an inflamed vagina. This causes pain during sexual intercourse. Psychologically, women may feel as if they are not as attractive while on interferon, as hair may become thinner and facial skin drier, giving the appearance of more wrinkles. All of the above result in decreased libido.

Vaginal dryness may be alleviated by using a vaginal lubricant such as K-Y jelly or any other water-soluble lubricant that contains glycerin. Avoid using petroleum-based lubricants such as Vaseline, as they may increase the likelihood of vaginal infections. Furthermore, petroleum-based lubricants may erode and damage latex, decreasing the effectiveness of condoms. The use of vaginal gels that contain both progesterone and estrogen may need to be prescribed by one's gynecologist. Kegel exercises (contracting the pelvic muscles) are important to do twice a day to strengthen the pelvic muscles and to increase the blood flow to the vagina (thereby naturally increasing vaginal lubrication). Vaginal fungal infections may be eradicated with mycostatin creams, which are available over the counter. Treatment of fatigue, depression, and hair loss are discussed elsewhere in this chapter. Treatment of dry skin is discussed in chapter 13 (side effects of ribavirin). Sexual dysfunction may also occur in men while on interferon. Treatment is discussed in chapter 24.

Menstrual Irregularities

Women with hepatitis C who are on interferon therapy have reported a variety of menstrual irregularities, including premature or delayed menses, diminished or prolonged days of menstrual flow, and clotting and spotting during menstruation. Women also often report having premenstrual syndrome symptoms (PMS) more frequently and with greater intensity while on interferon therapy. Women on interferon who have cirrhosis appear to have more menstrual abnormalities than women with less-damaged livers. Menstruation typically returns to normal within six months of discontinuing interferon therapy.

Other Side Effects

Elevated *triglyceride* levels can occur but are infrequent. Elevated levels typically return to normal once interferon is discontinued. People can develop a cough, nausea, anemia, dry skin, a rash, and/or itching while on therapy. These side effects are more commonly associated with ribavirin therapy. The reader is referred to page 191 for a discussion on managing these side effects.

DISCONTINUATION OF INTERFERON THERAPY DUE TO SIDE EFFECTS

All side effects experienced while taking interferon must be reported to one's doctor. If the side effects of interferon become too difficult to withstand and cannot be managed effectively, it is possible that the doctor may suggest discontinuation. Such a determination will depend on many factors. That is why a liver biopsy is so important to obtain prior to starting interferon therapy. For example, if the liver biopsy findings from a person with chronic hepatitis C reveal little scarring and/or inflammation, the doctor may recommend discontinuing interferon if the side effects are too overwhelming. Since chronic hepatitis C progresses so slowly, such a person may benefit from deferring treatment until the trial of a new drug becomes available.

On the other hand, if the liver biopsy findings on a person with chronic hepatitis reveal extensive scarring and inflammation, the doctor may recommend that this person attempt to continue therapy, despite the side effects.

FINANCIAL ISSUES CONCERNING INTERFERON

There are three financial issues that people must consider prior to beginning interferon or any other treatment regimen: the cost of the drug, the cost of the doctor visits, and the cost of the blood tests. This section will discuss each of these financial issues.

The Cost of the Drug

As noted on page 145 of this chapter, three types of alfa interferon have been approved in the United States for treating chronic hepatitis C, and one type has been approved for treating chronic hepatitis B. Treatment regimens vary as to duration (can range from six months to greater than a year), number of injections administered per week (can range from once a week to daily), and the dose of injection (can be weight-based or one-dose-fits-all). Therefore, the cost of a full course of interferon therapy can vary widely. (These variables are discussed in detail in the next two chapters.) As an example, the cost of a one-month supply of PEG-Intron or PEGASYS (even without ribavirin pills), can range from $1,300 to $1,700!

The two most important cost variables are usually the pharmacy the person is using and the type of insurance she has. The bottom line is that it tends to be very expensive to treat chronic hepatitis B and C with interferon. However, the treatment is well worth the expense, as interferon can increase life expectancy and decrease the likelihood of liver-related complications. The cost of the FDA-approved alfa interferons is covered by most insurance plans, including most managed-care plans. Often the doctor's office will need to obtain an "authorization" from the insurance company allowing the patient to use interferon. On occasion, an insurance company will be unwilling to pay for treatment or, more frequently, re-treatment with interferon. In this situation, the patient's doctor must write an appeal letter to the insurance company to explain the necessity of the treatment. This letter is known as a letter of medical necessity. After receiving such a letter, the insurance company will typically reverse the decision and agree to provide coverage. If this still does not work, the patient and the patient's doctor can request a telephone conference with the insurance company's medical board. During this telephone conference, it is up to the patient and the patient's doctor to convince the board that interferon will reduce the likelihood of complications of the disease, that interferon is cost effective, and that the interferon will improve the patient's quality of life. It is rare for the insurance company to reject payment for the drug if a cogent argument is made.

If the person is unable to obtain coverage for treatment or if she does not have any insurance coverage, the pharmaceutical company that manufactures the drugs may be able to assist with the cost. However, the person may be required to supply her latest tax return and a list of expenses related to the cost of treatment. Not everyone in this situation will qualify for financial assistance.

Medicare will cover the cost of interferon therapy, but with one restriction—the interferon injection must be administered by a doctor or the doctor's staff in the doctor's office or clinic, or by a Medicare-approved nurse at the patient's home. (Non-Medicare patients may administer their injections to themselves in their own homes.)

Finally, if the person is still having difficulty covering the cost of treatment, she should search for an experimental trial to enter. Often, but not always, the medications in an experimental trial are provided free of charge.

The Cost of the Doctor Visits

A person with chronic hepatitis B or chronic hepatitis C who is starting therapy will require frequent visits to the doctor's office. She should therefore make sure that the doctor accepts her particular insurance or managed-care plan. If the doctor accepts the plan, then the visits are covered by the insurance company. Often a minimal copayment ranging from $5 to $20 is required. With some managed-care plans, the doctor will need to write a letter to the insurance company and/or the patient's primary care physician, explaining the need for multiple long-term visits.

If the doctor does not accept the insurance or managed-care plan, then it may be necessary to arrange a payment schedule with the doctor's office. Usually, a reduced fee can be arranged in view of the fact that multiple visits will be required. Remember, the doctor is there to help the patient get better and will usually be willing to work out some kind of reasonable reduced-fee payment plan—especially if discussed in advance. Also, as discussed in chapter 4, even if the doctor does not belong to a particular managed-care program, reimbursement for the doctor visits may still be arranged through the insurance company. Usually this requires a telephone call or a letter from the patient to the insurance company explaining the necessity for seeing that particular specialist. Once again, this is why it is important to be under the care of a knowledgeable hepatologist. The insurance companies will commonly reimburse a hepatologist if she presents evidence that she has expertise in liver disease not offered by any of the other specialists on the insurance plan.

For people enrolled in an experimental study, the visits to the doctor are often free of charge or at a reduced fee. The person should always inquire whether her doctor is conducting any clinical trials or is aware of any nearby trials that will cover the costs of treatment.

The Cost of the Blood Tests

As with medications and doctor visits, the cost of blood tests is usually covered by the insurance plan or managed-care plan. Managed-care plans typically contract with specific laboratories to process blood work. It is important for the doctor to be aware of the specific laboratory that the insurance company has contracted with. This will ensure that all blood work is covered by the insurance.

If a person does not have insurance, either she or the doctor's office staff should personally contact the supervisor of the laboratory to inquire about payment arrangements. Usually a reduced-fee payment schedule to cover the costs of blood work can be arranged.

If the patient is enrolled in a clinical trial, the blood work is often sent to a centralized laboratory. In such cases, the costs are usually, but not always, covered by the sponsor of the trial.

CONCLUSION

This chapter discussed some important issues concerning treatment of chronic viral hepatitis. Hopefully the information contained in this chapter will assist a person with chronic viral hepatitis in making a decision about treatment, whether she should stick with a time-tested, FDA-approved medication or instead enter a clinical trial of a promising new medication. As interferon is often an effective treatment for chronic viral hepatitis, most people with chronic hepatitis B and/or chronic hepatitis C will want to consider it as a treatment option at some point. However, interferon does have potential side effects. With that in mind, this chapter provided some helpful tips to assist people who are experiencing side effects from interferon. Financial issues are the last thing that a person wants to worry about when she is sick. Therefore, this chapter also provided some tips that will hopefully lessen money worries, with the ultimate objective being to focus on the more important issue—getting better!

Now that the groundwork has been laid on some basic treatment issues relating to chronic hepatitis B and chronic hepatitis C, the next two chapters will deal with specific treatment options for people with these diseases.

Twelve

TREATING HEPATITIS B AND D

Hepatitis B is one of the most common infections in the world. Almost 400 million people worldwide, including 1.25 million people in the United States, have hepatitis B. Chronic infection with this virus is the most common cause of cirrhosis and liver cancer worldwide. This leads to the death of approximately 1 million people each year from the complications of hepatitis B. However, early medical intervention can prevent many of these deaths. People with chronic hepatitis B must attempt to eradicate the hepatitis B virus (HBV) from their bodies before long-term complications develop and the disease can be transmitted to others. The ultimate goal of therapy, therefore, is to eliminate HBV from the body. If this cannot be achieved, a secondary goal is to suppress the replication of HBV. The less HBV replicates, the less damage will be done to the liver and the less infectious the person will be to others.

Hepatitis delta virus (HDV) is a virus that can only live in a person infected with HBV. Approximately 70,000 people in the United States are infected with HDV. Hepatitis D tends to be a particularly severe infection with significant long-term consequences, causing greater than 1,000 deaths each year. Therefore, treatment of people infected with HDV is crucial.

This chapter focuses on the medical treatment of people who have progressed to chronic hepatitis B and analyzes which individuals will benefit most from therapy. It also discusses the circumstances under which people do or do not require treatment. Interferon, the first treatment for chronic hepatitis B to be approved by the FDA, is discussed in detail. While eradication of HBV can occur with interferon, not everyone responds to this therapy. Therefore, other medications for chronic hepatitis B, specifically lamivudine and adefovir, are also discussed. In fact, many specialists choose either lamivudine or adefovir instead of interferon as the first line of treatment. Since there are many other therapies currently under investigation, this chapter also discusses some promising treatment options. In addition, the treatment of people infected with HDV is addressed.

Finally, appropriate monitoring of people who are not undergoing treatment is covered.

TREATMENT OF ACUTE HEPATITIS B

Fortunately, only a small percentage of adults with acute hepatitis B progress to chronic hepatitis B. Most adults have an immune system that is strong enough to battle the virus and completely eliminate it from their bodies during the acute stages of disease, without the help of any medical treatment. Consequently, people with acute hepatitis B are not treated with antiviral medications, such as interferon, lamivudine, or adefovir. There is no pill, vitamin, or vaccination necessary during the acute stage of the disease. Most people are managed conservatively, at home, based on how they are feeling. Home therapy involves drinking plenty of fluids and bed rest, if necessary. A person's level of activity should be judged on an individual basis. While some people are very fatigued and require long periods of inactivity and bed rest, others feel perfectly normal and are able to return to work and daily activities immediately. Therefore, bed rest is not a requirement for everyone. Many people report an aversion to cigarette smoking during this time, which is better off avoided in any case. Finally, people should avoid alcohol and eat a healthy, well-balanced diet. See chapter 23 for more information on diet, nutrition, and exercise.

APPROVAL OF MEDICATION FOR CHRONIC HEPATITIS B

The first medication found to be effective for chronic hepatitis B, interferon alfa-2a (Intron A; manufactured by Schering-Plough Corporation) was approved by the FDA in July 1992. Lamivudine (Epivir-HBV; manufactured by GlaxoWellcome) was approved by the FDA in December 1998, and adefovir (Hepsera; manufactured by Gilead) was approved in September 2002. Other antiviral medications are in the process of investigation and await FDA approval.

MONITORING A PERSON PRIOR TO AND DURING THERAPY

Prior to starting therapy, a complete physical exam and several blood tests are necessary. These blood tests should include a *complete blood count (CBC),* which includes a platelet count; thyroid profile, including thyroid stimulating hormone (TSH); alpha-fetoprotein (AFP); human immunodeficiency virus (HIV); and complete blood chemistries, including a liver profile (total bilirubin, transaminases, and GGTP), prothrombin time (PT), and *antinuclear antibody (ANA).* (See chapter 3 for an explanation of most of these tests.) A liver biopsy is typically performed in order to determine the severity of disease. (See chapter 5 for a complete discussion of liver biopsies.)

During therapy, the specialist monitors the patient's symptoms and blood tests frequently. This is done to determine whether the person has responded to therapy, which is assessed by eradication of the virus (HBV DNA), normalization of liver enzymes (AST and ALT), and/or hepatitis B seroconversion (eradication of HBeAg and formation of HBeAb). The specialist will also monitor for any side effects of therapy and will check for possible drug resistance. Prior to the eradication of HBV from the body, people often have a "flare" of the disease. This flare is noted by an increase of transaminase activity, which is sometimes as high as ten to twenty times the upper limit of normal, and also by the return or worsening of symptoms. While this course of events typically causes the person experiencing them some alarm, this "flare" is actually indicative of a favorable outcome, namely HBV clearance from the body. One way that antivirals work is by assisting the immune system in attacking the virus. Picture a war going on inside the liver between the enemy (HBV) and the soldiers (antiviral medication). Just before the enemy is kicked out of the body, there is a great deal of upheaval ("flare"). The hope is that this battle will conclude with the antiviral medication having conquered HBV.

When a person responds to therapy, HBV DNA will no longer be detectable, HBeAg will become negative, and HBeAb will become positive (known as seroconversion). In addition, transaminase levels (ALT and AST) will normalize. However, HBsAg only occasionally becomes negative and HBcAb will be positive lifelong. (See table 9.1 on page 100 for further clarification.) Symptoms associated with hepatitis B, such as fatigue, weakness, and loss of appetite, will be diminished or even totally gone. Symptoms associated with some of the extrahepatic manifestations of chronic hepatitis B, such as fever, rash, and/or joint pain, will also improve. Liver scarring and inflammation may be expected to improve for those who have responded to therapy. In fact, some people may even reverse severe scarring of the liver from therapy (especially those who have cleared the virus from their bodies). Refer to the sidebar on the following page for a list of indicators of successful treatment.

ALFA INTERFERON THERAPY FOR CHRONIC HEPATITIS B

People with chronic hepatitis have a defective immune response to the interferon that is naturally produced by their bodies. So, as early as the 1970s, researchers began investigating interferon therapy for people with chronic hepatitis B. However, it wasn't until 1992 that the FDA approved interferon therapy for the treatment of chronic hepatitis—at a dose of 5 million units of interferon alfa-2b (Intron A) daily, or 10 million units three times per week. Therapy may last a minimum of four months, but usually lasts for six to twelve months. The longer the therapy, the more likely the seroconversion rate.

Approximately 37 percent of infected people will eradicate the virus as a result of six months of interferon. This compares to an approximately 10 percent chance each year of virus eradication by spontaneous remission (i.e., virus eradication without treatment). The disappearance of HBeAg and the formation of HBeAb occur in approximately 33 percent of patients after six months of interferon

---

Summary of Indicators of Successful Treatment

HBV DNA will become nondetectable

HBeAg will become negative

HBeAb will become positive

HBsAg will only occasionally become negative

HBcAb will remain positive lifelong

Transaminase levels will become normal

Liver inflammation and scarring will diminish or resolve

Symptoms will improve

---

treatment. The normalization of elevated transaminase levels occurs soon there-after. Approximately 10 percent of these people will lose the carrier state (meaning they will no longer be carriers, as manifested by the loss of HBsAg) within one year of commencing therapy, and over time this percentage increases.

People who are HBeAg negative but who nevertheless have a replicating virus (HBV DNA) are considered to have precore mutant strains of hepatitis B. These patients typically do not respond as well to interferon therapy as those people with HBeAg present. Approximately 10 to 15 percent of people will have a sustained eradication of HBV DNA and normalization of liver enzymes after six months of interferon therapy. With longer interferon regimens (greater than or equal to one year), sustained viral eradication rates increase to approximately 20 percent.

People who have been treated with interferon may experience beneficial long-term results, if they do not eradicate the virus on therapy. Survival has been shown to be longer, and the development of liver cancer and liver decompensation (development of encephalopathy, esophageal varices, and ascites) has been shown to be less likely in patients treated with interferon compared with patients who did not receive therapy.

Studies using pegylated interferon (sustained-release, long-acting interferon administered just once a week) on patients with chronic hepatitis B are currently under way. Preliminary results on patients treated with PEG-interferon alfa-2a for six months have shown that 24 percent eradicated HBV DNA, normalized liver enzymes, and became HBeAg negative six months after discontinuation of therapy compared with only 12 percent of patients treated with conventional alfa interferon 2a. Furthermore, in recent studies, 43 percent of people taking PEGASYS compared with only 29 percent of people taking Epivir decreased their HBV

DNA levels. Therefore, pegylated interferon appears to be a promising treatment for chronic hepatitis B. FDA approval of PEGASYS for the treatment of hepatitis B is expected in 2005. (Please refer to chapter 13 for more information on pegylated interferon.)

Those Most Likely to Respond to Interferon Therapy

Although it is impossible to predict which people with chronic hepatitis B will respond to therapy, some indicators can identify the people who will be most likely to respond. The characteristics of these people include the following:

- Elevated levels of transaminases (ALT and AST) greater than 100 IU/ml

- Low level of HBV DNA, less than 200 pg/dl (picograms per deciliter)

- Liver biopsy findings of moderate to severe inflammation

- Short duration of the disease

- No evidence of decompensated cirrhosis (for example, no bleeding esophageal varices, ascites, etc.)

- Female gender

- Acquisition of infection as an adult

- No evidence of hepatitis delta virus (HDV)

- Non-immunocompromised (for example, HIV negative; not an organ transplant recipient)

- HBeAg positive (nonmutant form of HBV)

- Non-Asian origins

- (Possibly) those with genotype B

OTHER TREATMENT OPTIONS FOR CHRONIC HEPATITIS B

Interferon works well for many people with chronic hepatitis B. However, interferon is not without side effects. At times, the side effects may be so severe that discontinuation of the drug becomes necessary. (For a discussion of managing these side effects, see chapter 11.)

Alternatively, some people do not respond to treatment with interferon. Asian people who acquired hepatitis B at birth—especially those with normal transaminases; people with mutant strains of HBV (those people that are HBeAg negative but positive for HBV DNA); and liver transplant recipients are among those who tend not to respond to interferon. In addition, some people are at risk of serious complications if treated with interferon. An example is people with decompensated liver disease. These people may develop liver failure if treated with interferon. One other downside to interferon is that it must be given by injection, a route that is somewhat unpleasant to many people.

For all of the above-mentioned reasons, a number of alternative antiviral and immune-system–modifying medications are being used to treat people with chronic hepatitis B. The following pages briefly describe some of the most promising of these medications. Of these medications, only lamivudine (Epivir-HBV) and adefovir (Hepsera) are FDA approved for the treatment of chronic hepatitis B.

Nucleoside and Nucleotide Agents

Nucleoside and nucleotide analogues are oral antiviral agents. A *nucleoside* is a compound that forms the building blocks of *deoxyribonucleic acid (DNA)* and *ribonucleic acid (RNA)*—the compounds in which genetic information is stored. A *nucleotide* is like a nucleoside except that it has a phosphorus molecule attached to it. An *analogue* is a compound that resembles another compound in structure and function. Some of these drugs appear to be quite effective in suppressing HBV replication and disease activity. However, these medications often do not lead to long-term remissions. Moreover, the development of mutant strains of HBV, which are resistant to therapy, commonly occurs during treatment and, with even greater frequency, after treatment has been discontinued. Whether continuous long-term therapy with these drugs is necessary, and what, if any, side effects occur during long-term therapy are issues under investigation.

The following pages discuss nucleoside and nucleotide agents that have been, or are in the process of being, investigated for the treatment of chronic hepatitis B.

Lamivudine (Epivir-HBV) Therapy for Chronic Hepatitis B

Lamivudine is a nucleoside analogue manufactured by GlaxoWellcome, Inc. Lamivudine was initially evaluated in 1991 as a treatment for people with AIDS. It was found to be a potent inhibitor of HIV replication. As approximately 10 percent of HIV-infected people are also infected with chronic hepatitis B, it was observed that lamivudine was capable of inhibiting the replication of HBV as well. Lamivudine, marketed as Epivir-HBV, was FDA approved for treating people with chronic hepatitis B in December 1998. In fact, some experts recommend it as the first line of therapy.

In contrast to interferon, lamivudine appears to work well regardless of the individual characteristics of the patient. Therefore, people who notoriously respond poorly to interferon—those with normal liver enzymes, Asians, those with HBV mutations, those with high levels of viral replication (HBV DNA), those who are immunosuppressed, and those who acquired infection at birth—appear to respond well to lamivudine. Also, compared with interferon therapy, in which approximately one-third of individuals eradicate HBV DNA, virtually everyone treated with lamivudine becomes HBV DNA negative, and at a more rapid rate than the typical person who responds to interferon. Plus, it has been shown that almost 40 percent of people treated with lamivudine for up to three years eradicate HBeAg, and almost half of these patients develop HBsAb (HBsAg seroconversion). It should be noted that the longer patients are treated with lamivudine, the higher the seroconversion rate will be. As with interferon, patients with high baseline ALT levels are more likely to respond to lamivudine. Most important, it has been demonstrated that people treated with lamivudine experience a greater decrease in liver inflammation and are less likely to progress to scarring (as per liver biopsy samples) than similar people treated with interferon. Some patients may even reverse liver scarring (fibrosis) that is already present. Even in the absence of HBeAg seroconversion, inflammation and scarring may improve with lamivudine.

Furthermore, lamivudine may provide some benefit in circumstances in which interferon use is inadvisable (such as in people with decompensated cirrhosis) or ineffective (such as in treating HBV infection occurring after a liver transplant or treating people with normal liver enzymes who acquired infection at birth). In fact, a recent study showed that people who lack HBeAg but who have active viral replication (known as HBV precore mutant strains) not only respond well to lamivudine with evidence of HBV DNA loss but have a low incidence of viral resistance.

Because it is administered orally, lamivudine is easy to take. It is also very well tolerated. It is associated with very few side effects. The most commonly occurring ones include headache, diarrhea, fatigue, nausea, abdominal pain, muscle aches, coughing, and skin rashes. These occur infrequently, however. In fact, in one study, these side effects occurred with the same frequency in people with HBV who were not treated with lamivudine.

Unfortunately, lamivudine does have some drawbacks and does not appear to be the answer for everyone with chronic hepatitis B. Upon discontinuation of lamivudine, up to half of patients will relapse, as noted by a return of HBV DNA and a flare of ALT levels. But the major drawback of lamivudine is the frequent occurrence of lamivudine-resistant HBV mutations, known as YMDD mutations. YMDD mutations typically occur approximately nine months after treatment has begun. People treated for one year develop drug resistance (YMDD mutations) up to 32 percent of the time, and approximately two-thirds of people treated for four years develop drug resistance. People who develop drug resistance experience a return of HBV DNA, elevated ALT levels. Drug resistance neutralizes lamivudine's ability to reduce liver inflammation and scarring. In fact, some drug-resistant patients experience a severe flare of hepatitis and show a reversal of previous improvements on liver biopsy specimens. And the longer people are on lamivudine, the more likely it is that drug-resistant mutants will form. Lamivudine is often given to patients with HBV after liver transplantation. Emergence of lamivudine-resistant HBV strains after transplantation is associated with a poor outcome, and even liver failure, in some patients. Similarly, HBV patients who are also infected with HIV may experience liver failure, and even death, when lamivudine-resistant strains appear.

People most likely to develop lamivudine resistance include those with high HBV DNA levels and high ALT levels at the start of therapy, as well as those with advanced disease on liver biopsy specimens. Also people who are overweight have been noted to have an increased risk of lamivudine resistance.

The recommended dose of lamivudine is 100 mg, taken orally once a day. Treatment typically lasts one year, but this may vary, based on several criteria. In HBsAg positive patients, it is recommended that treatment be continued until HBV DNA is repeatedly nondetectable, HBeAg is negative, and (preferably) until HBeAb is positive. However, there are no definitive recommendations on how long to treat once seroconversion is achieved. In HBsAg negative patients (HBV mutants), it is recommended to continue treatment until HBV DNA is nondetectable and liver enzymes normalize. Since there is such a high HBV relapse rate after discontinuation of lamivudine, studies are evaluating long-term treatment for up to five years or even longer. Possibly the combination of lamivudine and an additional nucleoside analogue will delay or prevent the emergence of viral resistance. Studies are being conducted to test this.

Interferon Plus Lamivudine for Chronic Hepatitis B

Many studies have been conducted using a variety of regimens containing both interferon and lamivudine for patients with chronic hepatitis B. Some results suggest that *combination therapy*—given either sequentially or at the same time—works better than either therapy given alone. Further studies are currently being conducted to assess which regimens work best.

In addition, studies are being conducted using pegylated interferon with lamivudine for both HBeAg positive and HBeAg negative (precore mutants) individuals. It is suspected that results using this combination will be superior to those of conventional interferon combined with lamivudine. Patients who do not respond to interferon therapy alone respond better to lamivudine alone (given for one year) than they do to a combination of interferon and lamivudine. Studies of pegylated interferon in combination with lamivudine for chronic hepatitis B (both HBsAg positive and HBsAg negative individuals) are under way. However, preliminary results indicate that this combination is not significantly better than using PEGASYS alone.

Adefovir (Hepsera) Therapy for Chronic Hepatitis B

Adefovir is a nucleotide analogue that received FDA approval for treatment of chronic hepatitis B in September 2002. The standard dose is one 10-mg pill each day. Studies have shown that treating HBeAg patients for one year with adefovir results in an approximately 12 percent seroconversion rate (eradication of HBeAg and formation of HBeAb). And HBV DNA will drop to less than 400 copies/mL in approximately 21 percent of people. Significant improvement in liver inflammation and scarring (on liver biopsy specimens) has also been demonstrated. It appears that adefovir alone may be as effective as adefovir in combination with lamivudine. Efficacy has also been demonstrated as to HBeAg negative patients. Within this patient group after forty-eight weeks of therapy with adefovir, ALT levels normalize in approximately 72 percent of people, HBV DNA becomes nondetectable in 51 percent of people, and inflammation and scarring of the liver improve in 64 percent of patients. For treatment of HBV, adefovir appears to have the same advantages over interferon as lamivudine. For example, adefovir treatment achieves results similar to lamivudine for both HBeAg positive and HBeAg negative (precore mutants) people. Furthermore, neither race nor hepatitis B genotype has a significant impact on the efficacy of adefovir.

A major advantage of adefovir over lamivudine is that adefovir does not lead to the development of drug-resistant mutations. Adefovir has the ability to eradicate HBV DNA in people who have developed lamivudine-resistant mutations. This applies even to those people who developed these mutations after liver transplantation.

Once treatment with adefovir is discontinued, most people will relapse. Thus, going forward, long-term adefovir treatment will probably become the standard of care. So far, studies of people using adefovir for approximately three years have not noted any adverse consequences such as drug-resistant HBV mutant formation, severe side effects, or damage to other organs. The major side effect of adefovir is kidney damage, but this appears to be associated with dosages higher than 10 mg per day.

Lamivudine and Adefovir Combination Therapy

Studies combining lamivudine and adefovir are currently ongoing. Preliminary results appear promising. Patients who develop lamivudine-resistant HBV should not be treated with a combination of lamivudine and adefovir, but should discontinue lamivudine and be treated with adefovir alone.

Other Nucleoside Analogue Therapy for Chronic Hepatitis B

Some other nucleoside analogues, such as famciclovir and ganciclovir, have been tried, but have been found to be only temporarily effective, in addition to being less potent than lamivudine. Studies combining famciclovir and lamivudine may be promising, but further study is needed to confirm preliminary results. Emtricitabine ([FTC]—a derivative of lamivudine), clevudine (L-FMAU), Telbivudine (LdT), Elvucitabine (Beta-L Fd4C), and Valtorcitabine (Val-LdC) are undergoing investigation for use in people with chronic hepatitis B—both those with and those without HBeAg.

Preliminary studies using entecavir have revealed promising results on people who have developed lamivudine-resistant strains of HBV. Entecavir appears to be more potent than lamivudine and is likely to receive FDA approval in 2004 for treatment of HBV.

Thymosin

Thymosin is a *polypeptide* (a group of amino acids linked together) hormone that is produced by a gland located in the neck, known as the *thymus gland.* Studies have shown that thymosin can stimulate the immune system—thus, it has immunomodulatory properties. Studies suggest that thymosin can eradicate active hepatitis B viral infection from the body. In one study, thymosin alfa-1 treatment (Zadaxin; manufactured by SciClone Pharmaceuticals, Inc.) for twenty-six or fifty-two weeks (1.6 mg subcutaneously, twice a week) resulted in loss of HBV DNA and HBeAg from the blood in approximately 40 percent of people one year after completion of treatment. Furthermore, among the 40 percent of the people who responded, liver inflammation was significantly reduced.

Thymosin in combination with interferon appears to be quite beneficial for HBeAg negative (precore mutant) patients. Preliminary results have indicated that 71 percent of people treated with this combination achieved a sustained eradication of HBV DNA. Thymosin-alfa1 appears to be safe and to have few side effects. Further studies are being conducted to confirm these findings.

HBV Vaccine as Therapy

The immune system of most adults is strong enough to eradicate HBV from the body when exposure occurs. The failure of some adults to clear the virus is due to many factors, one of which is a poorly functioning or defective immune system. Researchers have sought to counter this circumstance by administering the hepatitis B vaccination to people with chronic hepatitis B in an attempt to stimulate an immune response against the virus. This strategy has been tried on a small group of people, and the results look promising. However, further research in this area is needed before it is offered as a therapy.

Interleukin-12

Interleukin-12 (IL-12) is a natural protein made in the body. This protein acts to regulate the intensity and duration of the body's immune response. Furthermore, IL-12 has been shown to induce interferon production in the body. Therefore, this agent can potentially assist the immune system in eradicating HBV from the body. Further study on this protein is needed before it can be offered as an effective treatment for individuals with chronic hepatitis B.

Other Therapies

Other agents, including gene therapies, are also under investigation for the treatment of HBV.

FACTORS THAT MAY ADVERSELY INFLUENCE RESPONSE TO ANTIVIRAL THERAPY

Unlike the factors that are beyond a person's control, there are some variables that a person does have control over that can influence her response to therapy. Alcohol use is one such variable. Alcohol is a potent liver toxin and can induce HBV to replicate. Therefore, total abstinence from alcohol consumption is recommended for people with chronic hepatitis B, especially those undergoing interferon therapy.

People with chronic hepatitis B who become infected with the hepatitis A virus (HAV) have been found to suffer from a particularly severe, and sometimes fatal, course of infection. Therefore, everyone with chronic hepatitis B should receive the vaccination against HAV if they have not already been exposed to this virus. Vaccination should preferably take place prior to the start of interferon therapy. (See chapter 24 for more information on vaccinations.)

It has been shown that marijuana use may decrease the effectiveness of interferon therapy and may inhibit the body's own natural production of interferon. Therefore, it is advisable for people with chronic hepatitis B to avoid marijuana, especially while on interferon treatment.

Immunosuppressed conditions, such as occur when one is undergoing treatment with corticosteroids (for example, prednisone), may cause activation of HBV. Therefore, unless absolutely required, people with chronic hepatitis B should avoid these types of medications when other treatment options exist.

ALTERING THE COURSE OF CHRONIC HEPATITIS B WITH TREATMENT

For people with chronic hepatitis B, treatment with interferon or lamivudine (and most likely adefovir) may decrease the incidence of long-term complications such as liver cancer, liver failure, and the subsequent need for liver transplantation. The result is a prolonged life expectancy. In some people, treatment totally eliminates HBV, and in others, treatment slows down the progression of the disease, although not eliminating it totally. Therefore, it makes sense for everyone with chronic hepatitis B to seek treatment (if they are candidates for treatment [see next section]). It should be stressed that even those people who eradicate HBsAg prior to the development of cirrhosis may still be at risk for the development of complications (such as liver cancer), but the risk of complications is probably significantly reduced. Therefore, even those people who have had a successful response to therapy should be monitored lifelong by their doctors.

IS ANTIVIRAL THERAPY FOR EVERYONE WITH CHRONIC HEPATITIS B?

Everybody with chronic hepatitis B should begin antiviral therapy if they are actively infectious—as indicated by the presence of HBV DNA in addition to elevated transaminase levels (AST and ALT more than two times the normal value) or moderate to severe inflammation on liver biopsy specimens.

People with chronic hepatitis B should not be treated if their transaminases are normal or less than two times the upper limit of normal, unless they have a significant degree of inflammation on their liver biopsy specimens. These people have only a minimal chance of eradicating the virus from their bodies. In fact, they may actually experience a worsening of the disease once antiviral treatment is stopped. Some liver experts have suggested initial treatment with a short course of steroids, such as prednisone, to stimulate viral replication followed by treatment with interferon. However, in many cases, this dual-treatment regimen has caused a worsening of the disease, and, as such, it cannot be recommended. These individuals should be observed and considered for treatment if liver enzymes elevate to more than two times normal.

People with chronic hepatitis B who have decompensated cirrhosis (see chapter 6) should refrain from treatment with interferon. People with decompensated cirrhosis who are treated with interferon are likely to experience severe complications such as liver failure, infection, and hemorrhage. If a person with decompensated cirrhosis opts to be treated with interferon, reduced dosages should be used. In addition, it is recommended that these people be placed on a list for and be prepared for liver transplantation (see chapter 22).

Therapy with lamivudine or adefovir therapy is typically recommended for people with decompensated liver disease awaiting transplantation, so as to reduce their HBV DNA levels. And the addition of high-dose hepatitis B immunoglobulin (HBIG) improves the efficacy of lamivudine or adefovir for these individuals. This combination has been shown to decrease the likelihood of HBV recurrence after transplantation. Maintenance of antiviral therapy after transplantation is typically recommended.

TREATMENT OF CHRONIC HEPATITIS D

Hepatitis delta virus (HDV) is a virus that can live only in a person who is infected with HBV. Approximately 70,000 people in the United States are infected with HDV. Hepatitis D tends to be a particularly severe infection, with significant long-term consequences. HDV causes more than 1,000 deaths each year. Compared with people who have chronic hepatitis B alone, those with chronic infections of both HBV and HDV have a more aggressive disease course, and they develop cirrhosis faster. In fact, approximately 15 percent of people with chronic hepatitis D develop cirrhosis within two years of initially becoming infected with this virus. Therefore, treatment of people with chronic hepatitis D is crucial.

Unfortunately, HDV appears to be a particularly stubborn virus, as the virus does not respond particularly well to interferon treatment over sustained periods of time. When treatment with interferon alfa-2a is undertaken at 9 million units three times a week for forty-eight weeks, about half of those being treated will show signs of response—normalization of transaminases, eradication of hepatitis delta virus from the blood, and improvement of inflammation on liver biopsy samples. Unfortunately, this response is short-lived, as most people will relapse when therapy is discontinued. Furthermore, lamivudine does not appear to be beneficial in eradicating hepatitis D. Since this is such an aggressive virus, everyone with chronic hepatitis D should undergo treatment with interferon.

Studies involving long-term treatment with interferon, including maintenance dosing and the use of pegylated interferon, are being conducted. Other therapies, such as special nucleotide agents (known as antisense oligonucleotides) and agents that may block the lifecycle of HDV, are also being researched. Of course, the only way to cure hepatitis D is to prevent it in the first place. Prevention of hepatitis D is possible by preventing hepatitis B with the hepatitis B vaccination, which will be discussed in chapter 24.

MONITORING THOSE WHO ARE NOT TREATED

People with chronic hepatitis D and/or chronic hepatitis B who are not treated should have periodic follow-up visits with their liver specialists. It is recommended that these visits occur from two to four times per year. During a typical visit, a physical exam will be conducted and blood work will be obtained. A sonogram of the liver will need to be obtained once or twice a year, depending upon the person's individual characteristics. The purpose of these visits is to assess the patient's status and to determine if she is stable or is progressing to cirrhosis, liver failure, and/or liver cancer. The specialist will seek to assess whether the patient has silently converted into an active stage of the disease, wherein she is highly infectious to others and consequently an appropriate candidate for treatment. A repeat liver biopsy is sometimes performed approximately every five years in order to assess disease progression—although intervals may vary at the discretion of the doctor.

CONCLUSION

Treatment options for chronic hepatitis B are increasing, and some are quite promising. The availability of two different orally administered medications each of which has little to no side effects represents a tremendous advance in the treatment of chronic hepatitis B. Treatment with available medications has been shown to slow, or even reverse, HBV in some cases. The best treatment, of course, is prevention. This is discussed in chapter 24.

The next chapter discusses the treatment of another chronic virus, the hepatitis C virus (HCV), which has several effective treatments presently available and some promising new ones on the horizon.

Thirteen

TREATING HEPATITIS C

Approximately 300 million people are infected with hepatitis C virus (HCV) worldwide. In the United States, where about 2 percent of the population is infected with HCV, chronic hepatitis C is the most common reason for a person to require a liver transplant. Approximately 730 liver transplants due to chronic hepatitis C are performed each year. It is estimated that approximately 8,000 to 10,000 Americans die each year from chronic hepatitis C. The National Institutes of Health (NIH) estimates that without effective treatment, this number could triple within the next few decades. However, chronic hepatitis C should not be viewed as inevitably leading to death. It is important to keep in mind that some effective treatments are available and that some new and improved treatments are being developed. So, if people with chronic hepatitis C seek appropriate medical care, it is unlikely that this estimated future death toll will be a reality. In fact, many people with chronic hepatitis C live a long and healthy life. Some do not even require therapy at all.

The goals of therapy are to suppress viral activity and replication, to decrease inflammation in and damage to the liver, to prevent future inflammation and liver damage, to decrease a person's chances of progressing to cirrhosis and liver cancer, and to diminish any symptoms that are present. These goals are capable of being achieved—but only through antiviral therapy.

Therapy for chronic hepatitis C has advanced greatly since the discovery of the hepatitis C virus in 1989. Response rates to interferon treatment, which hovered around 10 percent in the early 1990s, have increased to greater than 50 percent, thanks to the latest breakthrough in treatment—pegylated interferon and ribavirin combination therapy.

This chapter discusses the treatment of acute and chronic hepatitis C. It analyzes who will benefit the most from treatment and the circumstances under which people do and do not require treatment. Alfa interferon (Intron A) was the first effective treatment for chronic hepatitis C. It was approved by the FDA in

1991. People tend to vary greatly in their response to alfa-interferon based on a variety of factors. This chapter will discuss these factors. The different types of interferon and the different interferon treatment regimens are discussed in detail in this chapter. This chapter will also discuss a major advancement in the treatment of chronic hepatitis C—pegylation of interferon. The combination of pegylated interferon plus ribavirin, which has become the standard therapy since its FDA approval in 2001, will be discussed. The potential side effects of ribavirin will also be discussed. Finally, some promising experimental treatment options will be reviewed.

TREATMENT OF ACUTE HEPATITIS C

The incidence of acute hepatitis C has dropped dramatically in the past few years. In the 1980s, approximately 200,000 new infections occurred each year. Yet recent statistics show that only approximately 30,000 new infections are occurring each year. Since the symptoms associated with acute HCV are either nonspecific or nonexistent, only a small percentage of these people will be diagnosed during the acute stage of the disease. Still, in view of the extraordinarily high likelihood of progression to chronic disease (approximately 75 to 85 percent), it is important to identify and treat these people in an attempt to eradicate the virus at the acute stage.

As discussed in chapter 10, people who work in a hospital or other healthcare facility (e.g., doctor's office, medical lab, blood bank), as well as public-safety workers and emergency medical workers, are at increased risk for contracting HCV through a needle stick or mucosal exposure to blood of infected persons that may occur while on the job. When this type of incident does occur, there is a 0 to 10 percent chance of transmission of HCV. Should such an incident happen, the infected person should immediately be tested to confirm the presence of HCV (indicated by the presence of HCV Ab in the person's blood). In people who are immunosuppressed, such as those with HIV or those on dialysis, HCV RNA should also be determined. And the exposed person needs immediate testing for HCV Ab and ALT to determine if she has a prior HCV positivity. Ten days to six weeks after exposure, HCV RNA needs to be performed on the exposed person. Multiple determinations of HCV RNA are required to confirm infectivity, since the level of HCV RNA waxes and wanes after infection. For example, HCV RNA may drop to a level beyond detection, but this does not necessarily indicate that the person does not have HCV. And one positive HCV RNA result does not definitely confirm acquisition of infection. Six months after exposure, HCV Ab and ALT levels need to be tested. If HCV Ab is negative and ALT levels are normal, then one can be confident that they did not contract HCV.

Immunoglobulin administration after exposure to HCV-infected blood (as is routinely done after exposure to HBV) will not prevent acquisition of HCV. Similarly, interferon prophylaxis is not warranted. Interferon will not prevent the acquisition of HCV, as this medication only works in the presence of active infection (a positive HCV RNA).

Many studies have shown that when a short course of interferon therapy—lasting one to three months—is provided to people with acute hepatitis C, it significantly reduces the likelihood of progression to chronic liver disease. However, the optimal time to begin therapy, the optimal duration of therapy, and the optimal medications to use—interferon alone, interferon plus ribavirin, or pegylated interferon (with or without ribavirin)—are not well defined. Since approximately 15 to 40 percent of people clear HCV within the first six months of exposure even without any therapy, some experts do not recommend treatment during this time. Furthermore, it appears that patients who become jaundiced after exposure to HCV have a high rate of spontaneous (without treatment) viral eradication within a month of the onset of jaundice. Alternatively, some experts recommend treatment for all people exposed once it has been confirmed that they have definitely contracted HCV (determined via serial HCV RNA testing). Eradication of the virus has been reported to occur in as many as 98 percent of people treated with interferon alfa-2b within twelve weeks of exposure. Interferon treatment typically lasts for twenty-four weeks. Therefore, it seems prudent to begin interferon treatment in patients with acute hepatitis C who did not spontaneously eradicate the virus within one month of the onset of symptoms.

Studies are ongoing on the treatment of acute hepatitis C with pegylated interferon. It is anticipated that response rates will approach 100 percent with this treatment.

THE REASONS TO TREAT CHRONIC HEPATITIS C

Chronic hepatitis C will not go away on its own. In most people, it is a slowly progressive disease. Not only does HCV do its damage slowly, but it usually does its damage silently. This explains why many people with chronic hepatitis C (especially those who have no symptoms) react with confusion when advised by their doctors to start treatment with interferon—an injectable medication that has potential side effects. "Why should I be treated? I feel fine!" is a comment that liver specialists commonly hear. Well, the answer to this question is that the benefits of treatment far outweigh the risks in most cases.

People with chronic hepatitis C are at risk for developing cirrhosis, liver failure, and liver cancer. Once cirrhosis has developed, the likelihood of responding to treatment is greatly reduced. Once a person develops liver failure and/or liver cancer, conventional medical therapies are unlikely to help and may actually worsen the patient's condition. And, if a person with HCV experiences liver failure and/or liver cancer and is fortunate enough to receive a liver transplant, HCV recurs in the new liver if it was not eradicated from the body prior to transplantation. Thus, therapy for HCV would become necessary post-transplantation anyway (and this is in addition to a bunch of other medications required to suppress the rejection of the new liver). Therefore, it is of utmost importance to attempt to eradicate HCV from the body in order to stop or slow progression of the disease before any liver-related complications develop. The sooner a person seeks treatment, the more likely she is to reap its benefits—benefits that include long-term eradication of HCV from the body (i.e., cure) and a reduced incidence of progression to cirrhosis, liver failure, and liver cancer. And people who are treated in the early stages of the disease are less likely to experience the adverse side effects sometimes associated with interferon therapy.

Treatment with interferon not only slows progression of the disease, but may actually reverse liver damage that has already been done, even in the early stages of cirrhosis! So, with treatment, even people who have progressed to cirrhosis may eradicate HCV from their bodies and may achieve a resolution of scarring as well. Studies have demonstrated that people with symptoms due to HCV experience a significant improvement in their quality of life once the virus is eradicated from their bodies (see chapter 10 for a discussion of the symptoms associated with hepatitis C). It has been shown that patients treated with interferon are less likely to die due to liver-related complications than patients not treated with interferon. These results have been shown to apply to patients who achieved sustained viral clearance as well as those who did not.

THOSE WHO SHOULD OR SHOULDN'T START ANTIVIRAL THERAPY

Are there some people who are not candidates for treatment? Well, many variables must be taken into consideration in answering this question. The National Institutes of Health (NIH) Consensus Statement, promulgated in June 2002, concluded that all persons with chronic hepatitis C are potential candidates for antiviral therapy. However, not everyone with chronic hepatitis C needs to be treated with antiviral medication. Whether or not to start treatment for chronic hepatitis C is an important decision that should be made jointly by the doctor and the patient. All individuals with elevated ALT levels, elevated hepatitis C viral loads (elevated HCV RNA), and inflammation or scarring on liver biopsy specimens are advised to consider treatment—unless specific reasons to avoid treatment exist. The following is a discussion of whether people with persistently normal ALT levels should start antiviral therapy and of some specific instances in which antiviral therapy may not be indicated, or may even be harmful. This section ends with a discussion of the use of interferon in people who actively use intravenous drugs or ingest alcohol. You may also want to review chapter 11 for information about the side effects of antiviral therapy.

Those with Normal ALT Levels

Approximately one-third of all people with chronic hepatitis C have persistently normal ALT levels, despite having elevated viral loads (HCV RNA). The significance of this finding is not known and may vary from person to person. Some experts, including myself, believe that these people may never have serious liver disease, and thus refer to these people as "healthy chronic carriers" of HCV.

Other experts believe that some people with chronic hepatitis C who have normal ALT levels will eventually develop liver inflammation and scarring and that some will even progress to cirrhosis. To complicate matters further, the degree of elevation of HCV RNA does not correlate with the severity of inflammation or damage found on liver biopsy samples. This leaves the doctor without any specific parameters with which to judge severity or worsening of disease.

Some experts recommend treatment with interferon for people with chronic hepatitis C who have normal ALT levels regardless of their HCV RNA level. Initially, it was thought that this group of people might respond better to therapy than people with elevated ALT levels. However, most of these trials have shown that interferon, given alone, eradicates the virus in about 20 percent of these people—the same percentage that applies to people with elevated ALT levels. Yet some studies have concluded that treatment with interferon alone does not provide any significant benefit to these people. Studies of pegylated interferon in combination with ribavirin are currently ongoing. It is anticipated that these people will experience long-term sustained HCV eradication percentages similar to those of people with elevated ALT levels who have undergone treatment with pegylated interferon and ribavirin—approximately 56 percent.

So, should people with persistently normal ALT levels be treated? Well, in 1997 the NIH in its consensus statement regarding the management of hepatitis C recommended that people with persistently normal ALT levels refrain from treatment. However, since it appears that some people with normal ALT levels do progress to serious liver disease, an alternative option—that of undergoing a liver biopsy—should be considered. In this manner, the doctor is able to evaluate the amount of inflammation and scarring present in the liver. If little or no inflammation or damage is present (which is typically found), the person should refrain from treatment, as these people are unlikely to progress to serious disease. If significant damage has occurred, especially if cirrhosis appears imminent, individuals should be given the option of antiviral treatment or the opportunity to participate in an ongoing trial of antiviral medication for people with chronic hepatitis C and normal ALT levels. In fact, in its 2002 consensus statement, the NIH amended its recommendation from 1997. The 2002 consensus statement recommends that patient motivation, genotype, symptoms, age, and presence of other illnesses, in addition to liver biopsy findings, should be considered when deciding whether to treat patients with persistently normal ALT levels.

One point that is important to remember is that ALT levels in people with chronic hepatitis C typically fluctuate. So it is to be expected that people whose transaminases are elevated most of the time will occasionally have normal transaminase levels. These people must be distinguished from those with persistently normal transaminases. The temporary normalization of ALT levels should not be equated with improvement of disease nor should it be used as a justification for not seeking treatment.

Those for Whom Antiviral Therapy Isn't Always Advisable

For certain people, the risks of treatment with interferon outweigh the potential benefits. The following section discusses some instances in which interferon treatment may not be advisable.

Those with Psychiatric Disorders

Interferon, whether administered alone or in combination with ribavirin, may cause significant depression, anxiety, and altered thought processes. Therefore, people who suffer from a severe underlying psychiatric disorder (such as those with persistent suicidal thoughts or suicide attempts) should refrain from treatment with interferon. Interferon may cause psychiatric problems to worsen or perhaps even to become life-threatening. People who suffer from a temporary severe psychiatric problem (such as depression induced by the death of a spouse) should postpone interferon therapy until the disorder has been brought under control. If a person has a stable chronic psychiatric disorder but is motivated to begin treatment for chronic hepatitis C, treatment can succeed by having the person closely and carefully comanaged by a psychiatrist and a liver specialist. People with a history of any psychiatric or psychological disorder should begin antidepressant and/or antianxiety medication prior to beginning interferon therapy (for a discussion of the management of depression while on interferon, see chapter 11).

Those with Decompensated Cirrhosis

People who have decompensated cirrhosis—those who have experienced complications due to cirrhosis, such as bleeding esophageal varices, or ascites—are not considered appropriate candidates for interferon therapy. These people usually have low platelet counts (thrombocytopenia), which may get even lower when treated with interferon, thereby putting these people at risk for life-threatening bleeding. People with decompensated cirrhosis should be referred to a liver transplant center for evaluation (see chapter 22). For these individuals treatment with interferon should only be started in the context of a clinical trial and by those patients already listed for transplantation.

Those Who Have Undergone Kidney Transplantation

Approximately 20 to 30 percent of individuals on hemodialysis for kidney failure are infected with chronic hepatitis C. These people are often awaiting kidney transplantation. Undergoing treatment with interferon after kidney transplantation is risky, as it may cause rejection of the newly transplanted kidney. Therefore, people with chronic hepatitis C who are also undergoing dialysis for the treatment of kidney failure should be treated for hepatitis C prior to undergoing a kidney transplant. Studies have demonstrated that the response of these people to interferon treatment for chronic hepatitis C is comparable to that of people with normally functioning kidneys.

Those with Autoimmune Disorders

Interferon may worsen an underlying autoimmune disorder, particularly autoimmune hepatitis (AIH) (discussed in chapter 14). People who have both AIH and chronic hepatitis C, and in whom AIH is the predominant liver disease, should be treated for AIH first. Of course, prior to making treatment decisions, a liver biopsy must be performed to confirm that AIH is the predominant liver disease. After AIH has been successfully treated, treatment of chronic hepatitis C may be attempted; however the risk of a severe relapse of AIH exists.

Other autoimmune disorders, such as thyroid disease, may worsen as a result of interferon treatment. People with thyroid disorders may undergo interferon therapy; however, the dosage of thyroid medication needs to be closely monitored and often needs to be altered.

Treatment of Active Intravenous Drug Users

Recent studies have demonstrated that people with HCV who actively use intravenous drugs, a condition previously considered to be a contraindication to treatment with interferon, may be successfully treated with interferon. Since intravenous drug use is currently the most common mode of transmission of new HCV infections, treatment of these individuals is important, as it may potentially reduce the spread of HCV. Ideally, these individuals should be enrolled in a methadone maintenance drug treatment program. The use of methadone is not a contraindication to interferon treatment. Furthermore, the decision of the NIH consensus statement of 2002 concluded that active intravenous drug use should not be considered a contraindication to treatment with interferon.

Treatment of People Who Actively Ingest Alcohol

Active alcohol ingestion during interferon treatment may negate the beneficial effects of therapy and may significantly reduce sustained response to therapy. Alcohol ingestion may also cause liver disease to progress to cirrhosis and its complications, including liver cancer. Therefore, patients should avoid all alcohol ingestion while on interferon therapy.

People Coinfected with HCV and HIV

Approximately 200,000 people in the United States are infected with both HCV and HIV. The incidence of death for people with HIV has dramatically declined since 1996 due to the implementation of highly active antiretroviral therapy (HAART). Since this time, hepatitis C has emerged as a major cause of illness and death in coinfected people. People infected with both viruses have been shown to have a more rapid progression to cirrhosis, liver failure, and liver cancer. Thus, people in whom HIV infection is well controlled should undergo treatment for HCV. Studies are presently being conducted on treating coinfected people with pegylated interferon plus ribavirin.

TREATMENT OF CHRONIC HEPATITIS C

Major advances in the treatment of chronic hepatitis C have been made over the past decade. Treatment is now effective for more than half the people with chronic hepatitis C. This section reviews the evolution of treatment of chronic hepatitis C, from treatment with interferon alone to combination therapy—interferon plus ribavirin—to the current treatment of choice—pegylated interferon plus ribavirin.

Interferon Alone

Three years before the hepatitis C virus was identified, researchers already had established that alfa interferon was an effective therapy for some people with non-A non-B hepatitis—which was known after 1989 as chronic hepatitis C. In February 1991, Intron A (interferon alfa-2b) became FDA approved as the first treatment for chronic hepatitis C. Currently, three brands of alfa interferon—Intron A (interferon alfa-2b), Roferon (interferon alfa-2a), and Infergen (interferon alfacon-1 or consensus interferon)—are FDA approved to treat people with chronic hepatitis C. Each of these brands has been approved for treating people who have never been treated before (*treatment naive*); for those who have been treated with interferon and relapsed after therapy was discontinued (*relapsers*); and for those who did not respond to interferon therapy at all (*nonresponders* or *treatment refractory*). The three FDA-approved interferons—as well as some other not-as-yet-approved interferons (such as interferon alfa-n1, interferon beta, interferon alfa-n3)—appear to be roughly equally effective. Standard interferon is given as a subcutaneous (SQ) injection three times per week.

Interferon was initially approved by the FDA to be given three times a week for a period of six months. Using this treatment regimen, approximately one-half of patients initially respond to therapy—they will return to a normal ALT level and their blood has a nondetectable viral load (HCV RNA). However, within six months of discontinuing alfa interferon therapy, as many as three quarters of these people relapse—that is, their ALT levels become elevated, and HCV RNA becomes detectable in their blood once again. Thus, the long-term sustained response rate after an initial course of twenty-four weeks of alfa interferon given three times a week is only approximately 12 percent. (A sustained response to therapy is defined as a nondetectable HCV RNA [HCV RNA less than 50 IU/ml] six months after discontinuation of therapy.)

The next major advance in HCV therapy was the discovery that if the course of treatment with interferon is lengthened to forty-eight weeks, approximately 20 percent of people will have a sustained response to therapy. Thus, until 1998, the standard treatment regimen for HCV was to administer interferon three times per week for forty-eight weeks.

Interferon Plus Ribavirin

From knowledge gained by the medical profession in the treatment of people with HIV, it became clear that combining two or more antiviral drugs together can be a particularly effective form of therapy to fight viruses. This method of combining medications together has been referred to as *cocktail therapy* (not to be confused with an alcoholic mixed drink). The addition of ribavirin (manufactured by Schering-Plough as Rebetol) to interferon was a major advance in the treatment of chronic hepatitis C. This combination therapy, marketed under the name Rebetron, was approved by the FDA in 1998. Rebetron has been shown to be a more effective treatment than interferon alone.

Studies have shown that Rebetron, used for forty-eight weeks by treatment-naive people, achieves a long-term sustained response in approximately 38 to 47 percent of people. Studies have also shown that approximately 6 to 26 percent of nonresponders achieve a sustained viral eradication with Rebetron therapy. People treated with Rebetron consistently demonstrated greater improvement on liver biopsy specimens than those treated with interferon alone.

Pegylated Interferon

Anyone would prefer to take a drug just once a week, as opposed to three times a week or daily. *Pegylation* is a process that involves attaching a large substance—known as *polyethylene glycol (PEG)*—to a protein. In the case of pegylated interferon *(PEG-interferon),* PEG is attached to interferon. This enables it to stay in the body longer. By using the process of pegylation, the frequency with which interferon is required to be injected is reduced from three times per week to once per week. Since pegylated interferon stays in the body longer than regular interferon, the hepatitis C virus is suppressed longer than with regular interferon. This results in improved response rates, that is, long-term eradication of HCV occurs more frequently than with standard interferon.

Two pegylated interferons are currently FDA approved—PEG-Intron (pegylated interferon alfa-2b) and PEGASYS (pegylated interferon alfa-2a). PEG-Intron is manufactured by Schering-Plough and was FDA approved in January 2001. The dose of PEG-Intron is determined by a patient's weight. Weekly dosages typically range from 80 to 150 mcg. The medication is administered once a week via injection. PEGASYS is manufactured by Hoffman-La Roche and was FDA approved in October 2002. The weekly dose of PEGASYS is 180 mcg and is independent of a person's weight. Long-term response rates are similar for the two types of pegylated interferon. In October 2003, the FDA approved the first ever pen delivery system for administration of PEG-Intron, known as the REDIPEN. This disposable single-dose delivery system is much easier to use and is more convenient than using the vial-and-syringe method.

The two types of pegylated interferon differ in the type of PEG molecule that is attached to interferon. PEG-Intron uses a straight small molecule of PEG, while PEGASYS uses a large rounded molecule of PEG. However, results appear to be similar for the two types. Approximately 24 percent of treatment-naive people who take either form of pegylated interferon for a period of forty-eight weeks demonstrate sustained virological response—that is, their HCV RNA is nondetectable (less than 50 IU/ml) six months after completion of therapy.

Studies are currently being conducted on pegylated-Infergen (PEG-alfacon-1) (consensus interferon), a product manufactured by Intermune.

Pegylated Interferon in Combination with Ribavirin

In August 2001, PEG-Intron was FDA approved for use in combination with ribavirin (ribavirin is marketed by Schering-Plough under the name Rebetol). In December 2002, PEGASYS was approved by the FDA to be taken in combination with ribavirin (ribavirin is marketed by Roche under the name Copegus). Combination therapy with pegylated interferon and ribavirin is the most effective treatment for patients with chronic hepatitis C. Long-term response rates appear to be similar for the two combinations of pegylated interferon and ribavirin. Schering-Plough has initiated a study aimed at comparing the efficacy and safety of the Peg-Intron's individualized weight-based dosing versus flat (that is, non-weight-based) dosing of PEGASYS. The results of this trial, named the IDEAL trial, are eagerly anticipated.

Long-term sustained response occurs in approximately 54 to 56 percent of people who take either form of pegylated interferon combined with ribavirin for forty-eight weeks. Response rates, dosage of ribavirin, and length of therapy vary with HCV genotype as follows:

- Genotype 1: Sustained response in people with genotype 1 ranges from 42 to 44 percent. Treatment should last for forty-eight weeks, using ribavirin at a daily dose of 1,000 to 1,200 mg.

- Genotypes 2 and 3: Sustained response in people with genotypes 2 and 3 ranges from 78 to 80 percent. Treatment should last at least twenty-four weeks. However, people who have severe scarring or cirrhosis (as per liver biopsy specimens) should be treated for forty-eight weeks. A daily dosage of 800 mg ribavirin may be used.

- Genotypes 4, 5, and 6: Studies on people with genotypes 4, 5, and 6 are limited. However, it appears that response rates are similar to those with genotype 1. Therefore, forty-eight weeks of therapy using ribavirin at a daily dose of 1,000 to 1,200 mg is recommended.

DETERMINING A RESPONSE TO THERAPY

Response to therapy is indicated by the normalization of alanine transaminase (ALT) and the eradication of HCV from the blood. Eradication, if achieved, is manifested as a nondetectable level of HCV RNA on blood tests. An HCV RNA level of less than 50 IU/ml is typically equated with nondetectability of HCV RNA. However, as discussed in chapter 10, HCV RNA levels may be tested at a level as low as 2 to 5 IU/ml. I advise the use of HCV RNA testing at this low level, as it provides a more precise measure for determining response to therapy.

A nonresponder is a person who does not normalize ALT levels and who continues to have detectable levels of HCV RNA in the blood while on therapy. These individuals are also known as being refractory to therapy. A responder is a person who normalizes ALT levels and eradicates HCV RNA while on therapy. Responders fall into one of two categories.

First, some fortunate people have a sustained response, meaning that the virus has remained undetectable for more than six months beyond the date therapy was discontinued. People who have a sustained response to therapy are unlikely to have a relapse of disease in the future. This has been demonstrated to hold true for at least fifteen years beyond the discontinuation of therapy. However, studies ranging from thirty to forty years still need to be conducted in order to assess the actual stability of this long-term response. However, I believe that if an HCV RNA level of less than 2 to 5 IU/ml still holds at six months after discontinuation of therapy, relapse will never occur. In essence, people who have achieved this are cured.

Second, some responders are known as relapsers, meaning that when they are taken off therapy, HCV RNA again becomes detectable in their blood and their ALT levels again become elevated. The reason why people relapse is not known. It may be due to the continued presence of the virus in their blood beyond the level that current tests for HCV RNA can detect. Alternatively, it may possibly be due to the virus "hiding" in parts of the body where it cannot be detected.

A relapse, when it happens, typically occurs within the first three months after therapy is discontinued and can be noted as early as one month after discontinuation of therapy. If a person has not relapsed three months after the discontinuation of therapy, their probability of a sustained response is greater than 90 percent. Once a person has eradicated HCV RNA from her blood for more than six months beyond the discontinuation of therapy, it is highly unlikely that the virus will ever return. Again, this is synonymous with a cure.

The last category of patients that needs to be mentioned is perhaps the least understood. There is a small group of people who initially respond to therapy—as manifested by nondetectable HCV RNA levels—but as therapy continues, the virus returns (that is, it again becomes detectable in the blood). This is known as a breakthrough response. Its cause is unclear but may result from the formation of mutations of HCV that make it resistant to further interferon treatment. More research needs to be done on this group of individuals to define the nature of these mutations and to determine further treatment options.

Certain characteristics are common to these people who are most likely to have a long-term response to therapy. Out of all characteristics, genotype is the most predictive of a response to therapy—people with genotypes 2 and 3 respond best to any antiviral therapy. In addition to genotype, the following patient characteristics are favorable:

• a low body weight (less than approximately 165 pounds or 75 kg)

• a low viral load (HCV RNA less than 2,000,000 IU/ml)

• the absence cirrhosis

• non African Americans

• lack of excessive iron on liver biopsy specimens

• the female gender, especially young women (may be due to the typically lower body weight of females compared to males, or to estrogen's effect on the liver).

• age less than forty years old at the time of infection

However, it should be kept in mind that people to whom these characteristics do not apply may still respond to therapy. As such, lack of these characteristics should not, in and of itself, dissuade a person from starting interferon therapy.

Response to alfa interferon can usually be determined after three months from the start of therapy—although some experts believe that as little as one month is enough time to judge whether or not a person will respond. A patient's response to therapy three months after its commencement is known as an early virological response (EVR). People who fail to achieve a significant drop in initial HCV RNA levels (defined as a 2-log, or 100-fold, drop—for example 2,000,000 IU/mL dropping to 20,000 IU/mL) after three months of therapy are unlikely to have a sustained response to therapy with further treatment. Another yardstick for measuring EVR is an undetectable HCV RNA level after twenty-four weeks of therapy. People whose HCV RNA is still detectable after twenty-four weeks of therapy are also unlikely to experience a sustained response to therapy with further treatment. EVR should not be used, unquestionably, as a reason for discontinuing therapy. Rather, EVR should be used to guide decisions about continuation of therapy after multiple factors are taken into consideration. These factors vary from patient to patient and include such variables as the degree of inflammation and scarring of the liver and the patient's motivation to continue therapy.

Everyone with chronic hepatitis C who is a candidate for therapy should consider treatment. People who respond to therapy have been shown to have decreased inflammation and scarring on liver biopsy specimens. In fact, people who achieve long-term sustained response to interferon therapy may even reverse cirrhosis in its earliest stages. Furthermore, it appears that people who do not respond to therapy still receive a benefit from treatment with interferon. Even in cases where interferon does not totally eradicate HCV, it may still decrease inflammation and scarring of the liver, thus potentially slowing the progression of the disease and decreasing the chances of developing cirrhosis and liver cancer. This is a crucial point to keep in mind while on therapy. Thus, even for those people who do not experience an early virological response (2-log or 100-fold drop of HCV RNA), continued treatment may still be beneficial. This is especially true for those people with significant scarring or cirrhosis.

INDIVIDUALIZING THERAPY

One important question that has not been addressed in any clinical study is how long a person should be treated once HCV RNA becomes nondetectable. Not all people require the same length of therapy in order to be cured, as each person has many individual characteristics that can affect response to therapy. My personal experience has been that some people require as little as six weeks of therapy in order to achieve a sustained viral clearance, whereas others need as long as two to three years on continuous therapy to achieve viral eradication. Clearly, treatment needs to be approached on an individualized basis. The standard approach of assigning people to a twenty-four- or forty-eight-week treatment regimen based primarily on the HCV genotype will not yield optimal results for many people. Going forward, this is an important issue that pharmaceutical companies and hepatologists must focus on to optimize treatment results for the highest possible percentage of patients.

RE-TREATMENT OF PATIENTS

Major advances in the treatment of chronic hepatitis C over the past decade have given rise to a quandary as to those patients who did not respond to earlier, less effective, treatment regimens. Whether to re-treat these individuals with pegylated interferon plus ribavirin is a difficult decision that can only be made after taking into account many variables. Foremost among these variables is the severity of the underlying liver disease. Therefore, a current liver biopsy is often needed to determine if re-treatment is advisable. People whose liver reveals severe inflammation and scarring should strongly consider being re-treated with pegylated interferon plus ribavirin in an attempt to eradicate the virus or, at the least, to slow advancement of the disease to cirrhosis and liver failure. For people with only mild disease, re-treatment may not be necessary. In addition to considering the severity of underlying liver disease, it is also important to take into consideration the patient's motivation to be re-treated.

Another important variable is the likelihood of response to re-treatment. People most likely to respond to re-treatment with pegylated interferon plus ribavirin include the following:

- People who previously relapsed

- People who were nonresponders but who achieved a significant decrease in HCV RNA levels on prior therapy (known as partial responders)

- People who were treated with interferon therapy alone

- People with genotypes 2 and 3

- Non-African Americans

The following statistics on re-treatment of people with pegylated interferon plus ribavirin are from preliminary results. (Studies are ongoing to confirm these percentages.)

- Approximately 35 percent of patients who were nonresponders to interferon therapy alone will achieve a sustained response when re-treated with pegylated interferon plus ribavirin

- Approximately 11 percent of nonresponders to interferon and ribavirin combination therapy will achieve a sustained response when re-treated with pegylated interferon plus ribavirin

- Approximately 60 percent of people who relapsed after interferon therapy alone will achieve a sustained response when re-treated with pegylated interferon plus ribavirin

- Approximately 40 percent of people who relapsed after interferon and ribavirin combination therapy will achieve a sustained response when re-treated with pegylated interferon plus ribavirin

People who do not respond to or relapse after treatment with pegylated interferon plus ribavirin still have some options, although they are limited at present time. Studies are ongoing to evaluate the effectiveness of PEGASYS plus ribavirin in people who did not respond to PEG-Intron plus ribavirin. Preliminary findings reveal that some patients who did not respond to PEG-Intron respond to PEGASYS. Some researchers believe that PEG-Intron must be given twice a week in order to obtain maximum effectiveness. Thus, biweekly PEG-Intron plus daily ribavirin may be a viable option for some people. Results of studies are currently pending on twice-a-week PEG-Intron administration. Many other medications are currently undergoing clinical trials (see discussion on page 195).

MONITORING PATIENTS BEFORE AND DURING THERAPY

Before starting therapy, a person should have a full series of blood tests. These should include transaminases, HCV RNA, HCV genotype, bilirubin, prothrombin time, and complete blood count with differential and platelets (CBC), thyroid tests, antinuclear antibody (ANA; see chapter 14), glucose (blood sugar) level, alpha-fetoprotein (AFP), and human immunodeficiency virus (HIV). (See chapter 3 for an explanation of some of these tests.) An EKG should be obtained in all men over forty and all women over fifty years old. If risk factors for cardiac disease are present, or if the patient has a history of cardiac disease, a more extensive cardiac evaluation may be required prior to starting therapy. A liver biopsy is highly recommended prior to beginning therapy (see chapter 5). It is not necessary to repeat a liver biopsy at the end of therapy—unless as part of a clinical study protocol. A complete physical exam—including an eye exam if a person has high blood pressure or diabetes—should be obtained. Other exams, such as a chest X ray, may be required on a case-by-case basis.

The patient should expect to see her doctor and to undergo blood tests monthly during therapy—although intervals may vary at the discretion of the doctor. On these occasions, the patient should discuss with her doctor any side effects of therapy she is experiencing and should feel free to ask the doctor any questions that pertain to the therapy. Typically, three months after starting therapy, the doctor will run blood tests to determine whether the person is responding to therapy. A response to therapy is indicated by a normal ALT and nondetectable HCV RNA in the blood. If the person is responding to therapy, repeat HCV RNA blood tests are typically done at the end of therapy—for example, twelve months from the commencement of treatment—to document end-of-treatment response. Other blood tests, as well as additional viral loads, may be drawn at the discretion of the doctor.

Side Effects of Ribavirin

Ribavirin is an orally administered synthetic antiviral agent. It is known medically as a guanosine nucleoside analogue—a component of DNA and RNA, the genetic building blocks of life. When used alone, it is ineffective against HCV—it may temporarily normalize ALT levels, but it has no effect on HCV RNA. However, when used in combination with alfa interferon, as so-called "cocktail therapy," it has been found to be quite effective against HCV. The recommended dose depends on the person's weight, but is usually about four to six tablets a day (each tablet is 200 mg), taken in two divided doses. As an example, a typical daily regimen might be two or three tablets in the morning and two or three tablets in the evening, for a total dosage of approximately 800 to 1,200 mg per day.

The exact way that ribavirin fights against viruses is not known. Also, it is not known why ribavirin works against HCV only when used in combination with interferon. However, it has been demonstrated that ribavirin works in tandem (and synergistically) with interferon and that it boosts interferon's antiviral and immune activity against HCV.

From the standpoint of mathematical probability, the more drugs a person takes, the greater the likelihood that she will experience adverse side effects. This is the downside of combination drug therapy. Therefore, it is not unexpected that discontinuation of therapy occurs with the highest frequency among people taking combination therapy. Out of those taking interferon plus ribavirin, approximately

10 to 14 percent discontinue therapy versus approximately 3 percent of those taking interferon alone. But not everyone experiences adverse side effects, and some people experience no side effects at all.

Newer improved drugs with a similar structure to ribavirin (known as ribavirin analogues) but less side effects are in the process of being developed. The most promising of these analogues is viramidine. The major advantage of this ribavirin analogue is its decreased incidence of associated anemia. Studies are currently ongoing.

The following is a discussion of the side effects most commonly associated with ribavirin—anemia, skin rash, cough, and birth defects (teratogenicity). The side effects associated with interferon are discussed in chapter 11. One side effect of ribavirin is actually advantageous. It is that ribavirin often causes an increase in the platelet count (this is known as thrombocytosis). Therefore, people who have low platelet counts—as is often seen in those with cirrhosis—may obtain this as an additional benefit from being treated with combination therapy. Furthermore, any ribavirin-induced platelet count elevation will help offset the platelet count reduction that interferon may cause.

Ribavirin-Induced Anemia

Ribavirin can accumulate in red blood cells (RBCs), destroying them. The destruction of red blood cells is known as *hemolysis*. Hemolysis results in a low red blood cell count—known as *hemolytic anemia*. This is detected on blood tests as a low hemoglobin (less than 12 g/dl). *Hemoglobin* is an iron-containing protein that is part of each red blood cell. A drop in hemoglobin level is perhaps the most serious side effect related to ribavirin. This side effect occurs in approximately 50 to 60 percent of people taking ribavirin in combination with interferon. And it is the most common reason for a patient to discontinue therapy. Symptoms associated with anemia include fatigue, shortness of breath, headaches, and heart palpitations. Overall this leads to a poor quality of life on therapy. Thus, if these symptoms are present, treatment of anemia will be necessary even if the hemoglobin is not under 12 g/dl but has nevertheless decreased from 16 to 13 g/dl, for example. In cases where anemia occurs as a result of ribavirin therapy, it will typically occur during the first few weeks of therapy, but it can occur at any time. Therefore, it is important to be diligent with follow-up visits to the doctor's office especially during the initial period of time after beginning therapy.

Ribavirin-induced anemia is both dose-dependent and reversible, meaning that if the ribavirin dose is lowered or discontinued, the anemia will resolve. However, it has been demonstrated that decreasing the ribavirin dose also diminishes the likelihood of eradicating the virus from the body. Studies have shown that even small reductions in ribavirin dosage result in a 50 percent decline in sustained response rate. And people who maintain therapeutic doses of pegylated interferon and ribavirin have the highest likelihood of attaining treatment success. Ribavirin-induced anemia is particularly dangerous for people with an underlying cardiac condition. Anyone with a prior history of heart disease should be evaluated by a cardiologist to determine if she is a suitable candidate for therapy, as anemia would put these people at increased risk for further heart problems. All men over the age of forty and all women over fifty should obtain an electrocardiogram (EKG) prior to beginning therapy.

Erythropoietin is a protein made by the body that can stimulate the formation of new red blood cells. Two forms of erythropoietin are currently approved for the treatment of anemia—Procrit (epoetin alfa) and Aranesp (darbepoetin alfa). However, only Procrit has been studied in anemic HCV patients undergoing interferon and ribavirin therapy. Preliminary studies have shown that Procrit, administered at a dose of 40,000 units, subcutaneously, once a week increases hemoglobin levels by about 2 to 3 g/dl. This enables therapeutic doses of ribavirin to be used, thereby increasing the likelihood of sustained viral clearance rates while improving the patient's quality of life while on therapy. Side effects of Procrit are infrequent. The most common side effects (occurring in approximately 10 percent of people) include high blood pressure, fatigue, headaches, fever, and seizures. As such, people with uncontrolled high blood pressure or uncontrolled seizure disorder should not be treated with any form of erythropoietin. Occasionally people are unresponsive to the effects of erythropoietin. In such cases, other causes of anemia should be searched for, such as iron, B_{12}, and folate deficiencies; active blood loss (due to gastrointestinal bleeding or heavy menstruation); and thalassemia—an inherited disorder that affects the production of normal hemoglobin.

I routinely start patients on a variety of supplements prior to the commencement of therapy. Foremost among these are the *antioxidants* vitamin C and vitamin E, which may delay the onset of, as well as reduce the degree of, ribavirin-induced anemia in some patients. Plus, vitamins C and E appear to provide numerous benefits to people with chronic hepatitis C (see page 200 of this chapter). However, larger studies will need to be conducted before this supplemental therapy is recommended by all physicians.

Despite the best efforts to counter it, patients may continue to suffer from anemia while on therapy, thereby necessitating either dose reduction or medication termination. In rare cases of severe anemia, a blood transfusion may become necessary.

Selenium has been found to increase both red and white blood cells in people with AIDS. Even though no studies have been conducted on the subject, it can be speculated that selenium may similarly decrease the incidence of low red and white cell counts, which are potential side effects of interferon and ribavirin therapy for chronic hepatitis C.

Birth Defects

Ribavirin is *teratogenic*—capable of causing birth defects. Therefore, people who are pregnant or contemplating pregnancy are not candidates for treatment. Furthermore, it is recommended to use two forms of contraception while on therapy and for six months following the discontinuation of therapy.

Nausea

Nausea occurs in approximately 24 to 43 percent of patients taking interferon and ribavirin. However, this side effect is believed to be primarily due to ribavirin. Nausea may be lessened by taking ribavirin with food. If this doesn't work, some additional strategies may help. Eat multiple small meals while on therapy. Large meals make nausea worse. Avoid mixing extremely cold and extremely hot foods. Fatty foods, such as red meat, as well as fried, spicy foods should also be avoided. Eat easy-to-digest foods such as crackers, broth, dry toast, and Jell-O. Ginger ale minimizes nausea. Do not lie down after meals, but it is important to rest after meals in a sitting or standing position. Excessive activity induces vomiting. (Remember what your mother told you—don't go swimming on a full stomach!) If a person still experiences nausea despite following these recommendations, antinausea medications may need to be prescribed. Metoclopramide (Reglan) 10-mg tablets taken orally half an hour prior to meals, as well as before going to sleep, usually relieves nausea. An antinausea suppository such as trimethobenzamide (Tigan) 200-mg suppository taken rectally may be helpful in situations when a person cannot tolerate anything taken orally. Ondansetron hydrochloride (Zofran) is an antinausea medication typically prescribed for cancer patients who are undergoing chemotherapy. This medication should be taken at a dose of 4 to 8 mg half an hour prior to taking ribavirin. If nausea still persists, a dose reduction of ribavirin in the amount of one or two pills per day may become necessary.

Dermatologic Side Effects

Skin problems occur in 10 to 30 percent of people undergoing combination therapy and are primarily caused by ribavirin. Dermatologic side effects include itching, rashes, and dry skin. Itching may be relieved by the use of antihistamines such as Benadryl or Claritin. Either Benadryl lotion or hydrocortisone cream may be applied directly to the itchy area. Some patients find relief using gentle anti-itching soaps and lotions. These products, made for sensitive skin, include Aveeno, Cetaphil soap, L'Occitane, as well as other brands containing an oatmeal base. (Itching is discussed in detail in chapter 20.) Rashes may occur anywhere on the body but are most common in sun-exposed areas and at the injection sites. It is important to protect the skin from direct sunlight. Sunbathing should be totally avoided while on therapy, as severe sunburns may occur. A sunscreen with an SPF of 30 or more must be applied to the face and any other exposed areas prior to going outside during daylight hours. In addition, women who wear makeup should use makeup containing a sunscreen with an SPF of 15 or higher. A hat with a brim is important to wear if going outdoors between 10:00 A.M. and 3:00 P.M. Tanning beds should be avoided. A person who is prone to rashes should take Benadryl half an hour before taking ribavirin. Either Benadryl lotion or hydrocortisone lotion applied directly to a rash usually provides relief. Treatment for dry skin entails drinking one gallon of water per day in addition to using topical moisturizers. Lachydrin (ammonium lactate) 12% lotion tends to keep the skin well hydrated, as it helps the skin hold water. This lotion requires a prescription from the doctor. Aquaphor, an over-the counter ointment, is helpful to protect particularly dry, chafed skin and lips. Bathing or showering less often and using warm rather than hot water in addition to using a body lotion with a lower water content will decrease skin dryness.

Pulmonary Side Effects

Shortness of breath occurs in approximately one quarter of people on ribavirin therapy. It is sometimes accompanied by a mild cough. A decrease in the dose of ribavirin will typically bring about a resolution of these symptoms. Any shortness of breath may also be due to anemia. As such, blood tests to check the hemoglobin level are typically obtained when this symptom occurs. If blood work is stable and if symptoms persist after a ribavirin dose reduction, a chest X ray should be obtained to eliminate other causes. Cough suppressants, whether prescription or over the counter, are sometimes helpful in treating this symptom. The use of a humidifier and air purifier may also reduce these symptoms.

Other Symptoms

Osteoporosis is a condition characterized by decreased bone mass and decreased bone density. This leads to a weakening of bones, thereby increasing the risk of bone pain and bone fractures. Some but not all experts believe that ribavirin may cause or worsen osteoporosis. Osteoporosis is discussed in chapter 20. Some other side effects of ribavirin include fatigue, pruritus, decreased appetite, insomnia, depression, and rash. The treatment of these symptoms is discussed in chapters 11 and 20. When these side effects do occur in connection with ribavirin therapy, they are usually not very severe, and they typically dissipate upon discontinuation of therapy.

OTHER TREATMENT OPTIONS FOR CHRONIC HEPATITIS C

For those who do not respond to the standard therapy for chronic hepatitis C, there are other choices available. The following is a discussion of some other treatment options available to those who have not responded to standard treatment regimens.

Infergen

Infergen (also known as consensus interferon or interferon alfacon-1), manufactured by Intermune, is a genetically bioengineered, synthetic form of alfa interferon. Compared to other Type 1 alfa interferons, it has significantly greater antiviral activity. It can be an effective treatment for some people who have relapsed or who did not respond to an initial course of treatment with alfa interferon. In fact, 58 percent of those who relapse after initially responding to treatment with alfa interferon experience a sustained long-term response when retreated with

15 mcg of Infergen three times a week for forty-eight weeks. And 13 percent of those who do not respond to an initial course of alfa interferon respond long-term to 15 mcg of Infergen three times a week for forty-eight weeks. Thus, Infergen can be a particularly effective alternative treatment option for those who relapse after an initial course of interferon therapy.

Studies are under way to assess the effectiveness of Infergen plus ribavirin for those who relapsed or who did not respond to pegylated interferon plus riba-virin combination therapy. One preliminary study has demonstrated that after twelve weeks of Infergen plus ribavirin combination therapy, 23 percent of peo-ple had a nondetectable HCV RNA and 60 percent experienced a 2-log drop of HCV RNA levels. The dose of Infergen being used in this study is 15 mcg given daily in combination with daily ribavirin. Another ongoing study is using a daily dose of Infergen in the amount of 18 to 27 mcg in combination with daily riba-virin. The preliminary results from this study are that 56 percent of those who did not respond to pegylated interferon plus ribavirin achieved nondetectable levels of HCV RNA after twenty-four weeks of Infergen plus ribavirin combination therapy. The preliminary results of these studies are encouraging, and the final results are being eagerly awaited.

Trials of pegylated-Infergen (also known as PEG-alfacon-1) plus ribavirin are expected to begin in 2004. This combination is expected to be quite promising.

Gamma Interferon

Gamma interferon-1b (also known as Actimmune), manufactured by Intermune, is another type of interferon. Although it has little antiviral activity, its antiscar-ring (antifibrotic) activity is significant. Gamma interferon is now being studied as a possible treatment for hepatitis C patients with extensive scarring. Study re-sults should be available in the near future.

Infergen and gamma interferon are currently undergoing studies to evaluate the synergistic effect of decreasing both the hepatitis C viral load and the scarring of the liver. It is expected that this combination of interferons will prove to en-hance the efficacy of drug treatment for hepatitis C.

Long-Term or Lifelong Suppressive Interferon Therapy— Maintenance Therapy

Long-term suppressive therapy of viruses involves long-duration, continuously ongoing therapy—possibly lasting lifelong. This approach to therapy has proven successful in treating people infected with HIV. The primary goal of suppressive therapy in people with chronic hepatitis C is to impede the progression of liver disease. Even when it cannot eradicate HCV from the body, long-term suppres-sive therapy may prevent cirrhosis, liver failure, and liver cancer.

It has been shown that there are substantial benefits to interferon therapy, even for people who do not eradicate HCV. Liver damage and inflammation are reduced in approximately 40 percent of those who undergo interferon therapy even without eradicating the virus. Furthermore, treatment with interferon may decrease the likelihood of developing liver cancer. In non-cirrhotic individuals who experience a sustained response to interferon, there is little-to-no likelihood of progression to cirrhosis and liver cancer. And in some people interferon therapy has even been shown to reverse cirrhosis! As such, those who have not eradicated HCV with conventional regimens of interferon treatment may still benefit from long-term, or possibly even lifelong, therapy. Two large studies—the HALT-C trial (an acronym for Hepatitis C Antiviral Long-term Treatment Against Cirrhosis) and the Co-Pilot trial (an acronym for Colchicine PegIntron Long Term Therapy)—are now under way to assess the effectiveness of long-term suppressive therapy with pegylated interferon.

Colchicine

Colchicine is an antiscarring (antifibrotic) drug. Its primary use has been in the treatment of people with gout. However, in one study, colchicine was shown to prolong the lives of some people with alcoholic cirrhosis. Colchicine is now undergoing trials to assess its antifibrotic capabilities in patients with HCV (part of the Co-Pilot trial).

Amantadine

Amantadine (also known as Symmetrel), manufactured by Endo Laboratories, is an oral antiviral medication used to treat people with influenza A (the flu), as well as people with Parkinson's disease, a neurological disorder. Only one study has shown amantadine to be an effective treatment for people with chronic hepatitis C. Minimal side effects were encountered in this study. Unfortunately, the effectiveness of amantadine has not been confirmed by other studies. Combination therapy using amantadine and interferon in chronic hepatitis C patients has been attempted. However, the results have been somewhat disappointing. Therefore, any initial enthusiasm for using amantadine to treat chronic hepatitis C has greatly diminished.

One recent study has concluded that approximately 20 percent of people who do not respond to treatment with interferon and ribavirin will respond to a combination of amantadine, Peg-Intron, and ribavirin. Although this result is preliminary and needs to be confirmed in additional studies, this triple combination therapy may prove to be of benefit to some nonresponders to standard therapy.

Ursodeoxycholic Acid

Ursodeoxycholic acid is a bile salt that has been shown to be beneficial in the treatment of some liver diseases. In people with primary biliary cirrhosis (see chapter 15), ursodeoxycholic acid can normalize transaminase levels and delay progression of the disease. Studies have monitored the effect of ursodeoxycholic acid, both alone and in combination with interferon, in people with chronic hepatitis C. When used as the sole agent for people with chronic hepatitis C, ursodeoxycholic acid appears to temporarily normalize transaminase levels. When used in combination with interferon, ursodeoxycholic acid results in a higher incidence of transaminase normalization compared with the incidence of transaminase normalization in people treated with interferon alone. However, it does not appear that ursodeoxycholic acid has any significant effect on reducing the hepatitis C viral load or in improving inflammation or scarring in the liver. Therefore, the long-term benefits of ursodeoxycholic acid appear limited.

Iron-Reduction Therapy

Phlebotomy—a form of iron-reduction therapy—involves taking blood out of the body via a catheter that is temporarily placed in a vein in the arm. This blood is then discarded. It cannot be used for blood donation or for any other purpose. Phlebotomy is the primary form of treatment for people with an iron overload disease, such as hemochromatosis (see chapter 18). People with chronic hepatitis C often have a high iron content in both their blood and livers. It is believed that such people may have a low response rate to alfa interferon alone. Some studies have shown that among this group of people, phlebotomy may improve the overall response to interferon therapy.

Chelation therapy—another form of iron-reduction therapy—involves the infusion of deferoxamine (Desferal) either into a vein or beneath the skin (subcutaneously). Deferoxamine works by binding to iron and promoting its elimination from the body. Its effectiveness as an adjunct to interferon therapy is being evaluated. So far, no definitive conclusions have been made concerning the long-term benefits of iron-reduction therapy for people with chronic hepatitis C.

Thymosin-alfa1 (Zadaxin)

Thymosin-alfa1 is a group of linked amino acids that is produced by the thymus gland, located in the neck. Thymosin-alfa1 is an important component of the body's immune system and helps fight off viral infections. Studies have shown that synthetic Thymosin-alfa1 (known as Zadaxin), manufactured by SciClone Pharmaceuticals, can stimulate the immune system to fight off viruses. Used by itself to treat people with chronic hepatitis C, Zadaxin produces no significant improvements. However, preliminary studies suggest that when used in combination with pegylated interferon, Zadaxin may lower or eradicate hepatitis C viral levels, in addition to improving inflammation and damage in the liver.

Preliminary studies pairing Zadaxin with pegylated interferon alpha-2a (PEGASYS) for those who fail to respond to interferon/ribavirin combination therapy look promising. In a recent study, 20 to 36 percent of people with hepatitis C who failed previous interferon treatment experienced significant decreases in viral load after three months of Zadaxin/PEGASYS combination therapy. Therefore, Zadaxin used in combination with PEGASYS may be of benefit to people with chronic hepatitis C who were nonresponders to previous interferon regimens. Further studies involving larger groups of people are under way. Zadaxin is administered at a dose of 1.6 mg twice a week by subcutaneous injection. So far, it appears that Zadaxin causes little, if any, side effects.

Other Promising Investigational Therapies

A major advance for potential future treatment strategies for hepatitis C was the discovery of the actual structure of two of the key enzymes involved in HCV replication. These enzymes are known as the NS3 protease and the NS3 helicase. Vertex Pharmaceuticals is attempting to develop a drug that will inhibit these specific enzymes—an HCV-protease and a HCV-helicase inhibitor.

Clinical trials are ongoing to evaluate the drug VS-497 (merimempodib), which is manufactured by Vertex Pharmaceuticals. VX-497 is an inhibitor of the enzyme inosine monophosphate dehydrogenase (IMPDH), which is essential for the production of a nucleotide—a compound that forms the building blocks of DNA and RNA. Therefore, blocking the production of IMPDH may slow or block HCV viral replication. In experimental trials, VX-497 has shown to be a potent antiviral, much more potent than ribavirin. And VX-497's antiviral activity appears to be even greater when it is combined with interferon.

Mycophenolate mofetil is another inhibitor of the enzyme IMPDH. This drug is currently used to prevent rejection of a newly transplanted liver. In one study, it was combined with PEGASYS, and some patients achieved sustained eradication. Further study is needed on this combination therapy before it can be recommended.

Histamine is a natural substance made by the body that may reverse the oxidative stress and free radical damage to the liver caused by HCV and may enhance the body's response to interferon. When histamine (manufactured by Maxim Pharmaceuticals as Ceplene) is combined with interferon, additional antiviral effects occur. The use of histamine in combination with peginterferon and ribavirin is being studied in ongoing trials.

Vaccines given to treat chronic hepatitis C, known as therapeutic HCV vaccines, and HCV antibody immunoglobulins given, alone or in combination with interferon, are in the preliminary stages of investigation.

Heptazyme (Ribozyme Pharmaceuticals, Inc.) is a type of *ribozyme*—a kind of RNA molecule with the unique ability to cut targeted genetic material. In the case of Heptazyme, the targeted genetic material is contained with HCV. When part of its key genetic material is severed, HCV, dies and, therefore, no further viruses particles can be produced. Unfortunately, initial studies have shown that blindness may be a possible side effect of Heptazyme. Further study is currently ongoing to determine if the benefits of this drug outweigh its risks. Other less toxic ribozymes are in the process of being developed.

The enzymes that are essential to HCV's replication—proteases, polymerases, and helicases—are all potential targets for drug therapy. So far, the protease inhibitor BILN 2016 appears to be the most promising *investigational drug* utilizing this approach. Preliminary results in people with genotype 1 have been impressive. Further studies on this promising new drug are ongoing, and the results are being eagerly anticipated.

ISIS-14803 is a synthetic antisense oligonucleotide that binds HCV RNA, thereby resulting in decreased viral replication. Initial studies have shown that ISIS-14803 (given intravenously) significantly reduces the level of HCV RNA in people who did not respond to previous interferon therapy. Studies are under way to determine the results of combining ISIS-14803 with peginterferon and ribavirin in people with genotype 1 who failed previous combination therapy.

ADJUNCTS TO THERAPY

Some researchers believe that vitamin E therapy may be a beneficial adjunct to the treatment of viral hepatitis. In some studies involving patients with chronic hepatitis C, response rates were improved by the addition of vitamin E (at a dose of 400 to 800 IU each day) to interferon and ribavirin. It has also been suggested that vitamin E may slow the progression of liver disease. In addition, vitamin E may help relieve leg cramps, diminish memory loss, and increase male sexual performance—benefits that are of particular relevance to those on interferon treatment. Finally, vitamin E may delay the onset of and reduce the degree of ribavirin-induced anemia in some patients.

Vitamin C has been shown to increase the production of interferon that is naturally produced by the body. Furthermore, some experts believe that vitamin C may delay the onset of and may reduce the degree of ribavirin-induced anemia in hepatitis C patients being treated with interferon and ribavirin. Therefore, supplementation with vitamin C, at a dose of 1,000 mg per day, may be beneficial for people being treated with interferon and ribavirin.

Some studies have concluded that the addition of zinc to interferon treatment may increase the likelihood of viral eradication. Although this benefit has not been proven, it is advisable that those on interferon therapy supplement their diets with one or two 30-mg tablets of zinc per day. While dosages of zinc up to 100 mg per day may boost the immune system and increase the likelihood of response to interferon, excessive consumption of zinc may be dangerous and may even depress the immune system.

The medication cimetidine (Tagamet) is a histamine-2 (H_2) blocker. Traditionally, cimetidine has been used to treat ulcers and heartburn. It has been postulated that cimetidine may also have antiviral and immune-modulating properties. Based on preliminary studies, cimetidine taken in combination with interferon appears to increase the likelihood of sustained viral eradication. But cimetidine may also result in elevated liver enzymes and decreased platelet counts. Therefore, further studies must be conducted to assess the utility of this over-the-counter medication as an adjunct to the HCV treatment regimen.

Readers should keep in mind that the above-mentioned potential benefits of vitamin E, vitamin C, zinc, and cimetidine are speculative—that is, they have not been proven in scientific studies. Yet even though such studies have not been conducted, it is advisable to consume these adjuncts to therapy, as long as there are no contraindications to do so.

MONITORING THOSE WHO ARE NOT BEING TREATED

People with chronic hepatitis C who are not treated (for whatever reason) should be monitored by a doctor at least twice a year. However, the frequency of these visits may need to be increased depending upon specific circumstances. For example, people with decompensated cirrhosis may need more frequent visits in order to manage complications, such as ascites. Visits consist of a history of new symptoms that have occurred, a physical exam, and some blood tests. If cirrhosis is present, an alpha-fetoprotein blood test and sonogram will be necessary once or twice a year. It is important to remember that blood work, symptoms, physical exams, and imaging studies are often inadequate to predict the progression of chronic hepatitis C. To best determine progression of the disease—the actual amount of new inflammation and scarring that has occurred—a liver biopsy, performed approximately every five years, may be necessary.

CONCLUSION

In this chapter, you learned about some of the remarkable advances that have been made in the treatment of hepatitis C since the virus was first identified. Advances in medications to treat people infected with chronic hepatitis C have made treatment with one drug alone largely a thing of the past. This applies especially to those people who are classically poor responders to therapy. We have learned that two drugs, each having a different mechanism of action against HCV, work better than one drug alone. Will the future of therapy for people who fail to respond to two medications be the addition of yet another agent? Will interferon always be included in the regimen? Only time will tell.

In the meantime, investigational trials of new drugs and new drug combinations are growing. It is to be expected that from this extensive research, some promising new treatment regimens will emerge. Since most people with chronic hepatitis C have a slowly progressive disease, many individuals will die with HCV rather than from HCV. Yet, it is not possible to predict with 100 percent accuracy which people will have a benign course of liver disease and which people will have an aggressive course of disease. Thus, treatment should be seriously considered by everyone with chronic hepatitis C.

The first chapter of part 3 discusses autoimmune hepatitis, a type of liver disease caused by an attack on the liver by a person's own immune system. The remaining chapters of part 3 cover other liver disorders and their treatments.

Part Three

Understanding and Treating Other Liver Diseases

Fourteen

AUTOIMMUNE HEPATITIS

Beth, a usually energetic twenty-two-year-old nurse, had been feeling relentlessly fatigued during the last few months. When her usually regular menstrual cycle stopped for three months, she became very concerned. The results of an at-home pregnancy test came up negative. So what was the problem? Maybe it was the extra shift she'd recently added to her already busy work schedule at the hospital. Or maybe the thyroid medication she just started taking to treat her recent diagnosis of hypothyroidism was to blame.

One day at work, a fellow nurse approached Beth and said in a concerned manner, "Beth, you look jaundiced. You should see a doctor right away." Beth looked in the mirror and was surprised to see that her eyes and skin were yellow.

Beth consulted with her family doctor, who referred her to a liver specialist. The specialist took a lengthy history from Beth, which included questions about exposure to viral hepatitis, medication history, and family history of liver disease. A physical exam was performed. In addition to jaundice, the doctor detected that Beth had an enlarged liver and spleen. A battery of blood tests was taken, which revealed that both her bilirubin level and transaminase levels were more than ten times the normal values. The test for viral hepatitis was negative, but some of Beth's autoimmune markers were positive. A liver biopsy was performed, which confirmed the suspected diagnosis of autoimmune hepatitis. The specialist placed Beth on two medications, and within three weeks she was back to her normal, healthy self.

Autoimmune hepatitis (AIH) is the subject of this chapter. Since this is a liver disease marked by a defect of the immune system, this chapter discusses the immune system as it relates to AIH. There is no single test that can accurately diagnose AIH. A combination of factors is used to arrive at the diagnosis. This chapter will discuss how the diagnosis of AIH is made and will discuss the course that should be taken when the conventional markers of the disease are absent. AIH responds remarkably well to treatment in certain people. Conventional treatments, which are generally quite effective, will be reviewed, as will their potential side effects. A discussion of long-term prognosis for people with AIH, some options when medical therapy fails, and some promising new therapies conclude this chapter.

WHAT IS AUTOIMMUNE HEPATITIS?

Autoimmune hepatitis (AIH) is an uncommon chronic liver disease that has the potential to lead to cirrhosis. It is characterized by inflammation of the liver and/or liver damage caused by an attack on the liver by a person's own immune system. This disease was first recognized in 1950, when it was noted that the condition primarily affected young women who stopped menstruating (a condition known as *amenorrhea*); who suffered from arthritis; who had a severe form of chronic hepatitis that rapidly progressed to cirrhosis; and who had an elevated protein (gamma globulin) found on their blood tests.

Some similarities between AIH and *systemic lupus erythematosus (SLE)*, another autoimmune disease, led to AIH being named lupoid hepatitis in 1956. Presently, much more is known about AIH. For starters, it has been confirmed that AIH and SLE are two totally separate disorders. Thus, the term *lupoid hepatitis* is no longer used. Furthermore, it has been established that despite a greater occurrence rate among young women—women account for approximately 70 to 80 percent of cases—AIH may also occur in men, and it may occur in either gender at any age. Finally, case studies have established that AIH has varying manifestations. It is not always a severe, rapidly progressive disease, as originally believed. In fact, it may have a mild, asymptomatic (without symptoms) natural history.

AIH occurs in about 100,000 to 200,000 people in the United States at any given time, and it accounts for approximately 10 to 20 percent of chronic hepatitis cases in the world. Approximately 6 percent of liver transplantations in the United States are performed due to AIH. It was originally believed that the disease most commonly manifested itself at either of two age intervals—peripubertally (around thirteen years old) or around fifty to sixty years old. It is now known that AIH can develop at any age and has been diagnosed in infants as well as in people in their seventies. However, in most cases, a patient with AIH is over forty years old at the time of the initial visit to a specialist.

THE IMMUNE SYSTEM AND AIH

The main function of the immune system is to protect the body against harmful substances. Many times each day the immune system is called upon to distinguish between substances that belong to the body, such as blood and internal organs, and substances that are foreign to the body, such as drugs, fumes, or viruses. In addition, it must distinguish between foreign substances that are potentially harmful and those that are safe. The immune system is hard at work protecting the body twenty-four hours a day.

Unfortunately, there are occasions when this vital and intricate system malfunctions. When the immune system fails to perform its duties properly, one of two scenarios may arise: either the body receives diminished protection, as occurs in immune-deficiency diseases such as AIDS or the immune system may fail to correctly distinguish between what belongs to the body and what is a foreign substance. The term *autoimmune reaction* is used to describe what happens when a person's body produces an immune response against its own tissues or organs. In other words, the body incorrectly identifies one of its organs (the liver, for example) as foreign, as not belonging to the body, or as the enemy. When this occurs, the immune system produces protective antibodies that actually attack the enemy organ. These antibodies are known as *autoantibodies*. (See chapter 7 for a brief discussion of the immune system as it relates to antibodies and antigens.)

Examples of common autoimmune diseases include Graves' disease, in which the thyroid is under attack; insulin-dependent diabetes mellitus, in which the pancreas is under attack; rheumatoid arthritis, in which the joints are under attack; and ulcerative colitis, in which the colon is under attack. Sometimes the body even attacks more than one organ, and a person can actually have more than one autoimmune disorder at a time. In the case of autoimmune hepatitis, the organ under siege is the liver. AIH is considered a type of chronic hepatitis because this autoimmune process typically continues indefinitely, or at least until cirrhosis and/or liver failure occur.

GENDER AND AIH

As stated above, AIH occurs predominantly in women. In fact, all autoimmune disorders disproportionately affect women. Although the reason for this is unknown, some researchers have speculated that a gene controlling the immune system may be located on the X chromosome. Since women have a double dose (XX) of the X chromosome (as opposed to men, who have one X and one Y chromosome), their immune response may significantly exceed the immune response of a man. Another theory involves estrogen and other female-related hormones. It is postulated that these female-specific hormones may be partly responsible for the increased immune response observed in women.

THE POSSIBLE CAUSES OF AIH

The exact cause of AIH is not known. However, it is believed that this disease arises when some factor occurs in a genetically predisposed person that triggers the body to initiate an autoimmune attack against the liver. Such triggering factors are not clearly established but may possibly include the following: viruses, such as hepatitis A, B, and C, the measles virus, and the Epstein-Barr virus (EBV); bacteria, such as salmonella and *Escherichia coli* (E. coli); medications, such as halothane (a type of anesthesia); or possibly even certain herbs, such as Dai-saiko-to and black cohosh. A long time may elapse between the exposure to the trigger and the onset of AIH. Presence of the trigger is not required for the continuation of AIH.

One specific gene does not predispose a person to AIH. Instead, it is most likely the interaction of multiple genes that makes a person susceptible to the development of AIH. The exact makeup of these genes has not as yet been defined. However, it is felt that the gene for female sex is most likely one of the genes contributing to a person's susceptibility to AIH. Much research is being conducted in this area. Furthermore, it is felt that multiple factors, both genetic and environmental, affect how severe the disease will manifest in a particular person. In summary, it is thought that the disease itself is not inherited, but that the predisposition (susceptibility) to have the disease is. In fact, AIH is rarely found in more than one member of the same family. However, other autoimmune diseases, such as rheumatoid arthritis or thyroid disease, are often present in a family member.

THE SYMPTOMS AND SIGNS OF AIH

There are a variety of ways in which a doctor may discover that a person has AIH. In its most clandestine form, AIH may be detected by accident upon the discovery of elevated transaminase levels on routine blood tests (see chapter 3) in a person who is asymptomatic. An asymptomatic presentation occurs approximately 15 to 20 percent of the time. These people often have a milder course of disease. At the opposite extreme, AIH may be discovered during an acute attack, usually characterized by grossly elevated transaminase levels, jaundice, severe itching, right upper quadrant pain, and fatigue. This occurs in up to 25 percent of the cases. Most of the people in these cases do not actually have acute AIH, but turn out to be having acute flare-ups of previously undiagnosed asymptomatic chronic AIH. Other people fall somewhere in between, having vague symptoms, such as a general sense of lethargy, muscle and joint aches, or mild abdominal discomfort.

Fatigue is the most common and often the sole symptom, occurring in approximately 85 percent of symptomatic people at presentation. The severity of fatigue does not always correlate with the degree of liver inflammation and damage. And some people continue to suffer from fatigue even when the disease is in remission.

In more advanced cases, symptoms and signs of decompensated cirrhosis, such as ascites, encephalopathy, or bleeding esophageal varices, may be the initial features of AIH. This is the initial presentation up to 30 percent of the time (see chapter 6 for a discussion of cirrhosis). About 40 percent of people may have symptoms due to other autoimmune disorders associated with AIH, such as a thyroid disorder, rheumatoid arthritis, ulcerative colitis, or others discussed on page 207. Menstrual irregularities are common in women with AIH; some stop menstruating altogether. Before a liver abnormality is discovered, often these people are first evaluated by another type of specialist, such as an endocrinologist when thyroid abnormalities are detected or a rheumatologist when arthritis is present, resulting in their referral to a hepatologist.

As with symptoms, signs of liver disease vary widely. On a physical exam, the doctor may detect jaundice (yellowing of the skin and eyes) and spider angiomatas (enlarged blood vessels), which are usually located on the upper body or face. The liver and spleen are often enlarged. Other signs include hirsutism (excessive hair growth) and acne.

People with AIH typically have a chronic fluctuating course. AIH is characterized by *exacerbations* (worsening) and remissions (abatement) of disease, which occur at varying intervals.

OTHER AUTOIMMUNE DISORDERS ASSOCIATED WITH AIH

Other autoimmune diseases may also occur in people with AIH. In fact, about 40 to 50 percent of people with AIH also have another autoimmune disease. In fact, the presence of one of these other autoimmune diseases in a family member may assist in making a diagnosis of AIH. The diseases most commonly associated with AIH include thyroid abnormalities, rheumatoid arthritis, and *ulcerative colitis.* These and other autoimmune disorders associated with AIH are listed below.

- Thyroid disorders—hyperthyroidism (overactive thyroid) and hypothyroidism (underactive thyroid)

- Rheumatoid arthritis—a chronic disease characterized by pain and swelling of the joints

- Ulcerative colitis—intestinal disorder characterized by inflammation of the large intestine (colon) and bloody diarrhea

- Diabetes mellitus and insipidus—glucose (sugar) abnormalities

- Blood disorders, including hemolytic anemia, a low blood count due to breakdown of red blood cells (hemoglobin and hematocrit), and thrombocytopenia (low platelet count)

- Celiac sprue—gluten (wheat) intolerance

- Myasthenia gravis—a neuromuscular disorder characterized by extreme muscle weakness

- Sjögren's syndrome—a chronic disease characterized by dry eyes and mouth

- Glomerulonephritis—a kidney disorder

- Vitiligo—a skin disorder characterized by patches of discoloration

DIAGNOSING AIH

There is no single test that will accurately diagnose AIH. However, many factors taken together can provide the basis for an accurate diagnosis. Most important, in order to have an accurate diagnosis of AIH, it is necessary to first eliminate all other causes of chronic liver disease, such as viral hepatitis, primary biliary cirrhosis, hemochromatosis, excessive alcohol consumption, and drug-induced liver disease including liver disease caused by herbal preparations.

In contrast to other liver diseases, such as chronic hepatitis C or hemochromatosis, AIH is a liver disease in which the degree of transaminase elevation and the severity of symptoms often (although not always) correlate with the degree of liver damage and inflammation. Many times, the dramatic improvement of symptoms and normalization of transaminase levels with treatment will essentially prove or confirm the diagnosis of AIH. However, liver function tests (LFTs), autoimmune blood tests, genetic markers, and liver biopsy findings, when evaluated together, in addition to response to therapy, more typically are used to confirm the diagnosis. These tests are discussed on the following pages.

Liver Function Tests (LFTs)

Typically, transaminase levels (AST and ALT) are predominantly elevated and GGTP and alkaline phosphatase (AP) are normal or close to normal. If the AP is very elevated in conjunction with normal or only slightly elevated transaminase levels, a diagnosis other than AIH should be considered.

In severe cases of AIH, transaminase levels are very elevated. Transaminase elevations may be as much as ten to twenty times normal values. For example, AST and ALT may be around 400 to 800 IU/l, and the bilirubin level may be around 10 mg/dl. In milder cases, the transaminase levels are only slightly elevated, around 60 to 200 IU/l, and the bilirubin level is normal. In any scenario, when liver function tests are elevated, other more specific blood tests for AIH should be run (see chapter 3 for an explanation of the liver function tests).

Specific Autoimmune Blood Tests

Specific autoimmune blood tests include a check for elevated immunoglobulin levels, specifically an elevated gamma globulin or immunoglobulin G (IgG) level. Gamma globulin or IgG levels greater than two times the upper limit of normal are highly suggestive of a diagnosis of AIH. In addition, the presence of *antinuclear antibody (ANA), smooth muscle antibody (SMA),* and the *liver-kidney-microsomal antibody (anti-LKMAb)* must be searched for. As mentioned previously, these antibodies are known as autoantibodies.

Autoantibodies do not cause AIH. However, many autoantibodies are produced by the body in people with AIH. ANA and SMA are the most common and are therefore considered "markers" of AIH. It should be noted that both ANA and

SMA are not specific for AIH. This means they may also occur in liver diseases other than AIH, as well as in diseases of other organs. Approximately 54 percent of people with AIH have both ANA and SMA present in their blood. Other people have one, but not both, of these autoantibodies. ANA occurs alone as a marker of AIH 13 percent of the time, and SMA occurs alone as a marker 33 percent of the time. The presence of both autoantibodies is not necessary for the diagnosis to be made. To make things even more confusing, it is possible for people to lack all autoantibodies and still have AIH. This occurs in about 10 to 20 percent of people with AIH. These people are known as autoantibody-negative AIH (type III AIH). (See page 214.)

It has been found that one or both of these autoantibodies, although not present initially, may appear later in the course of the disease. This is of importance for people who initially test negative for the presence of autoantibodies and thus have not been given a definitive diagnosis by their doctors.

When ANA and SMA are present in liver diseases other than AIH, their values tend to be very low and are thought to be of little significance. These autoantibodies are reported to doctors on blood work by dilution titers (the dilution of blood containing a specific antibody). A titer of 1:160 or greater is considered a high titer and is highly suggestive of a diagnosis of AIH. Titers of less than 1:80 are considered low titers and are not necessarily indicative of a diagnosis of AIH. Note that autoantibody titers can fluctuate from one blood test to the next, and during therapy for AIH, they may disappear altogether. Moreover, the levels of these autoantibodies do not correlate with the severity or prognosis of disease.

The liver-kidney-microsomal antibody (anti-LKMAb) characteristically occurs in the absence of ANA and SMA. LKM antibody has been found mainly in children in Europe and is rare in the United States, being found in only 4 percent of adults with AIH.

Approximately 60 to 90 percent of people with AIH have antibodies to peripheral antineutrophil cytoplasmic autoantibodies (pANCA), also known as peripheral antineutrophil nuclear antibodies (pANNA). PANCA is not a specific test for the diagnosis or prognosis of AIH but is a useful marker that may contribute to the diagnosis of this disease.

There are numerous other autoantibodies that are currently being studied. These include antibodies to soluble liver antigen/liver pancreas (anti-SLA/LP), antibodies to actin (anti-actin), antibodies to asialoglycoprotein receptor (anti-ASGPR), and liver-specific cytosol antigen type 1 (anti-LC1). Some of these autoantibodies may be shown to improve diagnostic accuracy or to be useful in predicting the prognosis of AIH. At the present time, however, these autoantibodies are investigational in nature.

Genetic Markers

It is believed that there is a genetic predisposition or susceptibility to the development of AIH. Research has focused primarily on genetic defects found on chromosome number 6. Chromosomes contain most or all of the DNA or RNA that make up the genes of an individual. *Human leukocyte antigens (HLAs)* are special antigens located on chromosomes that are believed to be factors in the hereditary predisposition of people to different diseases.

Certain HLAs found on chromosome number 6 are associated with AIH, which are known as HLA DR3 and HLA DR4. These HLAs can be detected by special blood tests, although these blood tests are not readily available in all laboratories. People with AIH who have HLA DR3 tend to be relatively young and typically have a very aggressive disease that is poorly responsive to medical therapy. People who have HLA DR4 tend to be relatively old and have a less aggressive disease that responds quite well to medical treatment. HLA typing is not usually performed during the routine evaluation of a person suspected of having AIH. However, these markers are particularly helpful in diagnosing AIH in people who lack conventional autoantibodies or whose diagnosis is otherwise in question.

Liver Biopsy

Liver biopsy, which was discussed at length in chapter 5, is the only test that will accurately determine the extent of inflammation and damage done to the liver by AIH. Moreover, there are findings on a liver biopsy that are highly suggestive of AIH and assist the specialist in making a diagnosis of AIH. Thus, a liver biopsy is an important tool for confirming the diagnosis of AIH and for determining its severity. Treatment decisions are usually based on the results of a liver biopsy.

THE OVERLAP SYNDROMES

Sometimes people will have features of AIH as well as the features of another autoimmune liver disease. These are known as overlap syndromes. The following is a discussion of these overlap syndromes. Overlap syndromes between different autoimmune liver diseases occur approximately 18 percent of the time. They may be difficult to diagnose and pose some treatment dilemmas. In general, the autoimmune liver disease with the predominant features should be the disease that is treated. People with equally mixed liver diseases usually respond well to a combination of therapies directed against both diseases.

AIH and Primary Biliary Cirrhosis

AIH overlaps with primary biliary cirrhosis (PBC) about 8 to 12 percent of the time. These people have the clinical features of AIH but have the presence of the autoantibody *antimitochondrial antibody (AMA)* in their blood, which is diagnostic of PBC. It has been suggested that those people who test positive for AMA should not be considered to have AIH. This is because there is such a strong association of AMA with PBC. It is important to always test these individuals for anti-LKMAb. If anti-LKMAb is positive, AIH is the most likely diagnosis. There is also a small group of people who are found to have AMA and who genuinely have AIH, not PBC. These individuals have very elevated transaminase levels with minimal elevation of alkaline phosphatase levels. AMA titers typically are low— less than 1:160 in most cases. These people typically respond well to conventional treatment for AIH. See chapter 15 for more information about PBC.

AIH and Primary Sclerosing Cholangitis

AIH may also overlap with a disease known as primary sclerosing cholangitis (PSC). This occurs about 6 percent of the time. PSC is an uncommon liver disease characterized by inflammation and damage to both the intrahepatic and extrahepatic bile ducts. PSC can lead to cirrhosis. PSC occurs most frequently in men and is commonly associated with ulcerative colitis. Therefore, people with AIH (especially men) who also have ulcerative colitis should undergo testing for PSC. People with both AIH and PSC typically have a poor response to steroid treatment. This type of overlap syndrome occurs most frequently in children. Rarely, people with long-standing, well-controlled AIH can develop PSC. Therefore, people with AIH who suddenly become resistant to standard therapy after being well controlled for many years, or who suddenly develop a *cholestatic liver enzyme* pattern—high levels of alkaline phosphatase and GGTP as compared to transaminase levels (see page 28)—should be evaluated for PSC. See chapter 15 for more information about PSC.

AIH and Autoimmune Cholangitis

Autoimmune cholangitis is an autoimmune liver disease characterized by inflammation of the liver and positive autoimmune markers (ANA and/or SMA), in addition to injury to the bile ducts. This disease has also been referred to as mitochondrial antibody-negative PBC. Treatment with steroids has different responses in different people. See chapter 15 for more information about autoimmune cholangitis.

Autoimmune Hepatitis and Viral Hepatitis

Autoantibodies (ANA, SMA, and anti-LKMAb) may occur in people with hepatitis B (HBV) and hepatitis C (HCV). Accurate diagnosis of the predominant disease is of crucial importance, as management strategies may otherwise be compromised. Approximately 20 to 40 percent of people with chronic HBV or HCV have low titers (less than 1:160) of autoantibodies. In the past, this situation was considered a dilemma for the treating physician. By focusing on the AIH and treating with prednisone (see page 216), the doctor risks increasing the replication of HBV and HCV. Yet, by focusing on the HBV or HCV and treating with interferon, the physician puts a person with AIH at risk for severe consequences, including possibly an episode of encephalopathy (mental confusion). Presently, the consensus is that administering interferon to people with chronic viral hepatitis with low levels of autoantibodies—a condition now termed "chronic viral hepatitis with autoimmune features"—is generally safe. Still it is recommended that all people be tested for autoantibodies prior to beginning interferon therapy. Those people found to have autoantibodies should be more closely monitored than those who lack autoantibodies.

The above situation needs to be distinguished from the rare case of a person who truly has the overlap syndrome of full-fledged AIH and chronic viral hepatitis. Such a person will have high autoantibody titers (greater than 1:320) and liver biopsy results consistent with AIH. These people tend to respond to steroid treatment as well as those people who have AIH alone.

CLASSIFICATION OF THE DIFFERENT TYPES OF AIH

Since there is no single test that accurately diagnoses AIH and since there is considerable variability in mode of presentation and severity of disease, the diagnosis of AIH is sometimes in question. Therefore, experts in this field have attempted to classify AIH into various parameters for the purposes of diagnosis, assessing prognosis, and planning treatment strategies. This section will discuss two proposed methods of classification—the autoantibody profile-based AIH classification and the "definite" and "probable" AIH classification.

Autoantibody Profile-based AIH Classification

In 1987 it was suggested that AIH be classified by the type of autoantibody present in the blood. Although subject to some debate among experts, under this method of classification AIH falls into three categories.

- Type I AIH, also known as classic AIH, was identified in the 1950s. It is characterized by the presence of the two autoantibodies: antinuclear antibody (ANA) and smooth muscle antibody (SMA). This is the most common form of AIH in the United States.

- Type II AIH was identified in the 1980s. It is characterized by the presence of the liver-kidney-microsomal antibody (anti-LKMAb). This autoantibody is present primarily in young women and in children with AIH. In these people, other autoantibodies, such as ANA and SMA, are characteristically absent. Untreated people with type II AIH are thought by some to have a rapidly progressive course of disease leading to cirrhosis. This type of AIH accounts for only about 4 percent of AIH cases in the United States.

- Type III AIH is also known as autoantibody-negative AIH. These people lack all autoantibody markers yet have all the other features of type I AIH. People with type III AIH respond to treatment in a manner similar to those people with autoantibodies. Antibody to soluble liver antigen/liver pancreas (anti-SLA/LP) appears to be a marker for the diagnosis of type III AIH. However, as stated on page 211, this autoantibody is currently investigational in nature and therefore cannot be readily obtained outside research protocols.

"Definite" and "Probable" AIH Classification

In 1999, an international panel of experts proposed that people should be classified as having either "definite" or "probable" AIH according to how similar their features are to classic lupoid hepatitis. People fulfilling either criterion should be treated with steroids. A good response to treatment is considered as confirmation of the diagnosis. This panel also recommended a scoring system in which positive or negative weighting factors are assigned to multiple parameters that either support or negate the diagnosis of AIH. The cumulative score is then used to classify people into having either "definite" or "probable" AIH. A very low score is inconsistent with the diagnosis of AIH altogether. Please see table 14.1 for a list summarizing the positive and negative weighting factors.

Table 14.1. Summary of the International AIH Panel Scoring System for the Diagnosis of AIH

Positive Weighting Factors	Negative Weighting Factors
Female gender	
High AST and ALT and low AP	High AP and low AST and ALT
High gamma globulin levels	
ANA, SMA, or anti-LKMAb positive	AMA positive
Negative for HBV and HCV	Positive for HBV or HCV
Negative drug history	Positive drug history
Low alcohol consumption	High alcohol consumption
Liver biopsy results consistent with AIH	Liver biopsy results inconsistent with AIH
Concurrent autoimmune diseases in the patient or family	
Positive for relevant HLAs	
Positive treatment response	

TREATMENT OF AIH

AIH was the first chronic liver disease in which medical therapy was proven to prolong a person's life. The goal of treatment of AIH is to ameliorate symptoms, to decrease the inflammation of the liver, to induce a long-term remission of the disease, and to prevent progression to cirrhosis. When treatment is successful, people have a normal life expectancy. This section discusses the medications used for AIH and includes information about the successes, relapses, and failures of treatment. The potential side effects of treatment and who is most likely to benefit from treatment are also covered.

Medications for the Treatment of AIH

People with AIH are typically treated with a combination of two medications: a steroid medication known as prednisone, a synthetic hormone similar to the hormones known as steroids (also known as corticosteroids) that the body produces naturally, and azathioprine (Imuran), a steroid-sparing agent that allows a person to be treated with lower dosages of prednisone. Both drugs have *anti-inflammatory* properties, meaning that they are capable of diminishing inflammation. Prednisone may be used alone in high doses (60 mg) or in combination with azathioprine. Both regimens are equally effective. The combination of prednisone and azathioprine is usually the preferred method of treatment. This is due to the lower incidence of prednisone-related side effects—10 percent versus 44 percent with higher doses of prednisone alone. Therefore, prednisone is typically used alone only in people who cannot take azathioprine. Azathioprine cannot be used in the following people: those with a low blood cell count, those with a thiopurine methyltransferase deficiency (such people are at high risk for the development of low blood counts if placed on azathioprine), pregnant women, and people who have any form of active cancer. A discussion of the side effects of prednisone and azathioprine begins on page 219.

The initial dose of prednisone is anywhere from 10 to 30 mg. This is usually combined with azathioprine, which is given in a dosage between 50 and 100 mg. Azathioprine is considered a steroid-sparing drug. This means that its anti-inflammatory properties allow for smaller doses of prednisone to be used. Therapy may last months or years or may even be lifelong. Generally, once remission is achieved, as judged by the resolution of symptoms, normalization or near normalization of transaminase elevations, and improvement of liver biopsy samples, dosages of medications are slowly decreased and eventually medication is discontinued. On average, it takes approximately twenty-two months' treatment before remission is achieved. Symptoms and enzyme abnormalities tend to resolve approximately three to six months earlier than the resolution of inflammation and scarring found on liver biopsy samples. Thus, it is important to repeat a liver biopsy prior to the discontinuation of medication. If a person should relapse after the medication is discontinued, lifelong therapy is advisable using low doses of prednisone (10 mg) and azathioprine (50 mg). Studies have shown that some of these people will remain in remission despite discontinuing prednisone, provided they continue the use of azathioprine.

Successes of Treatment

Early and aggressive treatment can slow or prevent progression of AIH to cirrhosis. In fact, some researchers feel that it may even reverse the course in some people with early stages of liver scarring. AIH generally responds very well to the combination regimen mentioned above, and remission is usually achieved in approximately 65 to 80 percent of the cases. It takes about a year and a half to two years for most people to go into remission. Some people respond quickly, sometimes in as little as six months, whereas others take years. Approximately 14 to 50 percent of these people remain in long-term remission after medications are discontinued. People who remain in remission usually have a normal life expectancy.

Successful response to treatment may be assessed from a combination of factors. For example, results of blood work will demonstrate a decrease of transaminase levels and immunoglobulin (IgG) levels. Liver biopsy specimens will show a decrease of inflammation and scarring. In some cases even cirrhosis has been reported to be reversed. Also, the resolution of symptoms is an indicator that treatment has been successful. It should be noted that many people feel better after only one to two weeks on therapy.

Relapse After Treatment

Relapse of AIH may occur between six months to three years after treatment is stopped. It typically is diagnosed by a transaminase elevation of about three times above the normal value. The chance of relapse within six months of medication discontinuation is approximately 50 percent. If a person has remained in remission more than one year after cessation of therapy, the probability of relapse at some future point during his lifetime is only approximately 10 percent.

Patients who relapse typically respond well to re-treatment. However, for relapsers, the likelihood of another relapse six months after medication withdrawal from re-treatment is almost 80 percent. Therefore, people who relapse benefit from long-term maintenance therapy with low doses of prednisone (10 mg) and azathioprine (50 mg). Compared with multiple rounds of treatment and withdrawal of medication, long-term maintenance therapy is actually associated with a lower incidence of side effects. Some people on long-term treatment with prednisone and azathioprine may eventually be tapered off the prednisone altogether and kept solely on azathioprine.

The reasons why some people relapse are unclear. Some researchers believe that people who have cirrhosis on initial liver biopsy specimens rarely remain in remission once treatment is discontinued. Discontinuation of medication prematurely may be another factor. Therefore, some doctors choose to perform a liver biopsy before discontinuing therapy to assess the actual degree of remaining liver inflammation. By proceeding in this manner, the rate of relapse diminishes to approximately 20 percent (as opposed to the 50 percent likelihood stated above), as premature termination of medication will be averted.

Treatment Failure

Up to 20 percent of people with AIH do not respond to conventional treatment. Treatment failure is defined as an increase in transaminase levels despite conventional doses of medication. It occurs most commonly during the initial two months of therapy. High-dose regimens such as prednisone 60 mg or a combination of prednisone 30 mg and azathioprine 150 mg should be tried for at least one month in people who have not responded during the initial two months of therapy. Seventy-five percent of people will improve within two years on this regimen and should be maintained lifelong on conventional doses of medication.

The reason why some people do not respond to conventional therapy is unclear and is subject to differing opinions among researchers. Some researchers believe that the types of people who are less likely to respond to treatment are those with cirrhosis as well as those who developed AIH at an early age. However, others believe that the presence of cirrhosis does not affect a person's response to therapy and that the presence of cirrhosis should not affect treatment decisions.

Some researchers believe that a genetic susceptibility accounts for the rapid disease progression and lack of response to treatment that apply to some people. Studies have shown that people who test positive for HLA DR3 are less likely to respond to treatment and are more likely to require liver transplantation than those people who tested positive for HLA DR4. Therefore, higher doses of conventional therapy, or perhaps the use of other drugs, may be advantageous for HLA DR3-positive people.

Incomplete Response

People who have been on therapy for over three years without achieving remission have a low probability (approximately 7 percent per year) that remission will ever be achieved. These people should probably discontinue medication so as to avoid developing medication-induced side effects. However, final treatment decisions should be determined on a case-by-case basis and involve weighing the risks versus the benefits of long-term therapy (see next section).

Treatment: Who Benefits and Who Doesn't

The benefits of treatment must always be weighed against the potential side effects and risks associated with treatment. People who will typically benefit from treatment include those with severe symptoms, those with severe damage on liver biopsy specimens, and those with severely elevated transaminase abnormalities of about five- to tenfold above the upper limits of normal. In all other cases, the decision to begin therapy should be made on a case-by-case basis.

There are some people who are not likely to benefit from treatment. For example, the initiation of treatment is usually unnecessary in people with mild hepatitis, as determined from results of a liver biopsy, along with liver enzyme abnormalities less than threefold above the upper limits of normal. In these people, the decision to initiate therapy is determined by the degree of symptoms. If symptoms are significant, then a trial of low-dose treatment should be attempted. If the person is asymptomatic, no therapy should be started. People without symptoms who do not require medication for AIH still require close monitoring. Visits to the hepatologist for a physical exam and blood tests are recommended twice a year. Liver biopsies at five- to ten-year intervals may be indicated in order to assess the progression of the disease.

Treatment is also not indicated for people who have cirrhosis without liver inflammation. People with decompensated cirrhosis, such as those with bleeding esophageal varices or ascites, should not be treated with medication, but should be evaluated for liver transplantation. Pregnant women may be treated; however, treatment should be with prednisone alone, as azathioprine may be toxic to the fetus.

Women who are postmenopausal are at increased risk for the development of osteoporosis while on prednisone. Therefore, some studies have concluded that the risks of treatment are outweighed by the benefits in these women. Yet many other investigators have found a similar occurrence of side effects from prednisone in postmenopausal and premenopausal women. Complications of prednisone primarily occurred in postmenopausal women when therapy was prolonged or when treatment after relapse was required. As always, the risks of treatment must be weighed against the potential benefits of treatment on a patient-by-patient basis.

Potential Side Effects of Treatment with Prednisone and/or Azathioprine

Approximately one-third of people undergoing treatment for AIH develop some side effects. Generally, side effects can be diminished by using lower doses of medications. However, approximately 10 percent of people on medications for AIH develop side effects that are so debilitating that they must discontinue therapy. These people may want to consider entering a clinical trial of an experimental medication. (See the section "Promising New Therapies for AIH" below.)

Side effects of both prednisone and azathioprine are dependent upon the dosage and duration of use. The higher the dose and the longer the duration of use, the greater the likelihood that side effects will be experienced. Note that people with cirrhosis appear to have more side effects from drug therapy than those without cirrhosis. See tables 14.2 and 14.3.

PROMISING NEW THERAPIES FOR AIH

When conventional therapy has failed, or when the side effects of conventional medicine limit its utility, other medications should be tried. There are some medications

Table 14.2. Potential Side Effects of Prednisone and Management Possibilities

Potential Side Effects	Management Possibilities
Psychiatric symptoms, such as mood swings, personality changes, depression, and irritability	Decrease dosage; consult with a therapist; reduce additional stress
Insomnia	Decrease dosage; take melatonin before bed
Fluid retention; high blood pressure; congestive heart failure	Low-sodium diet; blood pressure medication
Osteoporosis and other bone disorders	Calcium and vitamin D supplements; alendronate (Fosamax) or etidronate (Didronal); calcitonin nasal spray; sensible exercise program; hormone replacement therapy (HRT)
Gastrointestinal ulcers and inflammation	H_2 blocker, such as famotidine (Pepcid); pump inhibitor, such as lansoprazole (Prevacid), or omeprazole (Prilosec)
Impaired wound healing	Decrease dose prior to surgery
Muscle loss	Weight-training program
Headache	Low-sodium diet; acetaminophen in moderation
Diabetes	Insulin or oral hypoglycemic (sugar-lowering) medications
Glaucoma/cataracts	Frequent eye checkups
Weight gain due to increased appetite	Low-fat, low-sodium diet; exercise
Menstrual irregularities	Oral contraceptives
Acne	Acne medication

that are in use for the treatment of AIH but are still considered investigational. Clinical trials are being performed to assess their effectiveness in the treatment of AIH.

Cyclosporine and tacrolimus (FK-506) are two medications commonly used to prevent liver transplant rejection. These antirejection drugs, which are discussed in chapter 22, possess potent anti-inflammatory properties. Limited studies involving their use in people with AIH have revealed reductions of LFTs when taken for a period of one year. Further studies need to be conducted to clearly define the incidence of relapse and to determine whether the benefits of these medications outweigh their potential risks.

Budesonide is a steroid that is typically associated with fewer side effects

Table 14.3. Potential Side Effects of Azathioprine and Management Possibilities

Potential Side Effects	Management Possibilities
Nausea; vomiting; loss of appetite	Eat multiple small meals; take azathioprine with, or immediately after, meals; take azathioprine in divided doses
Diarrhea	Avoid dairy products; add white rice to diet
Rash and itching	Stay out of the sun; use over-the-counter anti-itching medication, such as the antihistamine Benadryl
Bone marrow depression	Have periodic blood work done; reduce dosage; temporarily withdraw azathioprine
Infection	Avoid people who are ill; wash hands carefully and frequently; reduce dosage
Cancer	Self breast and/or testicular exam; avoid excess sun exposure; use high-potency sunscreen; avoid smoking and drinking alcohol
Mouth sores	Attentively care for and clean mouth
Birth defects	Use birth control; discontinue if pregnant; avoid breast-feeding

than prednisone, especially that of bone loss. In some preliminary studies, people with AIH were treated with budesonide. Among people with AIH who are treatment dependent—those people who are unable to be withdrawn from medication without experiencing a relapse of disease—budesonide was not shown to be beneficial. However, for people with AIH who had not previously been treated (treatment naive), the results were promising. Further investigation is ongoing in this group of people. It is suspected that the major utility of budesonide will be in treatment-naive people with a mild form of AIH.

Deflazacort is another steroid that like budesonide has fewer side effects than prednisone. In some preliminary studies, deflazacort was substituted for prednisone in AIH people needing maintenance therapy. The results appear promising.

Ursodeoxycholic acid (Actigall; URSO) is a natural bile acid that is found in small quantities in humans, but is found in large quantities in bears. It is the standard therapy for people with primary biliary cirrhosis (see chapter 15). Studies in Japan have shown ursodeoxycholic acid to be beneficial as the initial treatment for AIH. However, similar studies conducted in the United States have not confirmed this finding. Ursodeoxycholic acid may be useful for people with mild AIH, or as an additional medication with prednisone and azathioprine for treatment for naive people with AIH, but further studies are needed to confirm this.

Both 6-Mercaptopurine (6-MP) and mycophenolate mofetil have been shown to be potential substitutes for azathioprine. These medications could be used by people who are unable to tolerate azathioprine or who are unresponsive to it. As a potential substitute for azathioprine, either 6-MP or mycophenolate mofetil may be of use as a conjunctive therapy along with prednisone. Further studies are needed to confirm the efficacy of these drugs.

Other medications that have shown to be potentially beneficial for treating AIH include *cytoprotective agents* (substances that can protect cells), such as polyunsaturated phosphatidylcholine and arginine thiazolidinecarboxylate; immunosuppressive drugs (medications that stifle the actions of the immune system), such as brequinar and rapamycin; and thymic hormone extracts. Studies performed using these medications are preliminary, and further study is required before any definite conclusions can be drawn. Future studies will likely focus on the identification of the specific antigens—autoantigens—of AIH. Once these autoantigens have been isolated, a vaccination or gene therapy may be feasible.

LIVER TRANSPLANTATION—WHEN ALL ELSE HAS FAILED

When all medical therapies have failed, or if complications from cirrhosis have developed, liver transplantation must be considered. The success rate of transplantation in people with AIH is excellent. See chapter 22 for information on liver transplantation.

THE LONG-TERM PROGNOSIS FOR THOSE WITH AIH

People who are appropriately and aggressively treated generally have a prolonged survival time. Treatment may reduce the chances of developing cirrhosis or at least slow its progression. Some researchers have shown that treatment can sometimes reverse liver scarring in those with the early stages of cirrhosis. Studies have also shown that people who are successfully treated have a life expectancy similar to that of the general population, even if cirrhosis was present at the time AIH was initially diagnosed. During the first three years of therapy, people with AIH have about an 11 percent probability each year of progressing to cirrhosis. After the initial three-year period, they have a 1 percent per year chance of developing cirrhosis. People with severe AIH who do not receive treatment have only about a 30 percent chance of surviving for five years. Many of these people will develop cirrhosis within two years of their diagnosis.

Any liver disease that leads to cirrhosis may potentially also lead to liver cancer. People with AIH and cirrhosis are at increased risk for the development of liver cancer. Fortunately, the incidence of liver cancer among people with AIH is much lower than it is among people with liver disorders such as hemochromatosis or chronic viral hepatitis. People with AIH in whom the development of cirrhosis is prevented by successful therapy will not be at risk for liver cancer.

CONCLUSION

As discussed in this chapter, autoimmune hepatitis is a liver disease that has a wide spectrum of severity. While some people are quite ill, others have a course so mild that no therapy is required. As there is no single test that definitively identifies people with AIH, multiple indicators are usually necessary to confirm the diagnosis. Determining who is a good candidate for treatment is crucial, as the medications used for treatment of AIH may have significant side effects. When people are treated promptly and aggressively, most have a relatively long-term survival rate. The next chapter discusses another liver disease—primary biliary cirrhosis (PBC). As noted in this chapter, PBC may occur in conjunction with AIH. While PBC is suspected to also be an autoimmune disease, the features and treatment of PBC differ drastically from those of AIH.

Fifteen

PRIMARY BILIARY CIRRHOSIS

Edith, a fifty-three-year-old homemaker, had been feeling somewhat fatigued for the past year. She had always been an energetic woman involved in two local benefit organizations while running a household, doing all the chores and errands, and taking care of four children. She blamed her uncharacteristic run-down feeling on her advancing age. But when Edith started feeling itchy all the time, she couldn't blame that on her age. She changed her brand of laundry detergent, thinking it could be an allergy and tried several over-the-counter topical creams that her pharmacist had recommended, but nothing worked. Finally, when her constant scratching started keeping her husband awake at night, he insisted that she see a dermatologist.

The dermatologist worked with Edith for two months, but none of the various medications and therapies he prescribed brought her relief. Another dermatologist told Edith that her condition was caused by her nerves and advised her to see a psychiatrist. Feeling frustrated and depressed by this point, Edith thought that might be a good idea. The psychiatrist concluded that Edith was suffering from depression and wanted to start her on a medication for depression; however, he required that she first get a checkup from her doctor. Edith's doctor conducted a thorough physical exam and drew blood for a comprehensive battery of blood tests. The tests revealed that Edith's liver enzymes were elevated, and she was referred to a liver specialist. The specialist ran additional blood tests and had Edith obtain a sonogram of her liver. After reviewing the test results, the liver specialist told Edith that she had a rare liver disease known as primary biliary cirrhosis. "This is most likely what has been causing your fatigue, itching, and depression," he told her. The results of a liver biopsy confirmed the specialist's diagnosis, and Edith began treatment.

Primary biliary cirrhosis (PBC), a relatively rare liver disease that occurs primarily in middle-aged women, is the topic of this chapter. You'll learn about the characteristics and possible causes of PBC. Also covered in this chapter are how PBC is diagnosed and what its associated symptoms are. In addition, the many other disorders frequently associated with PBC are detailed. The current medications that are used to treat PBC are discussed, and some promising new treatment strategies are reviewed. Finally, the natural history and prognosis of people with PBC, while somewhat unpredictable, conclude this chapter.

WHAT IS PRIMARY BILIARY CIRRHOSIS?

PBC is a chronic liver disease characterized by the slow destruction of the *intrahepatic* (within the liver) bile ducts. As discussed in earlier chapters, the term *chronic* connotes a duration of greater than six months. In fact, PBC may be accurately characterized as a lifelong illness. Like autoimmune hepatitis, which was discussed in chapter 14, PBC is also believed to be an autoimmune disorder. An autoimmune disorder is a condition in which the immune system malfunctions and produces an immune response (an attack) against its own organs. In PBC, as with autoimmune hepatitis (AIH), the organ under attack is the liver. However, unlike AIH, in which the immune system attacks liver cells, in PBC the immune system attacks the cells lining the bile ducts within the liver. A consequence of the autoimmune attack is that the bile ducts become damaged. Once the bile ducts have become damaged, the bile acids within the ducts spill out. Since bile acids are strong detergents, inflammation, damage, and scarring of liver tissue occur.

As discussed in chapter 1, bile ducts carry bile—a substance that aids in the digestion of fats and in the neutralization of poisons. When the bile ducts become inflamed and eventually destroyed, the surrounding liver tissue subsequently becomes damaged. This leads to scarring and cirrhosis. This explains the derivation of the name primary "biliary cirrhosis." This name can be a bit misleading since most people with PBC do not yet have cirrhosis at the time of initial diagnosis and some may never even progress to cirrhosis in their lifetimes. Because this is a disease wherein the bile ducts become inflamed (a condition known as *cholangitis*) by a process that is not due to an infection, the alternative name, chronic *nonsuppurative* (not pus-producing) cholangitis, has been suggested to be a more accurate description of this disease. However, this alternative name is not widely accepted and is therefore not in use.

PBC is known as one of the cholestatic liver diseases. Cholestatic liver diseases are characterized by cholestatic failure of bile flow. In PBC there is an eventual failure of bile flow within the liver, which is known as *intrahepatic cholestasis*. Cholestatic liver diseases are also characterized by a certain pattern of blood-test abnormalities (elevated levels of AP, GGTP, and bilirubin; see chapter 3). In addition, PBC is a liver disease that is commonly associated with many other disorders. A discussion of these disorders begins on page 231.

THE RISING REPORTS OF PBC

PBC was first described in 1851, but prior to the 1950s, very few cases of PBC were reported. Today, it is estimated that approximately 4 to 15 people per million each year are diagnosed with PBC and that there are approximately 20 to 250 people per million with PBC. The most likely explanation of why PBC is more commonly reported now involves the increased awareness of this disease among the medical profession and the improved methods of detection through routine blood work.

THOSE WHO ARE AT RISK FOR PBC

PBC occurs in all countries and among all races, although Caucasian people from Northern Europe appear to have a particularly high rate of occurrence. PBC appears to be very rare in Africa and India. First-degree family members—parents, siblings, and children—of a person with PBC appear to be approximately 1,000 times more likely to develop PBC compared with the general population. Therefore, family members should be checked for PBC. Family members have also been noted to have other autoimmune disorders, such as rheumatoid arthritis and thyroid disorders. Women are more likely to have PBC than men. In fact, approximately 90 to 95 percent of people with PBC are women. The reason for this disproportionate predisposition among women is unknown. However, as noted in chapter 14, all autoimmune diseases appear to be more common in women. PBC most often afflicts people between the ages of forty and sixty; however, people have been diagnosed with PBC while still in their twenties and even as late as their nineties.

THE CAUSES OF PBC

The exact cause of PBC is unknown. However, PBC is believed to be a disease of autoimmune origin occurring in people with a genetic susceptibility to the disease. The autoimmune nature of PBC is supported by its frequent association with other autoimmune disorders, such as rheumatoid arthritis. The laboratory findings of a special autoantibody known as the *antimitochondrial antibody* and an elevated immunoglobulin M (IgM) level lend additional support to this autoimmune characterization. As mentioned previously, the disease's autoimmune attack is targeted specifically against the cells lining the bile ducts within the liver.

Despite the accepted autoimmune and genetic aspect of PBC, the clustering of people with PBC in certain regions of the world suggests that one or more as-yet unknown environmental factors may trigger PBC. Once the autoimmune attack on the bile ducts is triggered, the process is not turned off but relentlessly continues until the bile ducts become destroyed and the liver becomes scarred. Many environmental factors have been cited as potentially triggering the autoimmune response that leads to the development of PBC. Such environmental factors include cigarette smoking; tainted well water; certain types of infections, either viruses or bacteria; and some medications, such as interferon (see chapter 12), estrogen, and chlorpromazine, an antipsychotic medication.

Many different types of infections have been implicated as possible triggers or causes of PBC. These include Epstein-Barr virus (EBV); herpes virus, the virus that causes shingles; *Escherichia coli* (E. coli), which can cause urinary tract infections; bacteria similar to the bacteria that causes tuberculosis, known as mycobacteria; chlamydia pneumonia; and retroviruses such as human immunodeficiency virus-1 (HIV-1), which is different from HIV-2, the retrovirus that causes AIDS.

THE SYMPTOMS AND SIGNS OF PBC

There is a wide spectrum of symptoms associated with PBC. At one end of the spectrum, a person with PBC can be asymptomatic (have no symptoms). These people are typically found to have PBC during evaluation of elevated AP and GGTP levels (see chapter 3) found on blood tests. However, some asymptomatic people with PBC have normal levels of AP and GGTP. In these instances, a positive antimitochondrial antibody (AMA) is the sole indication that the disease is present. Up to 60 percent of people discovered to have PBC have no symptoms. Diagnosis in such people has become more common due to routine blood tests that are performed during the course of a regular checkup. Note, however, that most people who are initially asymptomatic eventually do develop symptoms. This occurs in about three to four years from the time of initial diagnosis. However, symptoms can take as long as ten years to manifest. Interestingly, even in advanced stages of PBC, some people will still have no symptoms.

At the other end of the spectrum, a person with PBC may have severe symptoms. People with PBC and liver failure may experience upper gastrointestinal bleeding from esophageal varices, encephalopathy, or ascites. Most people fall somewhere in between these two extremes. In fact, the most typical presentation of PBC is that of relentless fatigue and pruritus (itching).

Fatigue is the most common symptom, occurring in approximately 65 percent of people with PBC. The cause of fatigue in people with PBC is not known, but depression and sleep disorders may be contributing factors. The degree of fatigue does not correlate with the severity of the disease and may be just as debilitating for a person in an early stage of PBC as it is for a person in an advanced stage of PBC.

Pruritus is the second most common symptom, occurring in approximately 55 percent of people with PBC. Generally, the itching becomes worse at night.

The severity of pruritus does not correlate with the severity of PBC. In fact, sometimes itching improves as PBC worsens. Although the cause of pruritus is not known, it can usually be successfully treated using cholestyramine, an orally taken bile-acid binder. Occasionally, itching may become so severe that it becomes an indication for liver transplantation.

Other symptoms associated with PBC may include unexplained weight loss, abdominal discomfort, bone problems, and depression. Urinary tract infections occur in approximately 20 percent of women with PBC. They are typically asymptomatic and may be recurrent. Often, people with PBC will have the symptoms of an associated autoimmune disorder, such as joint pains from rheumatoid arthritis or dry eyes and mouth from Sjögren's syndrome. The treatment of these specific symptoms will be discussed in chapter 20.

On a physical exam, the doctor may find an enlarged liver and spleen. Sometimes the liver is somewhat tender. A person's skin tone may be darker than usual due to excess deposits in the skin of a pigment known as *melanin*. This is a sign of advancing disease. Ironically, these people are often asked where they got their healthy tans. Dark skin tone may sometimes be a sign of jaundice, which is indicative of the final stage of PBC. Another sign of PBC is a condition known as *finger clubbing*—the tips of the fingers become enlarged and rounded like clubs.

There are two distinctive physical findings that occur frequently in people with PBC that immediately alert doctors to arrive at a diagnosis, and thus are considered hallmarks of the disease. The first physical finding is actually of two conditions— *xanthalasmas* and *xanthomas*. These are irregular fatty yellow nodules or patches on the skin due to disturbances in cholesterol metabolism. (They also occur in some people who have markedly elevated cholesterol levels from causes other than PBC.) Xanthalasmas occur in approximately 20 percent of PBC cases and are found around the eyes. Xanthomas commonly occur in the creases of the hands, arms, and legs, or on the elbows and knees. They may be painful and may cause difficulty with movement. Surgical removal is not advised, as they typically recur. Improvement of xanthalasmas formation may occur with medical therapy.

The second distinctive physical trait found in people with PBC is *excoriations* (severe scratch marks associated with breaks in the skin that often bleed) on the body due to intense scratching to relieve pruritus. These excoriations are commonly found in areas of the body that are easily accessible, such as the upper back, chest, and arms. Interestingly, in the later stages of the disease, both of these physical hallmarks of PBC occasionally improve.

DIAGNOSING PBC

PBC may be diagnosed by a combination of the symptoms that a person is experiencing, the physical findings detected on an exam, the results of blood work, the findings of a liver biopsy, and the results from imaging studies. These various diagnostic techniques are discussed below.

Blood Tests

PBC is most often diagnosed when abnormalities are found on blood tests. Usually, an isolated elevated alkaline phosphatase (AP) level is initially discovered. This typically leads to additional blood work testing for the antimitochondrial antibody (AMA). Additionally, cholesterol levels are usually elevated in people with PBC. The following is a discussion of these blood tests.

Liver Function Tests

In people with PBC, the AP and GGTP levels are elevated out of proportion to the transaminase (AST and ALT) levels. Thus, a typical person with PBC may have an AP and GGTP level around ten times the upper limit of normal, while their transaminase levels may be normal or only around one and a half to four times the upper limit of normal. This pattern of blood test abnormalities is referred to as cholestasis, specifically intrahepatic cholestasis. The bilirubin level is usually normal in the early stages of the disease (a condition known as anicteric cholestasis). However, the bilirubin level typically becomes elevated as the disease progresses. For more information concerning these blood tests, see chapter 3.

Autoantibodies

In 1965, it was discovered that people with PBC have an autoantibody known as the antimitochondrial antibody (AMA) present in their blood. This finding greatly advanced the diagnostic accuracy of this disease and allowed doctors to recognize the disease in its earliest and most treatable stages. In 1987, this diagnostic accuracy was further enhanced by the identification and cloning of specific antigens against AMA. The major antigen against AMA was discovered to be a component of *pyruvate dehydrogenase,* an enzyme involved in carbohydrate metabolism.

Approximately 95 percent of people with PBC have evidence of AMA. The finding of an AMA of a titer greater than 1:40 in a person almost always confirms the presence of PBC. The level of AMA is reported in titers, such as a titer of 1:160 or 1:640. However, the level of the titer does not correlate with the severity of the disease nor is it significant in regard to prognosis. A titer of less than 1:40 may not be diagnostic of PBC and may disappear when blood tests are repeated. Rarely, people are discovered to have a positive AMA yet lack all symptoms and have a normal AP and GGTP. It has been found that within approximately ten years, the development of symptoms and elevated AP levels occur. Thus, it is recommended that people who are AMA positive should be followed yearly by a liver specialist. Immunoglobulin M (IgM) is also commonly elevated in people with PBC. Other autoantibodies, such as SMA and ANA, may also be present, although their presence is not necessarily significant. See chapter 11 for more information concerning autoantibodies.

Cholesterol Levels

With PBC, cholesterol levels may become markedly elevated, especially in the later stages of the disease. In fact, levels of cholesterol may reach over 1,000 mg/dl, but there's no need to panic. As it turns out, people with PBC do not have an increased risk of heart disease or hardening of the arteries (atherosclerosis) due to this high cholesterol level. Furthermore, a person cannot reduce this elevated cholesterol level by adhering to a low-cholesterol diet.

Liver Biopsy

In cases of PBC, a liver biopsy (discussed in detail in chapter 5) is necessary in order to determine the extent of damage present and the exact stage of the disease. Furthermore, a liver biopsy confirms the diagnosis, gives an estimate of how long the disease has been present, and provides important information that will assist the doctor in determining appropriate treatment options. As opposed to other liver disorders, PBC has been neatly classified into four distinct stages that can only be determined by a liver biopsy. Stage 1 is characterized by the finding of damaged bile ducts. *Granulomas*—nodules filled with a variety of inflammatory cells—are often detected in this stage. Stage 2 is characterized by the finding of a proliferation of small bile ducts known as *bile ductules*. Stage 3 is characterized by fibrosis, and stage 4 is characterized by cirrhosis. Occasionally, a single specimen from a liver biopsy may show evidence of more than one stage of the disease. In such cases, the most advanced stage present should be considered the correct stage. People may progress through the different stages at varied and largely unpredictable rates. For example, a person may stay in stage 1 for many years and then rapidly progress from stage 2 to stage 3. Or a person may rapidly progress through stage 1 and then stay in stage 2 for many years.

Imaging Studies

Imaging studies generally do not add significant additional information concerning the status of a person diagnosed with PBC. However, imaging studies are important in cases when the diagnosis of PBC is in question, when there is a possible extrahepatic cause for elevated AP and GGTP, such as a bile duct blockage, or when a person is experiencing abdominal pain. As people with PBC are at risk for the development of gallstones, sonograms are useful in cases of abdominal pain. See chapter 3 for more information on imaging studies.

DISORDERS ASSOCIATED WITH PBC

PBC is frequently associated with autoimmune disorders of other organs. As a result, it is often a rheumatologist, dermatologist, or endocrinologist, rather than a liver specialist, who actually discovers that a person has a liver disorder. As many as 84 percent of people with PBC have been found to have an associated auto-immune disorder. The following is a discussion of these autoimmune disorders of organs other than the liver.

Thyroid Disorders

Up to 20 percent of people with PBC have some type of thyroid dysfunction. While the thyroid of a person suffering from PBC may sometimes be overactive (a condition known as hyperthyroidism), an underactive, slow-functioning thyroid (a condition known as hypothyroidism) is more common. Fatigue is a common symptom of hypothyroidism, which may be a contributing factor to the relentless fatigue experienced by many people with PBC. Therefore, it is important for the doctor to search for a thyroid disorder in people with PBC, especially in those who are experiencing fatigue. Treatment with thyroid medication often improves this type of fatigue.

Rheumatologic Disorders

Since many rheumatologic disorders have an autoimmune origin, it is not surprising that there is a high degree of association between rheumatologic disorders and PBC. People with PBC commonly have Sjögren's syndrome, which is characterized by *xerophthalmia* (dry eyes) and *xerostomia* (dry mouth). *Dysphagia* (trouble swallowing) occurs in approximately half of the people who have xerostomia, partly due to a lack of sufficient saliva. People with xerostomia are also at an increased risk for the development of dental cavities. In particularly severe cases, some people may even have difficulty speaking. *Scleroderma,* also common in people with PBC, is a disease characterized by thickening and hardening of the skin and even some internal organs due to excessive collagen deposits. When this disease affects the esophagus, it may cause dysphagia. Rheumatoid arthritis, which is characterized by joint aches and joint deformities, can also be seen in people with PBC.

Raynaud's phenomenon is another rheumatologic disorder that commonly occurs in people with PBC. Raynaud's phenomenon typically causes the fingertips to turn blue and become numb when exposed to cold weather or when the person is exposed to emotional stress. Sometimes this phenomenon is seen in conjunction with the following: excessive calcium deposits in parts of the body, known as *calcinosis*; abnormal movements of the esophagus, known as *esophageal dysmotility*; *scleroderma* of the fingers and toes, known as *sclerodactyly*; and small, thin, red spots on the skin or mucous membranes, known as *telangiectasia.* This group of disorders is collectively known as the *CREST syndrome* (Calcinosis, Raynaud's, Esophageal dysmotility, Sclerodactyly, Telangiectasia).

Finally, systemic lupus erythematosus (SLE), a disease affecting multiple organs and characterized by fever, skin rash, and arthritis, may also occur in people with PBC.

Dermatological Disorders

Many skin disorders are associated with PBC. As previously discussed, pruritus is the second most common manifestation of PBC. Xanthomas are also commonly seen in people with PBC. Vitiligo, a condition manifested by smooth, nonpigmented patches on various parts of the body, is believed to be an autoimmune phenomenon and is common in people with PBC.

Kidney Disorders

Recurrent urinary tract infections (UTIs) occur in approximately 20 percent of women with PBC. These UTIs are often asymptomatic and do not require antibiotic therapy. Other kidney disorders, such as renal tubular acidosis, have been noted to occur in people with PBC, but are usually not clinically significant.

Lung Disorders

Sarcoidosis is a disease characterized by the formation of granulomas in the lungs, skin, liver, lymph nodes, and bones. This disease resembles primary biliary cirrhosis (PBC) in that both diseases are characterized by the formation of granulomas. PBC and sarcoidosis occasionally coexist together.

Gastrointestinal Disorders

Many gastrointestinal disorders, including gallstones and diarrhea, occur in people with PBC. Right upper quadrant abdominal pain (pain over the area of the liver) has been noted in approximately 17 percent of PBC cases. The degree of pain typically does not correlate with the severity of PBC. Also, the cause of the pain is usually not discovered. In fact, in many cases, the pain resolves without any treatment at all.

Gallstones

Approximately 30 to 40 percent of people with PBC have gallstones. They are usually discovered by chance when a sonogram is obtained as part of an initial evaluation. Thus, while gallstones are the cause of right upper quadrant pain in some people with PBC, in others, they do not cause any symptoms at all.

Diarrhea

Diarrhea may have many causes in people with PBC. First, diarrhea may be a side effect of some medications used in the treatment of PBC, such as URSO and colchicine, or of cholestyramine, a medication used to control itching. (These medications are discussed in more detail further on in this chapter.)

Second, people in advanced stages of PBC who are cholestatic are unable to absorb fats efficiently, a condition known as fat malabsorption. This is caused by a failure to secrete bile salts necessary to absorb fats due to bile duct destruction that occurs within the livers of people with PBC. The fats that these people are unable to absorb are eliminated from their bodies in their stools, which tend to be light in color, loose in consistency, and frothy in texture. These stools are characterized by their ability to float on top of water, and it commonly takes as many as five attempts to flush them down the toilet. This type of stool is known as *steatorrhea.* People with fat malabsorption are unable to absorb the fat-soluble vitamins—A, D, E, and K. Thus, it is usually necessary to correct these vitamin deficiencies promptly. Other symptoms of fat malabsorption and how to treat it are discussed in chapter 23.

Third, an autoimmune disease known as celiac sprue can be the cause of diarrhea in people with PBC. *Celiac sprue* is a disease characterized by an inability to absorb *gluten* (a protein found in wheat, rye, oats, and barley). This is known as a *gluten intolerance.* Celiac sprue is approximately ten times more likely to occur in people with PBC than among members of the general population. The association of PBC with celiac sprue is important to recognize since people suffering from these diseases jointly can obtain relief from diarrhea and its associated weight loss by adhering to a gluten-free diet.

Diarrhea can also be due to ulcerative colitis, which may require treatment with prednisone, a steroid medication, or diarrhea may be due to a pancreatic disorder, which requires treatment with pancreatic enzyme replacement. Therefore, it is important to accurately diagnose why a person with PBC has diarrhea, as the treatment differs greatly dependent upon the cause.

Bone Disorders

People with PBC often suffer from severe bone problems, including bone loss, pain, and fractures. These bone disorders are often a source of great suffering and can severely disable a person. In fact, severe bone disease coupled with recurrent bone fractures in people with PBC may be an indication that liver transplantation is warranted.

Osteoporosis (a decrease in bone quantity) is the most common bone abnormality occurring in people with PBC. Some people with PBC may also have a genetic susceptibility for the development of osteoporosis. In others, the degree of osteoporosis correlates with the severity and duration of jaundice, possibly due to malabsorption of vitamin D, a fat-soluble vitamin. The hip and spine are the areas of the body most commonly affected by osteoporosis. Thus, people with osteoporosis are susceptible to hip fractures and often suffer from bad backs. It has been demonstrated that, after liver transplantation, osteoporosis often improves in people with PBC. Sometimes osteoporosis is the initial reason a person seeks medical care. An elevated AP in a person with osteoporosis without bone fractures should raise the physician's suspicion of PBC. The medical treatment of osteoporosis is discussed in chapter 20.

Osteomalacia—a softening of the bones similar to rickets—can also occur in people with PBC, but it is relatively rare. This condition is caused by a deficiency of vitamin D. Since people in advanced stages of PBC often have difficulty absorbing vitamin D, they are at risk for osteomalacia.

Since vitamin D deficiency results in calcium malabsorption, supplementation with vitamin D and calcium is recommended for people with either of these two bone conditions. In fact, vitamin D and calcium supplementation is recommended for all people with PBC. Note, however, that these supplements have not been shown to significantly prevent bone disease in people with PBC. Other potential therapies relating to bone disorders will be discussed in chapter 20.

FAT-SOLUBLE VITAMIN DEFICIENCIES

Fat-soluble vitamins include vitamins A, D, E, and K. They are absorbed by the body only with the help of fats or bile. In people with PBC, fat-soluble vitamins are usually poorly absorbed (malabsorbed) by the body due to impaired bile acid delivery to the duodenum. In such cases, vitamin supplementation is necessary. Vitamin A deficiency is noted most commonly, occurring in approximately 20 percent of people with PBC. It occurs more frequently in advanced stages of the disease, when cholestasis is worse. Occasionally it causes night blindness, but is typically asymptomatic. People with PBC are advised to take 25,000 to 50,000 IU of vitamin A two to three times per week.

Vitamin D deficiency is the next most common fat-soluble vitamin deficiency to occur. As discussed in the previous section, a vitamin D deficiency results in calcium malabsorption, and vitamin D and calcium supplementation is recommended for all people with PBC.

Vitamin E deficiency is rare and usually without symptoms, but replacement is recommended in all people with PBC. When symptoms do occur, a disturbance or a feeling of imbalance in walking, known as ataxia, may occur. Symptoms are more common in children than in adults with a vitamin E deficiency.

Vitamin K is used by the liver to manufacture the protein prothrombin. Prothrombin, as discussed in chapter 3, is essential for proper blood clotting. Without vitamin K, people would hemorrhage (continue bleeding) as the result of a cut. Vitamin K deficiency may sometimes be corrected by taking water-soluble vitamin K orally (5 to 10 mg per day). People with advanced stages of PBC tend to have a vitamin K deficiency that is impossible to correct with oral replacement. Vitamin K given by the subcutaneous route on a monthly basis should therefore be utilized. In situations where bleeding is a potential risk (such as for those people requiring surgery), intravenous infusions of fresh frozen plasma (FFP) must be given to temporarily correct this problem. Fat-soluble vitamins are discussed in more detail in chapter 23.

TREATMENT OF PBC

Since PBC cannot be cured, treatment is aimed at slowing the progression of the disease and controlling its symptoms. Treatment of the symptoms associated with

PBC will be discussed in chapter 20. The following is a discussion of the treatment of the disease itself. People with PBC who do not have any symptoms also have a decreased life expectancy, and progression to cirrhosis may occur prior to the development of any symptoms. Therefore, people suffering from symptoms as well as people who are asymptomatic require treatment in an attempt to retard disease progression. People with PBC may be treated with a single medication, a combination of medications, or will need to undergo a liver transplantation.

Single Medications

A variety of medications has been evaluated for the treatment of people with PBC, some of which have been found to be beneficial. Unfortunately, the adverse side effects of these drugs outweigh the potential benefits that they provide. Examples include prednisone, a steroid, which may accelerate the rate of bone loss associated with PBC; cyclosporine, an antirejection drug, which may cause high blood pressure and kidney dysfunction; and chlorambucil, a chemotherapy drug, which may be toxic to bone marrow.

Medications that have been studied but have not been shown to provide significant benefits to people with PBC include D-penicillamine, a copper-binding drug; azathioprine, an antirejection, immunosuppressive drug; and malotolate, an anti-inflammatory drug. The herb silymarin has also been tried on people with PBC, but did not appear to be of any benefit (see chapter 21 for more information on herbs).

There are other medications that appear to benefit people with PBC but are undergoing evaluation to confirm their effects. Examples of such medications include S-Adenosy-L-Methionine (SAMe), a type of amino acid; and tacrolimus, an antirejection, immunosuppressive drug.

Some investigators believe that PBC is caused by a type of virus, known as a retrovirus such as HIV-1. This retrovirus is different than HIV-2, the retrovirus that causes AIDS. Based on the assumption that PBC is caused by a retrovirus, pilot studies on people with PBC using antiretroviral therapy with either lamivudine or Combivir (lamivudine 150 mg plus zidovudine 300 mg, manufactured by GlaxoWellcome) are under way. Preliminary results suggest that Combivir may have some beneficial effects on people with PBC. Further study is anticipated on this provocative concept.

At present, the most effective drug treatment for PBC appears to be with one of the following three medications—ursodeoxycholic acid, methotrexate, or colchicine. The following is a discussion of these medications.

Ursodeoxycholic Acid

Ursodeoxycholic acid (also known as UDCA or ursodiol) is the drug most commonly used to treat PBC. In fact, it is the only drug that is FDA approved for the treatment of PBC. Ursodeoxycholic acid was initially found to be beneficial for people with PBC in the early 1980s and became FDA approved in 1998. It is manufactured by Axcan Pharma under the brand name URSO. URSO 250 is taken with food in oral pill form at a dosage of 13 to 15 mg/kg of body weight each day, administered in four divided doses. Each pill is 250 mg, making a typical dose two tablets twice a day. In November 2004, URSO 500 mg (URSO Forte) will be available. Therefore, the typical dose will now be one tablet twice daily. Actigall is another brand name for ursodeoxycholic acid. Actigall is marketed by Novartis in tablets of 300 mg. This drug is not FDA approved for the treatment of PBC; therefore, its use is considered "off label." Generic ursodeoxycholic acid is also available and known as ursodiol.

Ursodeoxycholic acid (UDCA) is a naturally occurring bile acid, but, unlike many other bile acids in the body, it is not toxic to the liver. It is found in humans in small quantities, but is found in large quantities in bears. UDCA was initially used to dissolve gallstones, a treatment that is no longer common. The exact mechanism by which ursodeoxycholic acid works in people with PBC is not known. However, it has been established that increasing the amount of UDCA in the body will generally decrease the amount of liver-toxic bile acids in the body. This, in turn, should diminish or prevent destruction of bile duct cells. In fact, in some studies, people treated with ursodeoxycholic acid have been shown to have decreased bile duct destruction. However, other studies have shown that UDCA does not prevent bile duct destruction. Instead, UDCA appears only to protect against the consequences of bile duct destruction. This finding explains that while UDCA can delay, it does not prevent, the progression of disease to cirrhosis in people with PBC.

UDCA provides significant benefits to people with PBC. Levels of liver function tests, IgM, AMA, and cholesterol typically show notable improvement. People find that UDCA, on occasion, relieves some of the symptoms associated with PBC, such as fatigue and itching. Most important, ursodeoxycholic acid has been found to slow the progression of PBC and to delay the occurrence of cirrhosis. Thus, people with PBC who are treated with UDCA have been found to live longer, have less liver-related complications, and need liver transplants less often when compared with those who are not treated with UDCA. UDCA may also have the additional benefit of decreasing the recurrence of colon polyps, although this finding needs to be confirmed by further studies.

Side effects of UDCA are minimal. Most studies have indicated that less than 3 percent of people develop adverse side effects from UDCA. When side effects are experienced, they include diarrhea, decreased white blood cell count, elevated glucose levels, elevated creatinine levels, peptic ulcers, and skin rashes. Overall, UDCA is a well-tolerated, safe, and effective medicine for the treatment of people with PBC.

The beneficial effects of ursodeoxycholic acid are experienced by approximately 80 percent of people with PBC who use this medication. These effects are most likely to occur the sooner a person is treated, for example, when the person is treated during the first or second stage of the disease. Higher doses than are currently used may work even better, but further study is needed. People who have PBC who do not respond to UDCA should consider combination therapy involving

UDCA with another medication, or they should consider trying a different medication. People whose bilirubin levels continue to worsen despite treatment with UDCA or any other medication should be evaluated for liver transplantation.

Methotrexate

Methotrexate is an immunosuppressive drug, meaning that it suppresses the immune system. When people with PBC are treated with an oral dose of 15 mg per week (0.25mg/kg body weight orally per week), liver enzyme levels have been shown to improve or decrease. In some people, fatigue and itching are relieved. Some studies have shown that methotrexate, taken alone or in combination with other drugs, may improve liver inflammation and intrahepatic bile duct injury. In other studies, while methotrexate was found to improve LFT abnormalities, it did not prevent the progression of disease or improve patient survival. Methotrexate may cause adverse side effects, and this serves to limit the drug's usefulness. In fact, in one study, approximately 14 percent of people taking methotrexate developed severe but reversible lung inflammation. The B vitamin folate (1mg per day) should be taken with methotrexate, since this medication may deplete the body's folate stores. Further studies are currently being conducted regarding the treatment with methotrexate in combination with other medications.

Colchicine

Colchicine is a medication with anti-inflammatory properties. It has been purported to reduce scarring (fibrosis, not cirrhosis) in some people with liver disease and, as such, may be said to have antifibrotic properties. Liver enzymes tend to improve in people with PBC who are treated with colchicine in two daily oral dosages of 0.6 mg each. However, liver enzymes do not improve to the same degree as with ursodeoxycholic acid or methotrexate. Colchicine has not been shown to reduce liver inflammation or bile duct damage. Colchicine's side effects are minimal. The most common of these, diarrhea, occurs in less than 10 percent of the cases. This symptom usually resolves once the dose of colchicine is decreased to once per day. Some researchers believe that colchicine may slow the rate of progression of PBC. Although the benefits of treatment with colchicine do not appear to be as substantial as those derived from treatment with ursodeoxycholic acid, colchicine is useful as an alternative treatment in those rare people who cannot tolerate ursodeoxycholic acid. Furthermore, colchicine may prove to be a useful additional therapy to ursodeoxycholic acid.

Medication Combinations

Many drug combinations have been tried in the treatment of people with PBC. The rationale is that the combined effect of two or more drugs, each with different mechanisms of action, might prove *synergistic* (complementary). Promising combinations that have been tested include ursodeoxycholic acid and methotrexate; ursodeoxycholic acid and colchicine; ursodeoxycholic acid and prednisone;

ursodeoxycholic acid and budesonide, a steroid similar to prednisone that also worsens bone problems in people with PBC; ursodeoxycholic acid, colchicine, and methotrexate; and ursodeoxycholic acid and mycophenolate mofetil, an immunosuppressive medication often used to prevent liver transplant rejection. While some studies using these combinations have shown some beneficial results in people with PBC, additional comprehensive studies involving larger groups must be done before any definitive conclusions can be drawn.

Liver Transplantation

Medical therapy has been shown to slow the progression of PBC, thereby delaying the need for a liver transplant in some people with PBC. Nonetheless, people with PBC continue to advance to cirrhosis and its complications or continue to have symptoms associated with PBC, such as severe fatigue, osteoporosis, or uncontrollable pruritus, any of which may render a liver transplant necessary. PBC has been one of the most common indications for liver transplantation in the United States. Occasionally, PBC has been demonstrated to recur in the new liver. When it does recur, progression is very slow. In general, people with PBC do very well after liver transplantation with excellent long-term survival. See chapter 22 for a complete discussion of this topic.

LIVER DISEASES THAT RESEMBLE PBC

Three other liver diseases resemble PBC in some respects. They are autoimmune cholangitis, primary sclerosing cholangitis, and PBC with "autoimmune features," also known as an overlap syndrome. As treatment and prognosis may differ in these diseases, it is most important to distinguish between them and PBC.

Autoimmune Cholangitis

Autoimmune cholangitis is characterized by liver enzyme abnormalities suggestive of cholestasis and biopsy results resembling those of people with PBC. However, the autoantibody AMA is not present in the blood of people with autoimmune cholangitis. Instead, other autoantibodies, namely ANA and SMA, are found in the blood. Accordingly, this disease is often referred to as "AMA-negative PBC." Some studies demonstrate that people with autoimmune cholangitis benefit from treatment with prednisone, either alone or in combination with azathioprine (see chapter 14). Other studies have found a greater benefit from the use of ursodeoxycholic acid on this group of people. In fact, there was no difference in the response to UDCA therapy in people with autoimmune cholangitis when compared to people with PBC who are AMA positive. Thus, it is usually more prudent to treat people with autoimmune cholangitis with UDCA, especially in light of the fact that prednisone therapy worsens osteoporosis in people with PBC.

Whether autoimmune cholangitis is a totally separate entity from PBC or simply PBC without the manifestation of a positive AMA on blood tests remains a subject of ongoing debate and research.

Primary Sclerosing Cholangitis

Primary sclerosing cholangitis (PSC) like PBC is a chronic cholestatic liver disease that results in damage to the intrahepatic bile ducts. Unlike PBC, PSC also results in damage to the extrahepatic bile ducts. Also unlike PBC, most people with PSC are male, and approximately two-thirds of people with PSC have an inflammatory disease of the colon (the large intestine) known as ulcerative colitis. Symptoms of PBC and PSC may overlap, as fatigue and itching are common to people with either disease.

There is a drastic difference in the way that the two diseases are diagnosed. Unlike the presence of AMA as a diagnostic marker in people with PBC, there are no diagnostic autoantibodies that occur in people with PSC. Instead, PSC requires a special procedure called an *endoscopic retrograde cholangiopancreatography (ERCP)* to be done in order for the disease to be accurately diagnosed. In an ERCP, a lighted tube (a special endoscope) is inserted into the patient's mouth and then is snaked through the stomach and into the small intestine. There is a tiny opening in the small intestine called the *ampulla of vater* that leads to the extrahepatic bile ducts. A thin wire is inserted into this opening and then into the extrahepatic bile ducts. This wire allows access into the extrahepatic bile ducts so that contrast dye needed to visualize the bile ducts on an X ray can be injected. An X ray can then be taken of the extrahepatic bile ducts to determine if they have suffered damage, thus making a diagnosis of PSC.

Complications from PBC and PSC are somewhat different. Extrahepatic bile duct blockages, due to bile duct damage and bile duct stones, occur in PSC but not in PBC, as only the intrahepatic bile ducts are damaged in PBC.

Medical treatment of people with PSC has been somewhat disappointing. Drugs that have been used with success in treating PBC patients have not shown an ability to slow the progression of PSC or to prevent its complications. Nor have these drugs exhibited much success at prolonging the survival of people with PSC. Liver transplantation is the best option for people with advanced PSC. For these people, results have been good with approximately 80 percent of transplant recipients surviving at least five years.

Primary Biliary Cirrhosis (PBC) and Autoimmune Hepatitis (AIH)— The "Overlap Syndrome"

About 8 to 12 percent of people who have PBC also have AIH. These people have the clinical features of AIH, such as very elevated transaminases and the autoantibodies of AIH—antinuclear antibody (ANA) and/or smooth muscle antibody (SMA). However, they also have the presence of antimitochondrial antibody (AMA) in their blood, which is diagnostic of PBC. It has been suggested by some experts that those people who test positive for AMA should not be considered to have AIH. This is because there is such a strong association of AMA with PBC. In fact, it has been demonstrated that features of AIH in people with PBC may be transient. Furthermore, response to UDCA appears to be similar in people with PBC with and without features of AIH.

It is important to always test people with the AIH/PBC overlap syndrome for the autoantibody-liver-kidney-microsomal antibody (anti-LKMAb). If anti-LKMAb is positive, the diagnosis of AIH is more likely. There is also a small group of people who are found to have AMA in their blood and who genuinely have AIH. These individuals have very elevated transaminase levels with minimal elevation of alkaline phosphatase levels. AMA titers typically are low, less than 1:160 in most cases. These people typically respond well to conventional treatment for AIH. See chapter 14 for more information about AIH.

THE NATURAL HISTORY AND PROGNOSIS FOR THOSE WITH PBC

PBC is a slowly progressive disease with a very long natural history. The average time span from initial diagnosis to death from complications of the disease is approximately twenty years. However, the rate of disease progression is quite variable, and therefore the natural history of PBC is typically unpredictable. Furthermore, the natural history of the disease may be altered by therapy. As noted above, ursodeoxycholic acid can slow down the progression of PBC and, therefore, can prolong a person's life.

Untreated asymptomatic people live approximately five years longer as compared to untreated symptomatic people—approximately ten to seventeen years versus approximately seven to twelve years, respectively. Some researchers have shown that asymptomatic people with associated autoimmune disorders have a worse prognosis than asymptomatic people without associated autoimmune disorders.

Once a person's bilirubin level becomes elevated, or once signs of liver failure—ascites, bleeding esophageal varices, and/or encephalopathy—appear, a poor prognosis is universal. Some studies have found that most people with PBC live less than two years once their bilirubin levels begin to progressively rise. Other studies have found that one-third of people will die within a year of the initial episode of bleeding esophageal varices. In any case, people with a poor prognosis should be promptly referred for liver transplantation. Liver transplantation is the only treatment that significantly alters the natural history of PBC. See chapter 22 for more information on liver transplantation.

PBC AND CANCER RISK

It is estimated that about 1 to 2 percent of deaths due to cirrhosis in the United States occur in people with PBC. Liver cancer can develop in anyone with cirrhosis, regardless of the cause. However, the chance that a person in the final stage of PBC (stage 4-cirrhosis) will develop liver cancer is rather low. In fact, a person in the final stage of PBC is much less likely to develop liver cancer than a person with chronic hepatitis B, chronic hepatitis C, or hemochromatosis. It has been estimated that only approximately 2 to 6 percent of people with PBC will develop liver cancer. Note, however, that the incidence of liver cancer among people with PBC appears to be significantly higher in men than in women. Furthermore, liver cancer has been shown to be a common cause of death in men with PBC, yet an uncommon cause of death in women with PBC. It has also been shown that an older age at the time of diagnosis, the male gender, and a history of a blood transfusion are all factors associated with an increased likelihood of the development of liver cancer. Thus, people, especially older males, in the final stage of PBC should probably undergo biannual screening for liver cancer. See chapter 19 for more information on liver cancer.

Some studies, although not all, have found an increased incidence of other cancers in people with PBC, especially breast cancer. However, since the likelihood that a person with PBC will develop a cancer outside of the liver is quite low, routine cancer surveillance—more diligent than that recommended for the general populations—is not mandatory.

CONCLUSION

In this chapter, you learned that PBC is a type of chronic cholestatic liver disease characterized by numerous associations with other autoimmune disorders that may affect virtually every organ in the body. PBC can have a varied presentation and unpredictable natural history. Unlike damaged liver cells, damaged bile ducts cannot regenerate. Consequently, there are no medical treatments that can cure PBC. However, progress in the treatment of PBC has been made, as some medications, in particular URSO, have been shown to slow the progression of the disease and to prolong survival. Unfortunately, some people do not respond to certain medications even though others with similar characteristics do. Future research is aimed at resolving this paradox and at finding better medical treatments.

The next chapter discusses nonalcoholic fatty liver disease and its two stages, a fatty liver and nonalcoholic *steatohepatitis* (NASH). Fatty liver is a disease that is commonly, but not always, associated with overweight people and has similarities to a fatty liver, but with the potential to lead to a serious outcome.

Sixteen

NONALCOHOLIC FATTY LIVER DISEASE

Muriel, a fifty-year-old paralegal, decided to join a gym to help her lose the thirty pounds she had gained since last year. When she joined, she received a free nutritional consultation and cholesterol check. Muriel was shocked to learn that her cholesterol level was greater than 300 mg/dl (normal levels being less than 200 mg/dl). Having just joined an HMO, she decided to make an appointment for an initial consultation. The doctor who examined Muriel found her liver to be somewhat enlarged. He drew some additional blood tests and gave her a low-cholesterol diet to follow based on his review of the cholesterol-level report that Muriel had obtained from the gym.

Muriel was feeling upbeat until she received a phone call a week later from the doctor, who informed her that her sugar levels were very high and that the blood work related to her liver (LFTs) was abnormal. The doctor told Muriel that she probably had diabetes and that she would need to begin taking medication as part of her treatment if additional testing confirmed this diagnosis. In addition, he advised her not to drink any more alcohol and to have her liver function tests (LFTs) repeated in approximately one week. (Apparently, the doctor suspected that Muriel had alcoholic liver disease.) Muriel was somewhat puzzled. The last alcoholic drink she had had was over three months ago at her nephew's bar mitzvah.

When Muriel returned to the doctor's office the following week to be retested, she stressed to him that she rarely consumed alcohol. However, the tests were abnormal again. More in-depth conversations with Muriel and her husband confirmed that she drank alcohol only on rare occasions. A sonogram of Muriel's liver revealed that she had a fatty liver. She was placed on a weight-reduction diet that

*was also low in cholesterol and was advised to continue her exercise
program at the gym. Over the course of the next few months, Muriel
lost twenty pounds. The LFTs were repeated, and this time they were
normal. In addition, Muriel's diabetes improved so much that she no
longer required medication for its treatment. The doctor concluded
that Muriel's elevated LFTs had been due to nonalcoholic fatty liver
disease (NAFLD).*

NAFLD is the most common liver disease in the United States. The two
stages of NAFLD—a fatty liver and NASH (nonalcoholic steatohepatitis)—will be discussed in this chapter. NAFLD is believed to be a disorder of insulin resistance. The definition of insulin resistance and how it relates to NAFLD will be discussed. Since being overweight is the most common cause of NAFLD, the definitions of overweight, obesity, and morbid obesity, will be provided. Some possible causes of fat accumulation in the liver, other than NAFLD, will also be discussed. The type of person who is at risk for development of these conditions will be identified, and the associated symptoms and physical findings will be described. The natural history and prognosis of a person with either a fatty liver or NASH will also be addressed. Finally, treatment options will be reviewed.

AN OVERVIEW OF NONALCOHOLIC FATTY LIVER DISEASE (NAFLD)

Nonalcoholic fatty liver disease is the most common liver disease in the United States. It consists of two stages—a fatty liver and nonalcoholic steatohepatitis (NASH). The only way to distinguish between these two stages is by looking at a sample of liver tissue under a microscope after a liver biopsy has been performed.

The medical term for a fatty liver is *hepatic* (liver) *steatosis* (fat). A fatty liver is considered a benign (harmless) condition characterized by fat deposits in liver cells (hepatocytes). This is a reversible condition and does not have the potential to lead to cirrhosis, liver failure, or liver cancer.

NASH is when a fatty liver has progressed to something worse—namely, inflammation (*steatohepatitis*) and scarring (*steatonecrosis*) of the liver. Unlike a fatty liver, NASH is not considered a harmless condition, but rather a liver disease with the potential to cause cirrhosis, liver failure, and liver cancer.

The reason that NAFLD is prefaced by the word *nonalcoholic* is because the results of liver biopsies from people with NAFLD are frequently identical to those from people with alcoholic liver disease. Yet people with NAFLD do not have a history of excessive alcohol use. "Excessive use" is commonly defined as greater than 80 grams per day for men and greater than 20 grams per day for women. (See chapter 17 for more information about alcohol and the liver.)

Medical authorities currently believe that most cases of NAFLD are caused by a condition known as insulin resistance. But, more about this later in the chapter. People with type 2 diabetes (adult onset diabetes), obese people, and people with hypertriglyceridemia (high level of fats [triglycerides] in the blood) are at risk for getting NAFLD. Excessive weight and an unhealthy diet, especially one high in fats and sugars, greatly increase the likelihood of someone getting NAFLD. A sedentary lifestyle will probably increase one's chance of getting NAFLD. Contrarily, regular exercise may reduce one's chances of getting NAFLD.

Now that you have a general idea of what NAFLD is, it will be easier to understand this chapter. Keep in mind two important points. First, NAFLD is an evolving disease and much research is going on in connection with it. Thus, there is some disagreement within the medical community as to the characteristics of NAFLD. And second, the terms *fatty liver, NASH,* and *NAFLD* are sometimes incorrectly interchanged and confused with one another. So, just remember, if you have either a fatty liver or NASH, by definition you have NAFLD.

INSULIN RESISTANCE AND NAFLD

Emerging trends in the study of NAFLD have supported the concept that most people who develop NAFLD have an *insulin resistance. Insulin* is an important hormone made by the pancreas. Insulin is released into the bloodstream in response to elevated *glucose* (blood sugar) levels that occur, for example, after eating a meal. Insulin keeps the glucose levels from becoming too elevated. To do this, insulin pushes glucose out of the bloodstream and into the cells of the body. The cells that are mainly involved with insulin are the fat, muscle, and liver cells (hepatocytes). When these cells receive glucose, it enables them to convert it to energy. When glucose is not metabolized properly (when the cells are insulin resistant), energy production is diminished, resulting in fatigue.

On the surface of the cells are little doors known medically as "insulin receptors." These doors (receptors) regulate the entrance of glucose into cells by opening and closing. People who are insulin resistant cannot utilize insulin efficiently. As such, they have poorly functioning cell doors, some of which open sluggishly and some of which do not open at all. With less doors open, glucose is unable to enter the cells and therefore accumulates in the blood. In order to try to clear excess glucose from the blood, the body signals the pancreas to produce additional insulin. This results in an overabundance of insulin in the blood, a condition referred to as *hyperinsulinemia.* By a complex mechanism, high levels of insulin in the blood also cause hypertriglyceridemia. This in turn causes fatty acids to be deposited in the liver. The result of all of these events—NAFLD! Approximately 10 to 25 percent of the population is insulin resistant, and almost all people with NAFLD are insulin resistant. However, it is believed that only a small percentage of people who are insulin resistant have NAFLD.

People who are overweight are more likely to show signs of insulin resistance than people who are of normal weight. But keep in mind that a sedentary lifestyle and a diet rich in sugars and fat may promote insulin resistance even among people who are not overweight. Thus, NAFLD can occur even in people of normal body weight. In fact, it is thought that most people with NAFLD have insulin resistance independent of weight.

It has been found that approximately 70 percent of diabetic people have some form of NAFLD and that approximately 5 to 20 percent of people with diabetes have cirrhosis due to NASH. In fact, diabetes in itself is believed to be a risk factor for development of cirrhosis.

THE "METABOLIC SYNDROME"

The combination of the findings of obesity, hyperinsulinemia, insulin resistance, diabetes, hypertriglyceridemia, and hypertension has been referred to as a *metabolic syndrome* or *syndrome X*. Recent research has determined that people with syndrome X also have a liver disease. NAFLD appears to be the liver component of this syndrome. In fact, people with syndrome X often have more advanced forms of NAFLD—for example, fibrosis or cirrhosis.

WHAT IS NAFLD?

People who are overweight are more likely to show signs of insulin resistance than people who are of normal weight. When a person gains weight, fat can accumulate everywhere on the body, including within the liver. As the term *fatty liver* suggests, a person can develop a liver that looks something like a rasher of raw bacon! In its worst-case scenario—in a morbidly obese person—almost the entire liver may become comprised of fat. This is in contrast to a person of normal weight, whose liver is usually (but not always) made up of less than 5 percent fat. The reason this statement is qualified by "but not always" is because a sedentary lifestyle and a diet rich in sugars and fat may lead to insulin resistance, and thus a fatty liver, even in nonoverweight people. Thus, although not as common, NAFLD can occur even in people of normal body weight.

Obesity-related NAFLD is most frequently seen in people who have central or abdominal obesity. Many people who have central obesity are insulin resistant and have NAFLD despite having a normal BMI. This demonstrates that the distribution of body fat is probably more important in the development of NAFLD than the total amount of fat on the body.

WHO IS AT RISK FOR NAFLD?

The association between fat accumulation in the liver and cirrhosis has been recognized for centuries. However, it was not until 1980 that the term nonalcoholic steatohepatitis was coined to describe a condition characterized by liver inflammation and damage occurring in people with a fatty liver who do not drink excessive quantities of alcohol. At the time NASH was initially described, the typical person diagnosed with this liver disease was a middle-aged, obese woman with noninsulin-dependent diabetes (also known as type 2 diabetes) and *hyperlipidemia*—high

How Is Obesity Defined?

In order to understand NAFLD and to appreciate how common it is in the United States, you will need to know how obesity is defined. Obesity is usually defined by a calculation known as the *body mass index (BMI)*. The BMI is calculated by dividing a person's weight in kilograms by his height in meters squared (kg/m^2). In the nonmetric system, BMI is calculated by dividing a person's weight in pounds by his height in inches squared and multiplying this number by 703 [BMI = (lbs/inches^2) x 703].

In adults, normal weight is defined as a BMI between 20 and 24.9, overweight from 25 to 29.9, obese between 30 and 39.9, and morbidly obese 40 and over. For example, a five foot three inch women is considered overweight at a weight of 141 pounds (BMI 25) and obese at a weight of 169 pounds (BMI 30). A man who is five foot nine inches is considered overweight at 169 pounds (BMI 25) and obese at 203 pounds (BMI 30).

The BMI ranges were conceived based on the effect that body weight has on certain diseases, primarily cardiovascular disease, high blood pressure (hypertension), diabetes, and premature death. It has been found that as BMI increases, the risk of the aforementioned diseases increases. Similarly, it has been determined that as the BMI increases, the risk of having NAFLD increases.

Some additional points about BMI need to be noted. First, BMI does not take into consideration a person's bone structure (small, medium, or large boned) or a person's muscularity. A large-boned bodybuilder may have a BMI of 35, falling into the obese category, even though his percentage of body fat may be very low. Thus, in many instances BMI is a poor estimate of body fat content. Second, the relation between BMI and the degree of fat varies with age and gender. Thus, at a given BMI, women and older people have a higher percentage of body fat than men and younger people, respectively.

Obesity can also be defined according to the distribution of fat on one's body. Fat is sometimes distributed predominantly to the hip area, known as a pear-shaped distribution; this occurs more commonly in women than in men. Other times it is distributed mainly to the abdominal area, known as an apple-shaped distribution (or as either abdominal obesity or central obesity); this occurs more commonly in men than in women. Abdominal obesity is defined as a waist circumference greater than 40 inches (102 centimeters) for men and 35 inches (88 centimeters) for women. Abdominal obesity is the type of obesity most commonly seen in people with NAFLD. Please refer to chapter 23 to learn more about obesity.

blood levels of triglycerides and cholesterol. However, as previously discussed, it is now recognized that NAFLD is not gender specific: It may occur at any age, and it often occurs in people who are not overweight, not diabetic, and not hyperlipidemic. In fact, some researchers believe that NAFLD is more common in men and that female hormones (estrogens) may act to protect a person from getting NAFLD. This theory is supported by the finding that NAFLD is more common among postmenopausal women than premenopausal women and is more common in postmenopausal women who do not receive estrogen replacement than in those who do.

People with NAFLD are typically overweight or obese. However, it is recognized that not all obese people have NAFLD and that not all people with NAFLD are obese. Some researchers have shown that obesity may increase the risk of developing NAFLD, particularly in cases where a person is exposed to another liver toxin (hepatotoxin), such as alcohol. In fact, it appears that obesity puts one at risk of developing alcohol-related liver disease. Thus, it is once again recommended that all people with any liver disease should avoid alcohol intake. Similarly, it appears that obesity increases the likelihood of liver enzyme elevations in people exposed to certain hepatotoxic (toxic to the liver) chemicals or medications. It is important to apprise your doctor of all the medications that you are taking (both prescribed and over the counter) and to inform him of any chemicals that you have been exposed to in the recent past.

High triglyceride levels (hypertriglyceridemia) are frequently found in people with NAFLD. However, whether hypertriglyceridemia causes NAFLD or whether NAFLD causes hypertriglyceridemia is not known. One study showed that people with triglyceride levels greater than 200 mg/dl are three times more likely to have NAFLD than people with normal triglyceride levels. Furthermore, this study found that people with low high-density lipoprotein (HDL) cholesterol levels are twice as likely to have NAFLD as people with normal HDLs.

As noted above, it has been found that approximately 70 percent of diabetic people have some form of NAFLD and that approximately 5 to 20 percent of people with diabetes have cirrhosis due to NASH. All people with type 2 diabetes should be aware that they are at high risk for NAFLD.

NAFLD has been found to run in some families, suggesting a genetic component to this disease. In fact, exciting new research has raised the possibility that NAFLD may be due to a gene mutation. Studies in this area have been limited, but they are ongoing.

THE PREVALENCE OF NAFLD

While the exact prevalence of NAFLD is unknown, it is believed to be the most common liver disease in the United States. It has been estimated that approximately 3 percent of the U.S. population have NASH and that 20 percent has a fatty liver. Furthermore, NAFLD is estimated to account for approximately 25 percent of all cases of liver disease in the United States.

There has been an alarming increase in the prevalence and severity of obesity in the United States in recent years. Why is this of grave concern? It is estimated that approximately one-third of Americans are obese and that approximately 75 percent of obese people have a fatty liver. This statistic probably reaches 100 percent among morbidly obese people. This is in contrast to statistics indicating that 3 percent of nonoverweight people have NAFLD.

NAFLD occurs in all age groups and races. In the United States, it appears to be more common among Caucasians and Hispanics than among African Americans. And a smaller percentage of the population of Japan as compared to that of the United States has NAFLD. This may be attributable to differences in diet as well as disparity in the prevalence of obesity. Some studies have attributed the above-mentioned disparities to genetic differences in body fat distribution. However, more research is needed to confirm this, since it seems at odds with recent statistics indicating that 50 percent of African-American women are obese, as compared with 40 percent of Hispanic women and 30 percent of Caucasian women.

OTHER CAUSES OF NAFLD

By now it should be clear that the liver is intricately involved in the breakdown (metabolism) of fat. This process can be disrupted by a number of factors, with the result being NAFLD. It should be mentioned that there are causes of NAFLD other than insulin resistance, type 2 diabetes, central obesity, and hypertriglyceridemia. With the exception of excessive alcohol intake, which is a common cause of fatty liver disease, most of these other factors are relatively uncommon causes of NAFLD and therefore will not be addressed in detail.

The term *drug-induced steatohepatitis* is typically applied to cases in which NAFLD stems from the use of a medication. Examples of drug-induced steatohepatitis include prednisone (a steroid), estrogen (the female hormone), tamoxifen (a medication used for breast cancer), and methotrexate (a type of chemotherapy). Drug-induced steatohepatitis may occur when these medications are used for more than six months. It should be noted that it is currently unclear whether these drugs by themselves cause NAFLD or whether they merely precipitate NAFLD in a susceptible person by exacerbating insulin resistance, central obesity, diabetes, and hypertriglyceridemia.

Occupational exposure to certain toxic chemicals (such as organic solvents and dimethlyformamide) and weight-reduction surgery (such as gastroplasty or jejuno [part of the small intestine] bypass surgery) can also lead to NAFLD. A rare disease known as Jamaican vomiting sickness can also lead to NAFLD. It is caused by ingestion of a toxin produced by the unripe fruit of the ackee tree. In cases where NAFLD was caused by a medication or toxin, discontinuation of the exposure will often reverse the condition. Celiac sprue (a disease of the small intestine characterized by gluten intolerance) and even other liver diseases such as hepatitis C are often associated with fat accumulation in the liver.

Rapid weight loss and starvation can also lead to NAFLD, in addition to worsening NAFLD that already exists. Thus, it is crucial to lose weight slowly and sensibly. It should be noted that people with end-stage liver disease often develop NAFLD. This is due to the fact that some people with end-stage liver disease develop a form of malnutrition known as protein-energy-malnutrition that is similar to the state of starvation (see chapter 23 for more about protein-energy-malnutrition).

THE SYMPTOMS AND PHYSICAL SIGNS OF NAFLD

Most people with NAFLD are asymptomatic (without symptoms). When symptoms do occur, they are usually nonspecific, such as fatigue and weakness. Occasionally, a person will complain of vague right upper quadrant discomfort (pain or discomfort over the area of the liver) or fullness. This may be due to fat stretching the liver. The presence or degree of symptoms has not been found to correlate with the severity of the disease. The development of ascites, encephalopathy, and/or jaundice are signs of advanced cirrhosis and only occur in the late stages of NASH.

During a physical exam, the doctor may detect an enlarged liver. Signs of cirrhosis and its complications, such as ascites (abnormal accumulation of fluid) or splenomegaly (enlarged spleen), may be present but only in people with NASH. These symptoms and physical findings often prompt further evaluation, including blood work, imaging studies, and possibly a liver biopsy.

DIAGNOSING NAFLD

There is no single test that can accurately diagnose NAFLD. The elimination of other causes of liver abnormalities, especially excessive alcohol use, is crucial in order for an accurate diagnosis to be made. Normalization of liver abnormalities upon elimination of the causative factor—for example, weight reduction where obesity is the causative factor—is often sufficient to confirm a diagnosis. When the diagnosis continues to be in doubt, a liver biopsy is necessary. The following section discusses blood tests, imaging studies, and liver biopsy findings in people with NAFLD.

Blood Tests

Blood test results are usually, but not always, abnormal in people with NAFLD. In fact, referral to a hepatologist is usually prompted by abnormal liver enzymes found on routine evaluation or during evaluation for an unrelated problem. There are no specific blood tests that are diagnostic for NAFLD. And there are no specific blood tests that can reliably distinguish between a fatty liver and NASH or that can determine either the extent of fat deposits or the severity of disease. In fact, the entire spectrum of NAFLD, from a fatty liver to cirrhosis, may occur in people with normal blood tests.

In general, transaminases (AST and ALT) are usually not higher than four times the upper limit of normal (upper limit of normal = 40 to 45 IU/l). In fact, in about one-third of people with NAFLD, these liver enzymes may even be normal. The degree of elevation does not correlate with the extent of fat accumulation, inflammation, or scarring found on the liver. However, the level of ALT elevation is usually higher than the level of AST elevation. This is the opposite of that seen in people with alcoholic liver disease (in which AST is higher than ALT), which is discussed in chapter 17. Thus, the recognition of this pattern of transaminase elevation is one manner of distinguishing between NAFLD and alcoholic liver disease, which often mimics the former condition. In NAFLD, the GGTP level is often elevated, and the degree of elevation has been found by some investigators to correlate with the extent of fat deposits in the liver. It should be noted that NAFLD is the most common cause of liver enzyme elevation among adults in the United States. Elevated levels of immunoglobulin A are being investigated as a possible means of measuring inflammation. In the absence of cirrhosis, the bilirubin level is normal (see chapter 3 for more information concerning these blood tests).

Many people with NAFLD, especially men, have evidence of iron overload (elevated transferrin saturation and serum ferritin levels). In some studies, an increased incidence (compared to the general population) of carrying one or two genes for hereditary hemochromatosis—a genetic disease of iron overload (see chapter 18)—was found among people with NAFLD. The presence of excessive iron is thought by some, but not all, experts to be associated with increased liver scarring.

Insulin levels are often elevated in individuals who have both NAFLD and insulin resistance. As such, testing one's insulin level after a twelve-hour fast may be helpful in making a diagnosis of NAFLD.

Carbohydrate-deficient transferrin (CDT) is a blood test that is being evaluated as an indicator of excessive alcohol use. *Transferrin* is a protein that transports iron through the body. It contains about 6 percent carbohydrate. In people who drink alcohol excessively, the carbohydrate content of transferrin decreases. CDT's validity as an indicator of excessive alcohol use has not been fully established. But if future studies can confirm its validity, it will be a valuable tool for physicians in distinguishing between NAFLD and alcoholic liver disease. CDTs present use is limited as it is currently strictly a research tool.

Imaging Studies

Most imaging studies, including ultrasound, CT scan, and MRI, can detect the presence of fat in the liver. In fact, the diagnosis of a fatty liver is sometimes discovered incidentally from an imaging study obtained during the evaluation of an unrelated problem. However, there are no imaging studies that can reliably distinguish between a fatty liver and NASH, or that can determine either the extent of fat deposits or the severity of disease. And since fat accumulation can also resemble cirrhosis and/or a liver tumor, the results of imaging studies are often a source of unnecessary confusion and distress. As always, when the diagnosis is in doubt, a liver biopsy is necessary.

Liver Biopsy

A liver biopsy is the only test that can reliably diagnose NAFLD. Furthermore, a liver biopsy can determine the amount of fatty deposits, the degree of inflammation, and the extent of damage to the liver. Liver biopsy findings for people with NAFLD often mimic the findings seen in people with alcoholic liver disease. Consequently, a thorough questioning of the patient, and if possible of the patient's family members as well, should be performed by the doctor in instances where the amount of alcohol intake is in question.

Granted, this method of investigation may appear somewhat intrusive. But since there is no single test that can accurately confirm or eliminate excessive alcohol consumption, this line of questioning is often necessary in order for the doctor to arrive at an accurate diagnosis and to offer appropriate treatment options. When NASH has progressed to cirrhosis, liver biopsy findings often reveal relatively few fatty deposits and often no fatty deposits at all. This sometimes causes additional difficulty in arriving at a correct diagnosis. However, it has been estimated that approximately 80 percent of instances of cirrhosis of unclear cause are probably due to NASH. Specific guidelines on the need for and timing of a liver biopsy have not been definitively established. Thus, decisions as to liver biopsy should be made on a case-to-case basis (see chapter 5 for a complete discussion of liver biopsies).

TREATMENT OF NAFLD

The following section discusses the treatments for NAFLD. It should be noted that there is no specific therapy for NAFLD that has clearly been proven effective. Treatment has focused on weight reduction and liver-protective (hepatoprotective) medications. As with all liver diseases, avoidance of alcohol—before, during, and after treatment—is essential. This is especially true for people with NAFLD, as alcohol may worsen the severity of fat deposits, fatty inflammation, and fatty scarring in the liver.

Weight Management

Overweight or obese people with NAFLD can usually normalize the elevations in liver enzymes, decrease some of the enlargement of their livers, and diminish the amount of fat in their livers merely through weight reduction. A weight loss of approximately 10 percent can significantly correct these abnormalities. If weight reduction is achieved early in the disease, progression to scarring and cirrhosis can possibly be prevented altogether. In fact, in one study, weight reduction actually reversed some scarring (fibrosis, not cirrhosis).

Three points need to be emphasized concerning weight reduction. First, weight loss must be sustained, or the disease will recur. Second, weight reduction must be achieved through reasonable methods, and it must occur at a slow pace. This means that people should aim for a one- to two-pound weight loss per week. Excessively rapid weight reduction or starvation techniques can actually worsen or even precipitate progression to cirrhosis and liver failure. Obviously, this is at odds with the purpose of the weight reduction. Furthermore, rapid weight loss has been shown to put people at risk for gallstone disease and can adversely affect a person's overall health. Third, an exercise routine must be incorporated into any weight-reduction routine.

There are numerous weight-loss diets on the market. However, their effects on NAFLD are unknown. Any diet should be evaluated by a knowledgeable hepatologist as to its likely effectiveness as a tool against NAFLD. In general, a diet low in saturated fat, low in simple carbohydrates, and high in fiber should be used. This type of diet may improve insulin resistance. Supplementation with polyunsaturated fatty acids has also been shown to improve insulin resistance, in addition to decreasing the risk for coronary artery disease. However, the effect of this type of supplementation on NAFLD needs to be studied.

Weight reduction is particularly important for those overweight people who have both NAFLD and an additional liver disease—for example, hepatitis C. In these people, a 10 percent weight loss will also lower elevated liver enzymes, although they may not revert to totally normal levels. It has been shown that people with chronic hepatitis C who also have excessive fat deposits (seen most commonly among people with genotype 3) are especially likely to experience a quick progression to cirrhosis.

A combination of aerobic and weight-bearing exercises is recommended as the most beneficial exercise regimen. It has been shown that improvement in insulin resistance correlates with the intensity of one's exercise program. It is well established that substantial benefits are obtained from exercise even when there is no accompanying weight reduction. Yet, ideally, some weight loss should be achieved as well. See chapter 23 for more detailed guidelines regarding weight loss and exercise.

Other Weight-Reduction Methods

Overweight patients who cannot lose weight from diet and exercise are sometimes treated with aggressive strategies such as surgery or weight-loss medications.

Surgery

Surgery should be reserved solely for obese individuals who are at least eighty to one hundred pounds overweight (BMI between 35 and 40 kg/m^2). Surgery can improve most obesity-related medical conditions, such as type 2 diabetes. However, studies have not yet been conducted to determine whether surgery is an effective strategy for treating NAFLD. People with NASH who have already progressed to cirrhosis should not have weight-reduction surgery performed since the ensuing rapid weight loss puts them at risk for liver failure.

The first operation that was used for severe obesity was the jejuno intestinal bypass. This operation, first performed in the early 1960s, produced weight loss by causing malabsorption. This meant that patients who ate large quantities of food would have difficulty digesting them. Thus, the food would be passed along the digestive tract too quickly for the body to absorb the calories. The problem with this surgery was that it caused a loss of essential nutrients. In addition, approximately 40 percent of patients developed liver function abnormalities after the operation, and severe NASH accompanied by liver failure developed in approximately 6 percent of patients. Therefore, this form of bypass surgery is no longer performed.

In vertical-banding gastroplasty—also known as stomach-stapling—the surgeon uses both a band and staples to create a small pouch at the top of the stomach where food enters from the esophagus. The lower outlet of the pouch has a small opening that delays the emptying of food from the pouch. If these people consume food in excess of the pouch's capacity, a sensation of fullness, discomfort, and nausea will occur. Although this operation leads to weight loss in almost all patients, it is less successful than gastric bypass surgery.

Gastric bypass surgery is superior to the vertical-banding gastroplasty as this operation restricts both food intake and the amount of calories the body absorbs. This surgery typically results in the loss of approximately two-thirds of excess weight within a two-year period. This type of surgery does carry a risk of nutritional deficiencies, and patients are advised to take nutritional supplements to prevent this complication.

Weight-Loss Medications

There are three FDA-approved medications for weight loss: phentermine (Adipex-P), sibutramine (Meridia), and orlistat (Xenical). The effectiveness of these medications in the management of NAFLD has not been studied. These medications have multiple side effects, including elevated heart rate and blood pressure (Adipex and Meridia) and gastrointestinal problems (Xenical). In addition, Xenical may cause fat-soluble vitamins (A, D, E, and K) to be poorly absorbed by the body. This may result in a deficiency of these vitamins. Since vitamin E may be beneficial in the treatment of NAFLD, malabsorption is a particularly unwelcome side effect. In general, weight-reduction medications are not recommended as a treatment for NAFLD.

Treatment of NAFLD in Those Who Are Not Overweight

The French delicacy pâté de foie gras is made by force-feeding geese or ducks a diet high in fats. "Foie gras" is French for fat(gras) liver(*foie*). By feeding geese a fatty diet, a fatty liver results. The same cause-and-effect scenario may be applicable to humans. Thus, dietary alterations, such as avoiding fat and excessive carbohydrates, may be a potentially effective treatment for people with NAFLD. This theory will require controlled studies to confirm its validity. It is important to understand that the distribution of fat on one's body is more important than the number of pounds one weighs. Thus, a person may be normal weight but have an excessive amount of weight around the midsection. This abdominal (or central) obesity, as discussed on page 247, may cause NAFLD even in individuals of normal weight.

Treatment of NAFLD in Those with Diabetes

In people with insulin-dependent diabetes, close control of sugar levels is crucial for minimizing the amount of fat in the liver. However, for noninsulin-dependent diabetics (the group more likely to have NAFLD), controlling sugar levels, while important for overall health, will generally not improve liver abnormalities. For noninsulin-dependent diabetics who are overweight, weight reduction is the only effective treatment option.

Treatment of NAFLD with Medications or Supplements

Many medications are presently being evaluated for people with NAFLD. The most promising one appears to be ursodeoxycholic acid (UDCA). UDCA, also known by the brand names Actigall, URSO, and ursodiol, is a naturally occurring bile acid that, unlike many other bile acids in the body, is not toxic to the liver. It is found in a small quantity in the human body, but in a large quantity in a bear's body. UDCA was initially used to dissolve gallstones but is now commonly used to treat many different liver diseases, specifically primary biliary cirrhosis (see chapter 15). Initial studies involving people with NASH have shown that treatment with UDCA can lead to improvements in liver enzymes and to a reduction in the severity of fatty deposits in the liver. UDCA may possibly decrease the risk of developing gallstones during weight reduction. Further studies are ongoing as to the effects of UDCA on NAFLD.

Metformin (Glucophage) and rosiglitazone (Avandia) are oral glucose-lowering (also known as hypoglycemic) medications used to treat type 2 diabetes. These medications work by correcting insulin resistance. Therefore, these types of drugs may potentially benefit people with NAFLD and insulin resistance. In fact, preliminary studies have shown that treatment with metformin can improve liver enzyme elevations in people with NAFLD. However, improvement in the amount of fat and inflammation in the liver has thus far been established only in studies involving animals. Studies on humans will be required before these medications can be recommended for people with NAFLD.

Clofibrate, a triglyceride-lowering drug, has been tested as a treatment but has not shown to be beneficial. Gemfibrozil, another triglyceride-lowering medication, was able to improve liver enzyme elevations in a small group of people with NAFLD, but its effects on liver fat and scarring were not tested. Further study is needed on gemfibrozil. Polymixin B is an antibiotic that can reduce the amount of bacteria in the intestines. This medication may be characterized as a form of "bowel decontaminate." Studies have shown that administering polymixin B to people on intravenous feedings (total parenteral nutrition [TPN]) can reduce the amount of fat in their livers. This treatment option needs further study before definite conclusions can be drawn about its effectiveness in treating people with NAFLD.

Betaine is a precursor of S-adenosyl methionine (SAMe), a derivative of the amino acid methionine. SAMe is purported to promote the health of the liver. In two studies, some patients who were treated with betaine experienced decreased liver enzyme elevations and a decreased amount of fatty deposits in their livers. The mechanism by which betaine exerts its beneficial effect on the liver is not clear, but it is believed that it may assist in transporting fat away from the liver. More research is needed in this area.

Certain nutritional deficiencies that are common among people with NAFLD may provide a clue in the search for a successful treatment. Some people who receive intravenous feedings for prolonged periods of time develop fatty liver in addition to a choline deficiency (choline is a B vitamin). Correcting the choline deficiency in these people has been shown to resolve the fatty liver as well. Choline supplementation in people with NAFLD is a promising treatment option, but is one that requires further study. Coenzyme A is a substance that is essential for the metabolism of carbohydrates, fats, and certain amino acids. It contains pantothenic acid, a B vitamin that is necessary for growth. In some studies, people with NAFLD were supplemented with a form of coenzyme A, and this caused the extent of fat deposits in the liver to decrease. More research must be done to confirm the efficacy of this type of nutritional supplementation.

One preliminary study has indicated that vitamin E (alpha-tocopherol) supplementation may be a beneficial adjunctive treatment for people with NAFLD, but more research is needed in this area. Biotin, a B vitamin, has been shown to decrease insulin resistance. Studies on people with NAFLD have not been conducted at this time, but biotin supplementation would be an interesting area of exploration for people with NAFLD.

Treatment of NAFLD with Phlebotomy

Some experts have found that people with both NAFLD and elevated amounts of iron in their livers appear to have an increased incidence of progression to scarring. This is particularly true for people with one or two gene mutations for hereditary hemochromatosis (see chapter 18). Therefore, treatment with phlebotomy (the removal of blood through a vein) for these people is a potential option. Preliminary studies involving people treated with serial phlebotomies have shown that they experienced a decreased insulin resistance. This is a controversial area, as some studies have found no correlation between the presence of iron and the existence of liver scarring in people with NAFLD. More research is needed in this area before routine phlebotomy can be recommended for people with both NAFLD and iron overload.

Treatment of NAFLD in Those Who Have Developed Decompensated Cirrhosis

If a person with NAFLD develops complications of cirrhosis, he should be evaluated for liver transplantation. NAFLD is said to account for approximately 2 to 3 percent of transplantations in the United States, although this may be an underestimate. People often gain weight after transplantation, as a result of post-transplant medications (including corticosteroids) as well as a feeling of well-being. In one study of patients transplanted due to NAFLD, NAFLD recurred in approximately one-third of patients, 12.5 percent of whom had already progressed to cirrhosis. All transplant recipients, especially those prone to NAFLD, must be diligent about maintaining a normal weight, as NAFLD can recur and progress to cirrhosis as well after transplantation. See chapter 22 for more information concerning liver transplantation.

THE NATURAL HISTORY AND PROGNOSIS FOR THOSE WITH NAFLD

Fatty liver is a relatively harmless condition that does not lead to any significant short- or long-term consequences. Thus, people with fatty liver rarely, if ever, experience liver-related complications or a decreased life span due to this condition. However, there is some controversy as to whether an increased amount of fat in the liver actually does increase the liver's susceptibility to injury. In fact, it has been recognized that people who receive a fatty liver in a liver transplant have an increased complication rate as compared to people who receive a normal liver. This realization has led to the discontinuance of using livers with more than 30 percent fat for liver transplantation. Furthermore, whether fatty liver can progress to NASH has not been definitively determined. However, since such a progression most likely can occur, people diagnosed with a fatty liver should attempt to eliminate the condition.

The natural history of NASH is somewhat unclear. It appears to be a progressive disease, but the actual risk of progression to cirrhosis is unknown. Some studies have noted that as many as 50 percent of people with NASH will likely progress to cirrhosis. Other studies have concluded that there is only a minimal risk of progression to cirrhosis. The risk of progression to cirrhosis probably lies somewhere between these two extremes. In any event, NASH appears to be a slowly progressive disease, but a disease that can lead to cirrhosis and its complications. One study showed that factors such as age of greater than forty to fifty years old, obesity, diabetes, hyperlipidemia (especially high triglycerides), and possibly female gender and high blood pressure increase the risk for progression to cirrhosis. However, more research is needed to conclusively prove that these factors are reliable predictors of progression to cirrhosis.

People with NASH whose biopsies reveal high iron deposits on their livers appear to be at increased risk for scarring and therefore for progression to cirrhosis. These people often carry a single gene mutation for the liver disease known as hemochromatosis (see chapter 18 for more information about hemochromatosis). One study found that 59 percent of people with NASH were alive ten years after being diagnosed. Thus, it appears that the life expectancy for people with NASH, while somewhat lower than that of the general population, is not significantly shortened.

It is unclear how often NASH leads to hepatocellular carcinoma (HCC). However, studies have shown that people with both HCC and cirrhosis of unclear cause often are found to have features of the metabolic syndrome (type 2 diabetes, obesity, high triglycerides, and insulin resistance) as well. It is believed that the cases of cirrhosis of unknown origin that led to HCC most likely occurred among people with undiagnosed NASH.

CONCLUSION

In this chapter you learned that while excess fat deposits in the liver can be relatively harmless, there is the possibility that fat may increase the liver's susceptibility to injury. This has led researchers to consider whether a fatty liver is perhaps the initial stage of NASH. The perspective on NAFLD has changed dramatically in recent years. Initially believed to be a benign disease limited primarily to middle-aged, obese women with diabetes, it is now recognized as a progressive disease that may lead to cirrhosis and liver cancer and that can affect virtually anyone. Furthermore, the consensus among experts is that most cases of NAFLD are due to insulin resistance. NAFLD is now considered to be the most common cause of elevated liver enzymes and is probably the most common liver disease in the United States. Future research will be targeted at identifying who is at risk for NAFLD and at developing therapies that can stop or slow the course of this disease.

The next chapter discusses alcoholic liver disease, a liver disease that closely resembles NAFLD on liver biopsy specimens, but is otherwise—as you will soon learn—very different.

Seventeen

ALCOHOL AND THE LIVER AND ALCOHOLIC LIVER DISEASE

Adele, a fifty-four-year-old administrator, noticed that for the past month she was gaining weight rapidly. In fact, the only clothes she could fit into were her maternity dresses from twenty-five years ago. She noticed that her stomach was quite distended and that her legs were swollen. She made an appointment with her family doctor to find out what was going on.

After asking her some questions, the doctor examined Adele and noticed that she had spider angiomatas on her upper chest and arms. He also noted that her palms were bright red. Even though she had gained almost thirty pounds since her last checkup two years ago, her muscles looked wasted. The exam further revealed that Adele's abdomen was distended from ascites and that her legs were swollen from edema. The doctor reviewed Adele's medical records and noted that on her patient questionnaire, she claimed to drink wine only on social occasions. When he asked Adele about this, she asserted that she only drank socially or when dining out. After giving her a prescription for diuretics (water pills) and a low-sodium diet to follow, the doctor asked Adele to return in two weeks with her husband.

Two weeks later, Adele's ascites had significantly improved, and she had lost twelve pounds due to the diuretics and low-sodium diet. In the consultation room with Adele and her husband, the doctor asked again how frequently Adele consumed alcohol. When she replied as she had two weeks earlier, Adele's husband was surprised and exclaimed, "Adele! What about the wine you drink every night with dinner and the martini you have as soon as you get home from work?" From this additional information, the doctor concluded that Adele had alcoholic cirrhosis and advised her to go into an alcohol rehabilitation program.

A lcohol and the liver and alcoholic liver disease (ALD) are the subjects of this chapter. Topics covered include how alcohol is processed by the body, the liver's role in rendering alcohol harmless, and why the liver more than any other organ in the body is susceptible to harm from alcohol. Also discussed are the multitude of factors, including genetics and gender, that contribute to the development of ALD. In addition, the adverse effects on the liver of combining alcohol and other drugs, such as acetaminophen, are addressed. This chapter also explains how a diagnosis of ALD is made. It discusses the various stages of ALD and its treatment. In addition, this chapter addresses which organs, besides the liver, are adversely affected by alcohol consumption. Finally, the natural history and prognosis of people with ALD are addressed.

THE PREVALENCE OF ALCOHOLIC LIVER DISEASE

Medical problems due to excessive alcohol intake occur in approximately 10 percent of the U.S. population. About 25 percent of these people develop alcoholic liver disease (ALD), one of the most common causes of liver disease in the United States. In fact, ALD is the fourth most common cause of death among middle-aged Americans. ALD may affect people from any country, any socioeconomic background, or any religion or race. One reason why ALD is so common is that alcohol—a potentially toxic substance with significant abuse potential— may be obtained inexpensively and with ease. In fact, alcohol use is encouraged in our society, as is evident in the many advertisements, movies, and television shows that portray the consumption of alcohol as sophisticated and fun.

ALCOHOL AND THE LIVER

It is common knowledge that drinking too much alcohol can be harmful to many of the organs in the body, especially the liver. But most people do not know that it is, in fact, the liver that is primarily responsible for protecting itself and the rest of the body from the harmful effects of alcohol.

The liver provides the body with two separate ways to metabolize (break down) alcohol. By metabolizing alcohol into less toxic by-products, the liver prevents dangerously high levels of alcohol from accumulating in the bloodstream. One way the liver renders alcohol harmless is with the assistance of *enzymes* (proteins that induce chemical changes in other substances while remaining unchanged by the process). These particular enzymes are known as *alcohol dehydrogenase* and *aldehyde dehydrogenase*. They literally turn alcohol into a form of vinegar that is totally harmless to the liver and the rest of the body. Alcohol can also be broken down by an alternative method, a pathway in the liver known as the *microsomal ethanol oxidizing system (MEOS)* that contains a group of enzymes known as the *cytochrome P-450 system*. The cytochrome P-450 system is a complex group of specialized enzymes within the liver that are responsible for the conversion of fat-soluble substances to water-soluble substances. Liver damage occurs when one of these mechanisms of alcohol breakdown either fails to function properly or is overwhelmed by an excessive amount of alcohol ingestion. This can happen due to a variety of other factors, in addition to drinking too much alcohol, which are discussed in the next section.

There are many misconceptions that people typically have about alcohol and the liver. The following lists some of these common misconceptions:

- Social drinking is unlikely to cause liver damage

- If a person's liver disease was not caused by alcohol, there is no need to limit alcohol consumption

- If a person does not drink any alcohol, they can't get liver disease

- All alcoholics eventually get liver disease

- If a person with ALD abstains from alcohol, he no longer has to worry about his liver

- Alcohol provides some nutritional value

- Beer and wine cannot cause liver damage

When the liver has been damaged by alcohol and can no longer prevent dangerously high levels of this toxin from accumulating in the bloodstream, other body parts can become damaged. One reason why alcohol can so easily damage other organs is that alcohol is soluble in both water and fat. This enables it to readily enter any organ and negatively affect its vital functions.

FACTORS THAT CONTRIBUTE TO THE DEVELOPMENT OF ALD

Not everyone who drinks alcohol excessively develops ALD. In fact, only about 25 percent of alcoholics develop ALD, and only 10 to 15 percent of alcoholics are found to have cirrhosis during autopsy. So why are some people more likely than others to develop ALD? There is no single answer to this question, as many variables contribute to the development of ALD. The following is a discussion of some of these variables.

Dose and Duration of Alcohol Intake

People who drink large quantities of alcohol over a long period of time are generally at greatest risk of developing ALD. But remember, the alcoholic content differs among different kinds of alcoholic beverages. Therefore, the likelihood of developing ALD is affected by the alcohol content of the beverage ingested, not by the type of alcoholic beverage consumed.

In general, consumption of about 80 grams of alcohol daily for a significant length of time is required for men to develop ALD. Eighty grams of alcohol is roughly equivalent to a six-pack of beer or a liter of wine. (To convert grams to ounces, multiply by 20 and divide by 567.) Women are much more susceptible to the toxicity of alcohol than are men (see "Gender" on page 263). It has been estimated that it takes as little as 20 grams of daily alcohol ingestion over an extended period of time for women to develop ALD. The specific length of time it takes for ALD to develop is not known with any precision because so many different factors play a role in its development. Similarly, the amount of time that it takes for cirrhosis to develop is unknown. However, it appears that an average person must drink the above-mentioned amounts of alcohol daily for at least five years in order for cirrhosis to develop. That's right. A mere five years of excessive drinking puts a person at significant risk for developing cirrhosis! Moreover, remember that the above figures are just estimates and that the results may vary depending upon many other factors.

Genetics

Genetics play an important role in the development of ALD. Most people are familiar with the stereotype of the person who "can drink anyone under the table," or of the easily inebriated person colloquially referred to as a "cheap date." Well, it has been found that people who fall into the first category are the ones most likely to develop ALD. And the "cheap dates" are the ones least likely to develop ALD. These observations have, at least in part, a genetic basis.

It has been discovered that genetic differences regarding the efficiency of the enzymes (alcohol dehydrogenase and aldehyde dehydrogenase) that establish the rate of the metabolism of alcohol exist among people. Thus, fast metabolizers of alcohol have to drink more than everyone else in order to obtain the desired effects of alcohol. As compared with people who metabolize alcohol at a normal rate, they are less intoxicated after drinking equivalent amounts of alcohol. These people are the ones most likely to develop liver damage, as they are able to consistently consume high levels of alcohol for many years. On the other hand, slow metabolizers of alcohol become intoxicated rapidly when they consume alcohol. These people develop high levels of alcohol in their bloodstreams after consuming only small amounts of liquor. Since these people require relatively minimal quantities of alcohol in order to become intoxicated, they are unlikely to consume alcohol in great enough quantities to develop ALD and are therefore the least likely ones to develop ALD.

A similar characteristic is common among Asian people. Certain Asian populations have an impairment of the activity of an enzyme involved in alcohol metabolism—aldehyde dehydrogenase. This impairment results in accumulations of the toxin acetaldehyde in the body. Skin flushing, increased heart rate, and severe nausea and vomiting occur in these people when they ingest any alcoholic beverage. To some extent, this accounts for the low incidence of ALD in the

Asian population compared with the U.S. population. To take advantage of this reaction, disulfiram (Antabuse), a medication that inhibits aldehyde dehydrogenase and results in acetaldehyde accumulation, is used as a deterrent to consume alcohol.

Genetic markers (specific genes) have been searched for to further explain why certain people are more susceptible to the toxic effects of alcohol on the liver than others. While many candidate genes have been suggested, to date no specific gene has been proven to directly influence the development of alcoholic liver disease. However, specific genes located on chromosome #6 are most commonly implicated.

Gender

Gender differences play a role in a person's susceptibility to the effects of alcohol on the liver. While alcoholism is more common among men, it has been demonstrated that women are more susceptible to the adverse consequences of alcohol on the liver. In fact, women who develop ALD and cirrhosis due to alcohol do so at a younger age than men, and they have consumed less alcohol in total. It has been noted that women with cirrhosis due to alcohol have a shorter life expectancy than men with cirrhosis due to alcohol.

So why are women so much more susceptible to the toxicity of alcohol than men? Well, the most obvious explanation is that women generally weigh less and are smaller than men. Women on average have a smaller total body area throughout which any ingested alcohol can be distributed. But neither this fact nor the total amount of alcohol ingested completely accounts for why women are at a much greater risk of developing ALD. Hormonal differences between men and women have been suggested as a factor. It has been demonstrated experimentally that female rats are more susceptible to alcohol-induced liver damage than male rats, at least in part because of the higher levels of estrogen, the female sex hormone, in their bodies. However, this theory has not been proven in humans.

Probably the factor that most significantly differentiates the genders is that, as compared with men, many women (not all) have less of the enzyme alcohol dehydrogenase in the lining of their stomachs. This enzyme is the same one that is found in the liver that breaks down alcohol into the by-products that are less toxic to the liver. Thus, the reduced amount of alcohol dehydrogenase enzyme in women increases the likelihood that they will absorb nonmetabolized alcohol from their stomach linings directly into their bloodstreams. Hypothetically, if a man and a woman of equal size and weight each consumes an equivalent amount of alcohol over the same span of time, the woman will have a much higher blood-alcohol level than the man. Once in their bloodstreams, high blood-alcohol levels circulate in their bodies, placing women at increased risk for the toxic effects of alcohol on their livers and other organs.

In addition, studies show that women solicit treatment for alcohol-related problems only half as often as men do. Also, by the time a woman seeks help for her problems, she tends to be sicker and at a more advanced stage of liver disease. It is believed that one reason for this is that women may hide their addictions more successfully than men, and they are not as likely to suffer the adverse social and legal problems due to drinking alcohol. Therefore, their family members, friends, and doctors are less likely to suspect them of alcohol abuse. Studies have shown that after completing treatment in an alcohol rehabilitation program, women return to drinking alcohol more often than men. Unfortunately, statistics indicate that the incidence of alcohol abuse among women is increasing in the United States.

The Presence of Other Liver Diseases

Alcohol has been shown to worsen the course of many liver diseases. Since alcohol is a potential toxin to the liver, people with any type of liver disease should refrain from drinking alcohol.

There appears to be an added harmful effect to the liver when alcohol is consumed by a person who has one of the hepatitis viruses. Thus, for people with chronic viral hepatitis (see part 2), consuming alcohol is likely to lead to a worsening of liver disease. In people with hepatitis C, alcohol has been shown to promote the replication of the hepatitis C virus (HCV), thus resulting in elevated hepatitis C viral loads. Furthermore, it has been shown that for people with chronic hepatitis C, consumption of even minimal quantities of alcohol may accelerate the progression of liver disease to cirrhosis. In fact, HCV has been found frequently in people with ALD, especially in those people who have severe liver damage or cirrhosis, suggesting a causative relationship (that is, HCV contributed to the liver damage).

Evidence of infection with the hepatitis B virus (HBV) is more common among alcoholics than the general population. Furthermore, HBV is often found in people with cirrhosis due to ALD. People with ALD who become acutely infected with HBV typically have a much more severe course of infection than people without ALD. Therefore, as with all liver diseases, it is especially important for people with chronic hepatitis B and chronic hepatitis C to refrain from drinking alcohol.

Alcohol can increase iron absorption. Therefore, it is important for people with hemochromatosis and other diseases of iron overload (see chapter 18) to refrain from consuming alcohol, since alcohol may worsen liver damage. It is important to remember that for any person with liver disease, excessive alcohol consumption doubles (at the very least) the risk of liver cancer.

The Use of Other Drugs

As noted on page 260, the cytochrome P-450 system is one mechanism by which alcohol is broken down. This system is also responsible for the metabolism of a variety of other drugs and medications, some of which are regularly used by people who abuse alcohol. Since these drugs compete for the same pathway as alcohol to be broken down, the capacity of this pathway becomes strained. Thus, toxic levels of these drugs and/or alcohol accumulate in the body. This may lead to additional and often severe liver injury and may account for why some people develop a more rapidly progressive course of ALD than others.

The most well-established alcohol/drug toxicity is caused by the simultaneous use of alcohol with acetaminophen (Tylenol). Typically, one tablet of acetaminophen is 500 mg. A therapeutic dose for minor aches and pains can range anywhere from 2 to 6 grams per day (four to twelve tablets). In people without ALD, dosages greater than 7 to 10 grams (14 to 20 tablets) over a twenty-four-hour period may cause liver damage. But for people with ALD, dosages greater than 2 grams (4 tabs) over a twenty-four-hour period may cause additional and severe liver damage. Therefore, it is crucial for people with ALD to avoid taking more than four tablets of acetaminophen within a twenty-four-hour period. These people are advised to limit their intake to one to two 500-mg tablets per twenty-four-hour period.

People are often surprised to learn that for people with liver disease, acetaminophen within these limited dosages is actually safer than taking aspirin (ASA) or other nonsteroidal anti-inflammatory drugs (NSAIDs), such as Motrin or Advil. Aspirin and other NSAIDs may cause bleeding disorders (particularly in the gastrointestinal tract) and kidney disorders, in addition to liver injury. Therefore, people with ALD, especially those who already have a bleeding disorder, should always avoid even small doses of these medications. People should also be aware that other over-the-counter medications, as well as some prescription medicines, may contain acetaminophen or aspirin and other NSAIDs. Therefore, it is important to carefully read the label of any medication prior to taking it. Of course, labels should always be read carefully, and when in doubt, a person should check with his doctor or pharmacist concerning the presence of these substances in a particular medication. Another drug that increases alcohol's toxic effects on the liver is isoniazid—a drug used to treat tuberculosis. The effect of this drug and others on the liver is discussed in more detail in chapter 24.

When alcohol is ingested in combination with other medications, it often enhances the effect and/or side effects of that medication. For example, it may cause excessive sedation (sleepiness) when taken with an antianxiety drug, such as alprazolam (Xanax). Or alcohol may increase nausea, vomiting, and severe stomach cramping when taken with certain antibiotics, such as cefaclor (Ceclor). Many drugs such as the H_2 blockers—cimetidine (Tagamet) and ranitidine (Zantac)—can elevate blood-alcohol levels, thereby resulting in increased alcohol toxicity. A person should always consult with a doctor or pharmacist prior to ingesting alcohol in combination with any other medication.

Lastly, it is important for people with ALD to refrain from using cocaine. The combined ingestion of alcohol and cocaine can accelerate liver injury, and, at high enough levels, this toxic combination has the potential to substantially injure the kidneys and muscles and can even cause death. It is unwise for anyone with any liver disease, or anyone for that matter, to use cocaine, as there is evidence that cocaine in and of itself may cause liver injury.

Malnutrition

Poor dietary habits may also contribute to the progression of ALD. In fact, malnutrition—defined by the lack of calories and protein consumed—is noted in almost all people with advanced ALD. Deficiencies of vitamins and minerals are also virtually universal. In people with ALD, these substances are poorly absorbed from the stomach lining as a consequence of alcohol's harmful effects on the gastrointestinal tract. The prevalence of poor dietary habits in general among people with ALD also accounts for the nutritional deficiencies that they commonly exhibit. See chapter 23 for some helpful information on diet and nutrition.

Weight

Being overweight has been shown to be a risk factor for the development of another liver disease: nonalcoholic fatty liver disease (NAFLD) (see chapter 16). The influence of weight on people with alcoholic liver disease has been evaluated in research studies. It was found that alcoholic people who are overweight are more likely to develop cirrhosis as compared to alcoholic people who are of normal weight. Therefore, it is important that people with ALD maintain normal weight levels (see chapters 16 and 23 for more information on normal weight levels).

Diabetes

People with high blood sugar (glucose) levels and/or diabetes have been found to be at increased risk for developing liver scarring compared with people who have normal sugar levels. Thus, it is important for people with ALD to maintain low-sugar diets. Those with diabetes should be on sugar-lowering medications.

Other Factors

Some factors that are relevant to ALD come from within the body itself. These include:

- *cytokines:* substances that are secreted by cells of the immune system

- *endotoxins:* a component of the cell wall of certain types of bacteria

- *free radicals:* toxic, highly reactive compounds that are naturally produced by the body

- *oxidative stress:* oxygen in a deformed toxic state due to alcohol consumption

- *autoimmune reaction* (see chapter 14 for a discussion of autoimmunity)

THE SYMPTOMS AND PHYSICAL SIGNS OF ALD

Symptoms of ALD are nonspecific and may be vague or even absent altogether. They may include fatigue or weakness, both of which can be associated with any type of liver disorder. Symptoms are sometimes related to the stage of the disease. For example, if decompensated cirrhosis is present, a symptom may be encephalopathy or ascites. But more often, symptoms do not correlate with the severity of liver damage. Diminished sexual function, diminished sexual drive (libido), and infertility may be signs of ALD. In addition, a person with ALD may experience symptoms that are unrelated to the liver, such as depression, insomnia, lack of concentration, violent behavior, and tremulousness (shakiness).

On a physical exam, the doctor may find an enlarged spleen or a tender, enlarged liver. Physical findings, such as spider angiomatas, palmar erythema, parotid enlargement, Dupuytren's contracture (these were discussed in chapter 2), and, of course, the smell of alcohol on the breath are more common among people with ALD than with people who have other liver diseases. Men may display signs of feminization, such as gynecomastia, testicular atrophy, and muscle wasting. Many of these physical findings reflect altered estrogen (a female hormone) metabolism by the liver. While some of these signs are suggestive of ALD, none is diagnostic of this condition.

DIAGNOSING ALD

There is no specific test that can accurately diagnosis ALD. Therefore, ALD is typically diagnosed by a combination of self-recognition, doctor recognition, blood work, imaging studies, and liver biopsy. These methods of diagnosis are discussed below.

Recognition by Patient and Doctor

People with ALD often fail to realize that they have a drinking problem. In many cases, the nonrecognition of a problem may be attributable to self-denial (as with Adele at the beginning of this chapter). It can be difficult for doctors to diagnose ALD in cases where the patient is adamantly denying excessive alcohol use. A good way for a person to determine if he has a drinking problem is by answering a few simple questions honestly. See the inset "The CAGE Questionnaire" on page 269.

The first step toward a diagnosis of ALD is a doctor's high degree of suspicion that his patient drinks alcohol excessively. Anyone a doctor suspects of alcohol abuse usually will be asked to take the CAGE screening test. Doctors may also decide to have a meeting with the person's family or to speak with his friends or coworkers—always with his patient's informed consent—in order to better assess the actual degree of alcohol abuse. While this may seem intrusive, it is important to remember that the doctor's objective is to make an accurate diagnosis (not to punish or judge), so that appropriate treatment may be given, and so that the long-term consequences of ALD may, if possible, be avoided.

Blood Tests

There is no single blood test that can accurately diagnose ALD. However, the combined results of the following blood tests may suggest a diagnosis of ALD. Although these blood tests are not as accurate as the CAGE screening test, they are very useful in identifying people in severe denial and people who are unwilling to cooperate with a doctor's questioning.

Liver Enzymes

In people with ALD, transaminases (AST and ALT) may be elevated but are rarely higher than 300 to 400 IU/dl. The level of elevation does not correlate with disease severity. This point is underscored by the finding that some people with cirrhosis due to alcohol have transaminases that are totally normal. In people with ALD, the AST is often elevated to a level two to three times greater than the ALT. This is partly due to a vitamin B_6 (pyridoxine) deficiency, which is often found in alcoholics. If the transaminases are found to be greatly elevated (greater than 1,000 IU/dl), the most likely cause for this is that too much acetaminophen was taken during a drinking binge. This is indicative of a serious situation necessitating immediate hospitalization and emergency treatment.

In people with ALD, GGTP is almost always elevated. This liver enzyme is frequently used as a screening test for excessive alcohol intake. Unfortunately, this test is nondiagnostic for ALD since GGTP elevations may be attributable to numerous different causes. AP is also often elevated but is likewise nonspecific for ALD (see chapter 3 for information on these blood tests).

Blood-Alcohol Level

Measurement of alcohol in the blood is quite accurate. However, these levels typically reflect the amount of alcohol consumed only on the previous day. So, if a person went to a party and had a few social drinks or drank alcohol for any reason the evening before the test, his blood-alcohol level would be very high. One alcoholic beverage typically raises the blood-alcohol level by 15 to 20 mg/dl. This is the amount of alcohol metabolized by the liver in one hour. A blood-alcohol level between 20 and 99 mg/dl may cause impaired coordination and a feeling of euphoria.

Blood-alcohol levels are a poor indicator of chronic alcohol abuse and ALD. One exception is the finding of a value greater than 150 mg/dl in a nonintoxicated person, as this level is extremely high and typically causes difficulty walking, poor judgment, uncontrollable moods, and altered thought processes.

Other Blood Tests

In people with ALD, elevated uric acid levels—which are typically associated with *gout* (painful joint inflammation)—may occur. Triglyceride levels may be

The CAGE Questionnaire

People who drink alcohol on a regular basis need to ask themselves four questions. These four questions make up the CAGE questionnaire. Its purpose is to help determine whether or not there is an alcohol-related problem. Even if only one question is answered positively, the possibility exists that the person does have such a problem. If two or more questions are answered positively, then the presence of alcoholism is very likely. The CAGE questionnaire has been found to be accurate almost 90 percent of the time.

The CAGE Screening Test for Alcoholism

- Have you ever felt the need to **C**ut down on drinking?

- Have you ever felt **A**nnoyed by criticism of your drinking?

- Have you ever had **G**uilty feelings about drinking?

- Have you ever taken a morning **E**ye-opener (a drink first thing in the morning)?

elevated, whereas the minerals potassium, magnesium, and phosphorus may be low. Levels of glucose may be either high or low. Zinc levels may be low, characteristic of, but not diagnostic of, ALD. Thyroid abnormalities are often associated with ALD. The *mean corpuscular volume (MCV)* is the volume of the average red blood cell in a sample of blood. This value can appear on a routine complete blood cell count (CBC). In people with ALD, this value is elevated (greater than 95 μm^3 (micrometers cubed)) due to the toxic effect that alcohol has on the bone marrow. This condition is also referred to as *macrocytosis* (large red blood cells).

In people with ALD, immunoglobulin A (IgA) is sometimes very elevated, and occasionally there are some autoantibodies, such as ANA or SMA, present at low titers.

People with ALD often have vitamin deficiencies, which show up on blood tests when ordered by a doctor, as a result of poor nutrition and poor absorption of nutrients into their bodies. Most common are vitamin B_{12} and folate deficiencies. A deficiency of both vitamin B_{12} and folate is suggestive of ALD. Low levels of vitamin B_{12} and folate can also cause a person's MCV to be elevated. An elevated ammonia level, when present in a person with ALD, is often a sign of encephalopathy (mental confusion).

Imaging Studies

A sonogram or a CT scan may reveal a fatty liver or an enlarged liver or spleen. But these findings are not diagnostic of ALD. As with other liver diseases, imaging studies cannot accurately diagnose ALD, nor can they determine the extent of liver damage that has occurred.

Liver Biopsy

For people with ALD, symptoms, physical findings, and laboratory tests typically do not correlate with the severity of inflammation or damage found on liver biopsy samples. Furthermore, they are often not indicative of the stage of ALD. A liver biopsy is the only test that can accurately confirm the diagnosis of ALD and determine the extent of damage caused by the disease. Moreover, a liver biopsy can determine the stage of ALD. This helps predict the likelihood of reversibility and helps to determine long-term prognosis. The stages of ALD are discussed in the following section. For a complete discussion of liver biopsies, see chapter 5.

THE STAGES OF ALD

There are three stages of alcoholic liver disease—alcoholic fatty liver, alcoholic hepatitis, and alcoholic cirrhosis. A person will not necessarily be aware of his progression from one stage into another. For example, a person may have alcoholic cirrhosis (as confirmed by a liver biopsy specimen) despite never having had an apparent episode of alcoholic hepatitis. Furthermore, all three stages may be present at the same time. Fatty liver and alcoholic hepatitis are potentially reversible. Alcoholic cirrhosis in its early, compensated state may even in some lucky cases be reversible. But once the complications of cirrhosis have occurred—decompensated cirrhosis (esophageal varices, ascites, encephalopathy)—it is always irreversible. A liver biopsy is the only available method for accurately determining long-term prognosis.

Alcoholic Fatty Liver

If a person drinks about 10 ounces (240 grams) of alcohol—equal to about three 6-packs of beer or 3 liters of wine—daily for about a week, he will most likely develop a fatty liver. In fact, steatosis (fatty liver) may occur after as little as three days of excessive alcohol ingestion. Many people who consider themselves social or weekend drinkers probably have had a fatty liver on several occasions. These people are usually asymptomatic (without symptoms). Their LFTs may be normal or slightly elevated. A physical exam may reveal an enlarged liver due to fatty deposits. A liver biopsy will show only fatty deposits and no other abnormalities. When inflammation is present in the liver among these people, their condition is known as steatohepatitis. The above-mentioned findings may be indistinguishable from fatty liver and nonalcoholic steatohepatitis (NASH), which were discussed in chapter 16. Alcoholic fatty liver is generally a benign, reversible condition. If alcohol intake is discontinued at this stage, no long-term consequences will be suffered.

Alcoholic Hepatitis

Alcoholic hepatitis is inflammation of the liver due to the toxic effects of alcohol. A person may have either acute or chronic alcoholic hepatitis. About half of all alcoholics will develop at least one episode of alcoholic hepatitis in their lifetimes. The symptoms and signs of alcoholic hepatitis vary greatly from person to person. At one end of the spectrum, a person may be asymptomatic. For such a person, the discovery of alcoholic hepatitis is likely to be made when abnormal LFTs appear on a blood test done in the course of a routine exam. For these people, alcoholic hepatitis is totally reversible if the person immediately and completely stops drinking alcohol.

At the other end of the spectrum, a person with alcoholic hepatitis may be severely ill, with fever, nausea and vomiting, abdominal pain, or even signs of severe liver damage and liver failure. Between 20 and 50 percent of these people are likely to die from a bout of alcoholic hepatitis. Those who survive may take up to six months to totally recuperate. Of course, they must totally abstain from drinking alcohol for the rest of their lives.

It must be remembered that alcoholic hepatitis can occur in a person whether or not he has alcoholic cirrhosis—a potentially irreversible condition. A finding of alcoholic hepatitis on a liver biopsy indicates that a person is at risk for developing cirrhosis. People with alcoholic hepatitis who continue to drink alcohol have at least a 50 percent chance of developing cirrhosis within ten years from the onset of alcoholic hepatitis.

Alcoholic Cirrhosis

Alcoholic cirrhosis is severe scarring of the liver due to alcohol. It is a potentially irreversible condition. The development of alcoholic cirrhosis carries with it the risk of complications that typically pertain to cirrhosis (see chapter 6). Once the complications of cirrhosis develop, alcoholic cirrhosis is irreversible.

All people with cirrhosis are at risk for liver cancer. In general, people with alcoholic cirrhosis have about a 15 percent overall lifetime risk of developing liver cancer. Paradoxically, people with alcoholic cirrhosis who continue to actively drink are actually less likely to develop liver cancer than those who abstain. This should in no way be construed as an incentive for an alcoholic to continue to drink alcohol. People with alcoholic cirrhosis who abstain from alcohol have repeatedly been shown to have a healthier and longer life span compared with those who continue to ingest alcohol.

TREATMENT OF ALD

Many different medications and nutritional therapies have been tested for use in the treatment of ALD. Most therapies involve either inhibiting or modifying the action of one or more cytokines. While some of these therapies have yielded beneficial results, in general the use of these therapies for ALD remains controversial. Consistently, the most effective form of therapy and the most important step toward recovery has been abstinence from alcohol. Other crucial steps toward recovery involve seeking the assistance of a support group and entering an alcohol treatment program. No one is expected to go it alone, and there are a variety of well-respected support groups devoted to helping people with alcohol problems achieve and sustain abstinence.

Corticosteroids—for example prednisone, an anti-inflammatory medication discussed in chapter 14—have, in some cases, been shown to improve survival in certain people with severe alcoholic hepatitis, as defined by the presence of encephalopathy, very prolonged prothrombin times, and/or elevated bilirubin levels. Present recommendations are to treat people who have severe alcoholic hepatitis with a corticosteroid for one month. This is followed by tapering and discontinuation of the corticosteroid in the following two to four weeks. However, due to the potential side effects of prednisone (see chapter 14), which may worsen some of the complications of ALD, not all people are candidates for this therapy.

Pentoxifylline (manufactured by Hoechst Marion Roussel as Trental) is a medication that is FDA approved for the treatment of *claudication*—a lack of arterial blood flow to the muscles, usually the calf muscles, resulting in limping. Pentoxifylline works by reducing the thickness of blood cells. This in turn makes it easier for blood to flow to muscles, thus improving the oxygen content of muscles. As stated earlier in this chapter, an overabundance of cytokines in a person's body may cause injury and death of liver cells and has been implicated in the development of ALD. Tumor necrosis factor (TNF), a cytokine, has been found in high doses in people with alcoholic hepatitis. It is felt that pentoxifylline may decrease TNF production, thus reducing some potential adverse consequences of alcoholic hepatitis. In fact, initial studies have shown a significant increase in survival and a significant decrease in the incidence of kidney failure in patients with alcoholic hepatitis who were treated with pentoxifylline versus those patients who were not treated. Therefore, pentoxifylline appears to be a promising treatment for people with alcoholic hepatitis. Further studies are needed to confirm these results.

Colchicine (a medication with antifibrotic and anti-inflammatory properties discussed in chapter 15) and propylthiouracil (PTU) (an antihyperthyroid medication) are the only medications that have been shown in clinical studies to improve long-term survival of people with ALD. In more recent studies, however, colchicine failed to show any survival benefits in people with alcoholic cirrhosis. Therefore, further study needs to be conducted before these medications can be recommended for the treatment of ALD.

Antioxidants may protect the liver from toxins such as alcohol. One of the ways that alcohol damages the liver is by interfering with the body's natural ability to create glutathione, an antioxidant naturally produced by the liver, by decreasing the activity of the enzyme SAMe synthetase. S-adenosyl methionine (SAMe) is a precursor of cysteine, one of the amino acids that makes up glutathione. SAMe is formed in the body when the amino acid methionine combines with adenosine triphosphate (ATP), the major source of energy in the body. Thus, SAMe increases production of glutathione in the liver. It has been purported that SAMe helps prevent the depletion of glutathione in the liver by alcohol and possibly prevents the progression of alcoholic liver injury. In fact, one study demonstrated that patients with early stages of alcoholic cirrhosis who took SAMe 1,200 mg per day for two years were less likely to die or need a liver transplant as compared to patients with early stages of alcoholic cirrhosis who did not take this supplement. More studies are needed on SAMe to confirm these results.

Nutritionally, the liver actually favors alcohol as a form of fuel. Thus, alcohol typically supplants many important nutrients needed for a healthy diet. For example, when alcohol replaces fat as an energy source, the first stage of ALD results—fatty liver. This also causes triglyceride levels to rise in the body, which puts a person at additional risk of heart disease. People with ALD should adopt a diet of healthy, nutritious foods and should attempt to increase their caloric intake to at least between 1,500 to 2,000 calories per day. It has been shown that people with severe ALD who ingest less than 1,000 calories per day of nutritious foods have a very poor prognosis. If a person with ALD cannot tolerate a regular meal, he should attempt to utilize one of the many supplement beverages that are readily available—many of which are designed specifically for alcoholics. Vitamin deficiencies are common in people with ALD. Approximately 40 percent of people with ALD have a deficiency of two or more water-soluble vitamins—vitamin C and the eight B vitamins. Folate and thiamine (vitamin B_1) are the vitamins most commonly found to be deficient. These vitamins should be replaced with 1 to 5 mg per day of folate and 50 to 100 mg per day of thiamine. See chapter 23 for more information on diet and nutrition.

Herbal remedies are often used by people with ALD, including milk thistle and Liverite—a combination of amino acids, milk thistle, and vitamins. Chapter 21 addresses herbal remedies in detail.

THE NATURAL HISTORY AND PROGNOSIS FOR THOSE WITH ALD

If alcohol use is discontinued prior to the development of cirrhosis, any inflammation or injury that has occurred to the liver is potentially reversible. It has been noted that people with alcoholic cirrhosis who abstain from drinking generally have a better prognosis than people with other forms of cirrhosis. In fact, people with alcoholic cirrhosis who have not had complications of cirrhosis, such as jaundice, variceal bleeding, or ascites, typically have a 90 percent chance of living for at least five more years. In fact, survival rates for these people are actually only slightly below that of the general population of comparable age and sex. However, once complications of cirrhosis have occurred, the chances of living for five more years decreases to 60 percent. And people with alcoholic cirrhosis have approximately a 15 percent overall lifetime risk of developing liver cancer.

For people with ALD, the key to a positive prognosis may be summed up in one word: abstinence. Those who do not abstain from drinking have a very poor prognosis. A persistently elevated bilirubin level and a prolonged prothrombin time (signs of decompensated cirrhosis) are the most reliable indicators of a poor prognosis. The level of certain cytokines in the blood may possibly predict prognosis in people with ALD. Some studies have suggested that cytokine levels correlate with both the bilirubin level and with mortality rates. Further investigation is needed to confirm these findings.

ARE THERE ANY HEALTH BENEFITS TO ALCOHOL?

Many studies have demonstrated the beneficial effects of alcohol on the heart. Some medical experts have gone as far as to make a blanket encouragement to the adult population to consume two alcoholic drinks per day (either wine, beer, or hard liquor) so as to decrease their risk of having a heart attack. While the beneficial effects of moderate daily alcohol intake are well established, it remains that people with liver disease should not consume any alcohol. As stated in this chapter as well as throughout this book, alcohol, even in moderation, can speed the progression of liver disease to cirrhosis and its complications. And keep in mind that even among people with no underlying liver disease, alcohol intake of three or more drinks per day leads to alcohol-induced cirrhosis at the rate of 2 to 3 percent of people per year. While all types of alcohol entail an increased risk for the development of cirrhosis, it appears that wine poses a lower risk than beer and hard liquor. Lastly, it should be kept in mind that many people suffer from some type of liver disease that is silent in nature. In fact, millions of people in the United States have a liver disease, such as hepatitis C or obesity-related liver disease, without realizing it. For these people, consuming alcohol of any type, even if done in moderation, may have potentially disastrous health consequences.

CONCLUSION

The most important message in this chapter is straightforward: If a person has any type of chronic liver disease, he should not ingest alcohol. In addition, it is especially important for any person with ALD to immediately abstain from consuming alcohol. The dosage and duration of alcohol ingestion are among the many factors that contribute to alcoholic liver damage and to the progression of ALD. This explains why some people can consume substantial amounts of alcohol without suffering adverse consequences whereas others are very susceptible to the toxicities of alcohol. Future research is likely to focus on identifying genes that make a person more susceptible to alcoholic cirrhosis and on learning more about the role of cytokines in the development of ALD. Future therapies will likely be targeted at altering or blocking the production of liver-toxic cytokines. Other therapies may focus on utilizing antibiotics against endotoxin-induced liver injury. In this chapter, you also learned that alcohol in combination with excessive iron accelerates the progression of liver disease.

The next chapter discusses hemochromatosis, an inherited disease of iron overload. It also discusses other diseases of iron overload that a person may acquire.

Eighteen

HEMOCHROMATOSIS
AND OTHER DISEASES
OF IRON OVERLOAD

*Patrick, a thirty-five-year-old construction worker, began to experi-
ence a lack of energy while working at his job. But what led him to
make an appointment with his doctor was his diminished interest in
sex. Patrick, who was well built and had a dark ruddy complexion, had
a long history of various muscle and joint pains, which he blamed on
the physical nature of his work. He also had a mild case of diabetes,
which he kept under control by watching his diet. He attributed his
bronze complexion to the long hours he spent working outdoors in
the sun. Patrick's doctor performed a physical exam and drew some
blood for routine blood tests. A week later, the doctor notified Patrick
that his iron level was elevated, as were some of his liver enzymes,
and he should return to the office for additional blood work. The doctor also asked him if anyone in his family had ever had liver disease.
After speaking to his mother, Patrick learned that both his aunt and
great grandfather—neither of whom drank much alcohol—had died
from cirrhosis. After some additional tests, the doctor confirmed that
Patrick had inherited hemochromatosis. He was referred to a liver
specialist who performed a liver biopsy, the results of which confirmed the diagnosis. Patrick's liver was loaded with iron. He was
sent for treatment with phlebotomies.*

Chances are many of you have seen Popeye gulping down a can of spinach
in order to get his muscle-producing supply of iron, and most of you have
probably heard that iron can "pep you up" or that it's just plain good for
you. Perhaps this explains why so many people take iron supplements expecting a boost of energy. For iron-deficient people, supplementing with iron may
be okay. But for people with iron-rich blood, taking iron supplements may be so

harmful that it can put them at risk for cirrhosis, liver cancer, impotence, and heart failure. Hemochromatosis—a genetic disease of iron overload—is the subject of this chapter. As the main repository for iron in the body, the liver is among the first organs to be affected by hemochromatosis and often suffers the greatest adverse consequences. This chapter covers hemochromatosis, its symptoms and signs, and how it is diagnosed and treated. In addition, it reviews exciting new advances made in this area. Toward the end, this chapter provides information about iron-overload diseases other than hemochromatosis.

WHAT IS HEMOCHROMATOSIS?

Hemochromatosis is a term that is used to describe an excessive deposition of iron in the body. Excess iron deposits may occur in the liver, heart, pancreas, joints, pituitary gland, or other organs. When this happens, the affected organ ceases to function properly and becomes damaged. Hemochromatosis can either be inherited at birth or may be acquired at some point due to a variety of causes.

Hereditary Hemochromatosis

If a person has inherited hemochromatosis, it is termed hereditary (or genetic) hemochromatosis (HH). These people have inherited the defective gene for the disease from their parents in an *autosomal recessive* manner. This means that in order to display the manifestations of hemochromatosis and to be at risk for its long-term complications, a person must inherit one gene from each parent. People with two hemochromatosis genes are known as *homozygotes*. People who inherit the hemochromatosis gene from only one parent are known as *heterozygotes*. Heterozygotes will not exhibit signs of the disease, nor are they at risk for complications of the disease. They are, however, carriers of the hemochromatosis gene and can pass the gene to their children. Carriers may also have a slight increase in iron absorption. The hemochromatosis gene is known as *HFE* and will be discussed later in this chapter.

Noninherited Iron Overload

A person can also have too much iron in the body due to nonhereditary causes, such as taking excessive amounts of iron supplements. Some medical literature refers to this as *secondary* or *acquired hemochromatosis*. However, it is more accurate to refer to this group of people as having a *secondary iron overload disease*. Therefore, the term *hemochromatosis* will be used in this book only in reference to those people who have inherited the disease. Secondary iron overload diseases and other nonhereditary liver diseases associated with elevated iron levels will be discussed beginning on page 286.

HOW COMMON IS HEMOCHROMATOSIS?

Hemochromatosis is a very common disorder. In fact, it is the most common genetic disease in the United States and among people of northern European descent. It is estimated that 1 in 250 to 300 Caucasians of northern European descent have this disease (approximately 1.5 million Americans). One in ten people are carriers of the disease (approximately 32 million Americans). Carriers have one copy of the mutant HFE gene. Although all ethnic groups are at risk for hemochromatosis, it has been found to be more prevalent in those of Irish, Scottish, Nordic, Celtic, or British ancestry.

AN OVERVIEW OF IRON

Hemochromatosis is a disorder of iron metabolism. Therefore, to understand hemochromatosis, it is crucial to understand what iron is, how iron is absorbed and stored, and what the effects are of having too much iron in the body.

Iron (Fe) is a mineral. A *mineral* is a substance that originates in the soil and water and eventually becomes incorporated into all animal and plant life through the food chain. While iron has many important functions in the body, an excess of iron may lead to liver damage and cirrhosis. Iron is a substance that contradicts the popular saying, "If a little is good, then more is better."

How Iron Damages the Liver

One way that iron damages the liver is by promoting the formation of harmful free radicals in the body. *Free radicals* are toxic, highly reactive compounds that are naturally produced by the body. The number of free radicals increases when the body is exposed to foreign substances (such as alcohol, cigarette smoke, radiation, or excessive iron) that it perceives as hazardous. Most free radicals in the body are toxic oxygen molecules. Oxygen in its toxic state can oxidize molecules in the body, corroding them—similar to the way rust forms on an iron fence, which is actually just oxidized iron.

Iron-induced oxidation of the cell walls is known as *lipid peroxidation.* The by-products of lipid peroxidation, such as hydrogen peroxide, are believed to be toxic to the liver. Anyone with any form of liver disease should bear this in mind, as iron has been shown to speed the progression and worsen the course of many liver diseases. This is especially true for alcoholic liver disease, as alcohol and excess iron have been shown to have an additive harmful effect on the liver.

How Iron Levels Are Determined

Normal iron levels routinely found on blood work range between 30 and 160 mcg/dl. Iron is stored in the cells of the body as *ferritin.* The normal ferritin level found on blood tests is 15 to 200 mcg/l. *Transferrin* is a protein that is made by the liver and transports iron through the body. The percentage of transferrin that is saturated with iron at any given time is known as the *transferrin saturation percent*. Normal transferrin saturation values range from 15 to 50 percent. Iron, ferritin, and transferrin saturation percent together are referred to as *iron studies*. If a person's iron studies are above the upper limit of normal on any of these tests, he should be checked for hemochromatosis. See "Diagnosing Hemochromatosis" on page 279.

How Iron Is Stored and Replaced

The amount of iron lost from the body on a daily basis is approximately 1 to 2 mg. People must replace this daily iron loss through the foods they eat. However, the average American diet contains about 10 to 20 mg of iron per day, an amount that greatly exceeds the average loss. Humans do not have a major route of elimination of iron from the body. Therefore, the content of iron in the body is determined by how much iron the body actually absorbs from food. For example, heme iron, which is obtained from animal meat, is better absorbed than nonheme iron, which is obtained from vegetables. So, with all due respect to Popeye, a juicy steak supplies the body with far more iron than does spinach. In people who are not at risk for iron overload, approximately 10 percent (1 to 2 mg) of dietary iron is absorbed by the lining of the duodenum. When the body's internal sensors detect an iron deficiency, more iron is absorbed from the diet. Conversely, if there is a surplus of iron already in the body, less iron is absorbed. Any excess iron that is not absorbed or eliminated from the body is stored predominantly in the liver as ferritin. In hemochromatosis, there is a defect in the body's ability to absorb iron. Moreover, the body's ability to sense an iron overload is lost. Thus, too much iron, approximately 3 to 6 mg per day, gets absorbed by the duodenum. The excess iron accumulates in the liver and other organs, such as the pancreas and heart, which can result in serious damage to these organs.

THE SYMPTOMS AND SIGNS OF HEMOCHROMATOSIS

As with most liver diseases, the symptoms of hemochromatosis are usually absent until the later stages of the disease and can be vague even when present. While this disease is present at birth, symptoms rarely appear before adulthood. This is because it takes time for an excessive amount of iron to accumulate in the body and cause organ damage. For example, up to the age of approximately twenty years old, an insignificant amount of iron—about 5 grams—accumulates in the body. About 10 to 20 grams of iron accumulate between ages twenty and forty years old. When more than 20 grams of iron accumulate in the body, organ damage typically occurs. Thus, men are usually over forty years old and women are usually over fifty years old when symptoms manifest. Men tend to have more pronounced symptoms than women. This is due to the greater amount of iron overload that exists in men because premenopausal women eliminate iron on a monthly basis through menstruation. Weakness and fatigue are the most common symptoms. Some people complain of a decreased appetite and weight loss.

Since the liver is the warehouse for the storage of excess iron, it is often damaged in the early stages of the disease. This may manifest as abdominal pain or a nondescript discomfort over the right upper quadrant (over the liver). Abnormalities due to excessive iron deposits in other organs or glands of the body occur late in the disease and may include decreased body hair, reduced interest in sex, impotence in men, and a lack of menstruation in women. Glucose intolerance or overt diabetes can also develop. Occasionally—approximately 8 percent of the time—a thyroid disorder will develop. Painful joints and arthritis occur in approximately one-fourth to one-half of people with hemochromatosis, usually beginning in the hands, but it can progress to the knees, back, and neck. People with hemochromatosis are also prone to osteoporosis.

Some people notice that they have developed what appears to be a "healthy" tan. This skin discoloration is anything but healthy. It is actually due to a combination of iron deposits in the skin and an increased production of the pigment melanin. This bronze coloration of the skin, known as *hyperpigmentation,* is most obvious in the sun-exposed areas of the body. In fact, hemochromatosis was originally called *bronze diabetes* because most people with hemochromatosis were first seen by a doctor in the later stages of the disease—after they had already developed grayish-bronze skin coloring and the symptoms of diabetes, including increased thirst and urination. Symptoms of more advanced hemochromatosis include heart failure, heart *arrhythmias* (an irregular heartbeat), and the manifestations of portal hypertension (discussed in chapter 6).

On physical exam, the doctor may detect an enlarged liver; *cardiomegaly* (an enlarged heart); bronze skin tone; testicular atrophy (shrunken testicles); swollen and tender joints; or signs of cirrhosis and/or liver failure. Any of these findings are suggestive of advanced hemochromatosis.

DIAGNOSING HEMOCHROMATOSIS

It has been shown that early detection and treatment of hemochromatosis can prevent the long-term, potentially fatal consequences of the disease. However, in the early stages of hemochromatosis, symptoms are usually absent or very vague. Symptoms in the later stages frequently mimic those of other more common diseases, such as heart disease, arthritis, and diabetes. Often, people go undiagnosed for many years. This may be because their iron studies appear normal or even low due to factors such as frequent blood donation, multiple pregnancies, menstruation, or gastrointestinal bleeding. Therefore, it is not surprising that about 90 percent of people with hemochromatosis go undiagnosed or misdiagnosed for so long.

So, how would a person normally discover that he has hemochromatosis in the first place? Well, the initial step is for the person to go to the doctor for a routine checkup and blood tests, despite feeling fine. In fact, the Iron Overload Diseases Association (IODA) recommends that all Americans eighteen years and older be routinely screened for iron overload. Another easy way to be checked for hemochromatosis is during blood donation. This is often free of charge at many local blood banks or hospitals. This section will discuss the utility of blood tests, a liver biopsy, and imaging studies in the diagnosis of hemochromatosis.

Iron Studies and Liver Function Tests (LFTs)

Hemochromatosis is often diagnosed in people when high or elevated iron studies are detected on routine blood tests. Iron studies commonly include three values—the iron level, the ferritin level (the level of iron stored in the liver), and the transferrin saturation percent (the percent of transferrin—a protein made in the liver that transports iron through the body—that is saturated with iron at any given time). The transferrin saturation percent is the first value to become elevated in people with hemochromatosis. In fact, it may even be elevated in people with hemochromatosis who have normal iron and ferritin levels. If the transferrin saturation percent is elevated to greater than 50 percent for women and 60 percent for men, the diagnosis of hemochromatosis is strongly suggested. The transferrin saturation percent is now the test recommended for screening the general adult population for iron overload states.

Serum ferritin levels may also be elevated in people with other liver diseases in the absence of hemochromatosis. In fact, approximately 50 percent of people with alcoholic liver disease, nonalcoholic fatty liver disease (NAFLD), or chronic hepatitis C have elevated ferritin levels. In addition, other diseases such as rheumatoid arthritis or certain types of cancers may cause elevated ferritin levels. Therefore, an elevated ferritin level does not indicate that a person has hemochromatosis. However, in people with confirmed hemochromatosis, a serum ferritin level of greater than 1,000 mcg/l usually correlates with the degree of liver scarring—fibrosis and cirrhosis. It should be noted that iron studies are more accurate when blood work is drawn after a person has fasted for about twelve hours.

Elevated LFTs are also commonly found in people with hemochromatosis. But don't be misled by normal LFTs. In the early stages of the disease, LFTs are rarely elevated.

The Hemochromatosis Gene (HFE)

When an elevated transferrin saturation percent is found, genetic testing is required. As discussed on page 276, a major advance in the diagnosis of hemochromatosis has been the identification of the gene for hemochromatosis known as HFE and the subsequent discovery of two specific gene mutations, C282Y and H63D, that are diagnostic for hemochromatosis.

More than 90 percent of people with hemochromatosis are homozygous for the gene mutation C282Y. The H63D mutation by itself is not as clearly associated with hemochromatosis. In fact, there are many people in the United States who are homozygous for the H63D gene mutation and rarely, if ever, develop iron overload. However, if a person inherits one H63D and one C282Y mutation—a condition known as a compound heterozygote—occasionally he will develop significant iron overload. Compound heterozygotes are found in approximately 4 percent of people with hemochromatosis. Two additional HFE gene mutations have been described, but their significance is unclear. Approximately 10 to 15 percent of people who do not carry either of these mutations still develop hemochromatosis. And there are some people who have been identified as having two C282Y mutations, yet have no evidence of iron overload. In fact, estimates vary considerably, from 1 to 50 percent, as to how many homozygotes actually develop clinically significant disease. Obviously, there are other unknown factors or other gene mutations not yet discovered that cause hemochromatosis and that cause people with two C282Y mutations to develop clinically significant disease.

The genetic DNA tests for identifying both C282Y and H63D are currently available and can be obtained simply by having some blood tests taken by the doctor. Also, there is a tissue-collection kit available that merely requires a person to swab the inside of his mouth with a cheek brush. This screening test can be performed at home. However, regardless of which screening method is used, a doctor must evaluate the results.

As discussed on page 276, hemochromatosis is an autosomal recessively inherited disease. Therefore, a person must inherit two copies of the hemochromatosis gene mutation in order to manifest the disease. If only one copy of the HFE gene is found to contain the C282Y mutation, the person is merely a carrier. Development of disease by such a person is unlikely; however, 15 to 25 percent of carriers have a slight increase in iron absorption.

Liver Biopsy

With the advent of genetic testing, a liver biopsy is no longer necessary to make a diagnosis of hemochromatosis. However, it is important for people diagnosed with hemochromatosis to have a liver biopsy in order to assess both the amount of iron stores in the liver and the degree of damage done to the liver by this overload of iron. A biopsy is the only reliable test for determining whether cirrhosis is present. This information is helpful for both the patient and the doctor as it will assist in determining long-term prognosis, for implementing screening procedures of esophageal varices and liver cancer, for assessing management and treatment, and for planning for possible liver transplantation.

There are some instances when a liver biopsy may not be necessary. These include people with hemochromatosis who are less than forty years old; who have normal LFTs and physical exam; whose serum ferritin level is less than 1,000 mg/l; and who have no evidence of other liver diseases. These people may forego a liver biopsy as they are unlikely to have significant liver damage. One study demonstrated that the combination of a ferritin level of greater than 1,000 mcg/l, a platelet count less than 200 x 10⁹/l and an AST level above the upper limit of normal is indicative of a diagnosis of cirrhosis in approximately 81 percent of people with C282Y hemochromatosis. This finding needs to be confirmed with further studies before it can be recommended as a means of diagnosing cirrhosis in lieu of a liver biopsy (see chapter 5 for detailed information about liver biopsies).

Imaging Studies

A sonogram is usually normal, but it may reveal an enlarged liver. While it will not reveal the degree to which the liver is damaged, it is a good screening test to evaluate for the presence or absence of liver cancer. Therefore, the doctor will most likely want a sonogram at some point in the evaluation. If a person's liver biopsy reveals cirrhosis, he will need to obtain a sonogram once or twice a year because such people are at high risk for the development of liver cancer.

CT scans may reveal evidence of iron overload in cases where the overload is very extensive. However, in milder cases of iron overload, the CT will be normal. MRIs can also detect a heavy iron overload. They are occasionally used to determine the amount of iron in the liver and the extent to which the liver has been damaged. It is important to remember that MRIs do not provide as much information as a liver biopsy. They should be substituted only for a liver biopsy in cases where it has been determined that a biopsy would be medically unsafe for a particular person. See chapter 3 for more information on imaging studies.

TREATMENT OF HEMOCHROMATOSIS

The goal of treatment of hemochromatosis is to remove the excess iron from the body to prevent the occurrence of organ damage. This can be easily and efficiently achieved by a method known as phlebotomy. Another way to remove excess iron is through a process known as chelation therapy. Finally, certain dietary restrictions also play a role in the treatment of hemochromatosis. The following is a discussion of these treatments.

Phlebotomy

Phlebotomy involves taking blood out of the body through a catheter that is temporarily placed in the arm. The blood that is removed from the body is discarded because it cannot be used for blood donation or for any other purpose. Approximately 500 ml (equal to one unit) of blood should be taken out each week. This will remove approximately 250 mg of iron on each occasion. For example, if a person has an excess of about 25 grams of iron, he will need to have approximately 100 units of blood removed. It usually takes about two years of weekly phlebotomies to deplete about 25 grams of iron. Prior to each phlebotomy, a person's red blood count, measured by hemoglobin or hematocrit, should be checked. Iron studies—

iron, ferritin, and transferrin saturation—should be checked about every three months. When the transferrin saturation falls below 50 percent and the serum ferritin falls below 50 mcg/l, the goal has been achieved. Mild anemia may develop at this point. Levels less than 25 mcg/l indicate iron deficiency anemia and require a temporary hold on further phlebotomies. Vitamin C supplements should always be avoided in people undergoing phlebotomy, as vitamin C enhances iron absorption in the body. This will be discussed in more detail on page 284.

If the results of a liver biopsy reveal excessive scarring, iron should be removed from the body at a quicker rate to attempt to avoid cirrhosis and its complications. These people should have blood removed at least twice a week. Removal of excess iron can stop the progression of hemochromatosis if cirrhosis is not present at the time of diagnosis. This point underscores the importance of early diagnosis and of prompt treatment as well as the need to consider evaluation with liver biopsy. Phlebotomy will not be able to improve cirrhosis. Yet despite the presence of cirrhosis, phlebotomy might alleviate some symptoms associated with hemochromatosis, especially fatigue and abdominal pain. Therefore, people with cirrhosis should still undergo phlebotomy. However, these people remain at risk for liver cancer and other complications of cirrhosis.

After the initial bulk of excessive iron has been removed, the frequency of phlebotomies is decreased to the level where 500 ml (one unit) of blood is removed approximately every three months. The goal should be to keep the ferritin level between 25 and 50 mcg/l at all times. The frequency of maintenance phlebotomies varies from three to twelve times a year, since people re-accumulate iron at varying degrees. Maintenance phlebotomy should continue lifelong.

Some symptoms totally resolve after successful phlebotomy. Fatigue improves in over 60 percent of people who have undergone phlebotomy. Hyperpigmentation also resolves in most people. Abdominal pain and enlargement of the liver, attributable to distention of the liver from iron overload, usually resolves after sufficient quantities of iron have been removed. Similarly, elevated LFTs usually normalize. Heart problems caused by hemochromatosis, such as congestive heart failure (CHF) and cardiomegaly (enlarged heart) also usually improve after excessive iron is removed.

Approximately 50 percent of people with diabetes due to hemochromatosis will be more easily managed. However, there will probably be a continued need for either insulin or *oral hypoglycemics*—sugar-lowering medications taken orally. Iron-depletion therapy has no effect on the course of hemochromatosis-associated arthritis. Treatment of joint pains should be with nonsteroidal anti-inflammatories, but in moderation, as these medications may also cause liver damage. In fact, arthritis may even develop after iron is depleted. Unfortunately, hemochromatosis-related impotence usually does not resolve. Furthermore, testosterone therapy for impotence should be avoided due to the potential additional risk factor for liver cancer, although this risk is not well documented. See chapter 24 for other treatments of sexual dysfunctions.

Chelation Therapy

Chelation therapy—involving the infusion of deferoxamine (Desferal, manufactured by Novartis Pharmaceuticals) either into a vein or subcutaneously—can also remove excess iron. This iron *chelator* (a binding agent) works by binding to iron and promoting its elimination from the body. This treatment takes much longer than phlebotomy, as only 10 to 20 mg of iron is removed each time—in contrast to 250 mg with phlebotomy. In addition, this treatment is more expensive than phlebotomy and is associated with some side effects, such as diarrhea, a rapid heartbeat, and hearing and visual disturbances. Therefore, deferoxamine infusions should be limited to people who otherwise cannot tolerate phlebotomy, such as those people with severe heart disease. Iron chelators taken orally, such as deferiprone, have been associated with significant toxicity and cannot be recommended at present.

Diet

While there is some disagreement as to how stringent a person needs to be in terms of dietary restrictions, it is probably a good idea to refrain from eating foods high in iron content. Such foods include all red meats—especially liver. Vegetable iron is not as efficiently absorbed into the body as animal iron. Therefore, total dietary restriction of green, leafy vegetables is not necessary or healthy. No iron supplements should be taken under any circumstances. People should avoid cooking with cast-iron cookware and utensils, which are often a source of hidden iron.

Vitamin C increases the body's ability to absorb iron from food. Therefore, no vitamin C supplements (including that found in multivitamins) should be taken, especially when undergoing phlebotomy. Some medicines contain iron, so labels should be read carefully. There are also many foods, especially cereals, that are fortified with iron. Some weight-gain and weight-loss products are loaded with iron and vitamin C. Furthermore, some herbs commonly taken to treat liver disease (milk thistle, dandelion, and licorice) may contain iron. Therefore, people with hemochromatosis should avoid all herbs. People must become informed consumers, carefully reading labels prior to purchasing foods, beverages, herbs, supplements, or any over-the-counter medicines from any supermarket, drugstore, or health-food store. There have been some reports of people with hemochromatosis who died due to eating raw shellfish that was contaminated with the bacteria *Vibrio vulnificus*. Thus, it is probably wise for people with hemochromatosis to avoid raw shellfish.

Lastly, alcohol should be avoided for two reasons. First, alcohol may increase iron absorption. Second, alcohol, in itself, is toxic to the liver. Thus, alcohol, even in moderate amounts, may worsen liver damage in people with hemochromatosis. In fact, it has been shown that people with hemochromatosis who drink more than 60 grams of alcohol each day are nine times more likely to develop cir-

rhosis and have a higher incidence of liver cancer as compared to people with hemochromatosis who drink less than 60 grams of alcohol each day. Thus, people
with hemochromatosis should not drink alcohol. See chapter 23 for more information on diet.

THE LONG-TERM PROGNOSIS FOR THOSE
WITH HEMOCHROMATOSIS

Hemochromatosis is a potentially fatal disease. However, if the disease is diagnosed
early and is treated promptly and aggressively, a person with hemochromatosis
will enjoy a normal life span. Once cirrhosis has developed, people are at increased
risk for the complications of cirrhosis and for the development of liver cancer—
even if iron stores have been successfully depleted through phlebotomy. In fact,
people with both hemochromatosis and cirrhosis are two hundred times more
likely (estimated at a 30 percent chance) to develop liver cancer compared with
the general population. Between 30 and 45 percent of deaths in people with hemochromatosis are due to liver cancer. Phlebotomy has been shown to somewhat
reduce the risk of liver cancer. See chapter 19 for more information on liver cancer.

There is potentially an increased risk of other types of cancers occurring in
people with hemochromatosis. Some studies have shown that people with hemochromatosis are more likely to develop colon, esophageal, lung, and skin cancers as compared with the general population. Also one study found that the
estimated risk of developing cancer in an organ other than the liver is twice as
great in people with hemochromatosis as compared to people with other types of
liver diseases. While these findings have not been confirmed, they suggest that
excessive iron has the potential to induce cancer in organs other than the liver.
Thus, phlebotomy is essential not only for reducing the risk of cirrhosis (and subsequently liver cancer), but also for reducing the risk of developing cancer in other
parts of the body.

Hemochromatosis may cause heart arrhythmias and heart failure. When heart
trouble occurs, aggressive treatment with phlebotomy and/or possibly chelation
therapy should commence promptly.

If complications of cirrhosis occur, the person should be considered for a
liver transplant. This option will be addressed in chapter 22.

Screening for Hemochromatosis

Screening family members for hemochromatosis is important since it is the most
common inherited disorder among Caucasians in the Western Hemisphere. Since
the gene for hemochromatosis is passed on recessively, successive generations
may include carriers, none of whom ever manifest the disease. All first-degree
relatives (children, siblings, and parents) of an individual with hemochromatosis
should be screened for this disease. Screening should be with a fasting transferrin saturation and ferritin level and/or the genetic markers C282Y and H63D.

Genetic screening is now being routinely performed at local blood bank donation centers. The likelihood of one's offspring getting hemochromatosis can be determined by testing the offspring's unaffected parent. If the unaffected parent does not have any C282Y mutations, the offspring can only be heterozygous (a carrier of hemochromatosis). If the unaffected parent is a heterozygote for the C282Y mutation, the offspring has a 50 percent chance of being homozygous (having hemochromatosis). As organ damage from hemochromatosis is extremely rare before adulthood, evaluation of first-degree relatives should begin when these people are approximately twenty years of age. In this way, the disorder may be detected early, long before injury to the liver has occurred.

The need for genetic screening of first-degree relatives is widely accepted. However, screening of the general population for hemochromatosis is a subject of ongoing debate. Those in favor of population-wide screening emphasize that the consequences of undetected hemochromatosis can be devastating—cirrhosis, heart disease, diabetes, and early death. Studies have confirmed that of people with hemochromatosis, 75 percent of men and 50 percent of women have elevated transferrin saturations and ferritin levels. Some studies have shown that between 50 and 95 percent of male C282Y homozygotes develop serious complications as a consequence of hemochromatosis. Add to the fact that treatment by phlebotomy is relatively simple and very effective. By identifying the disorder early on, before complications occur, the screening process can provide significant benefit to a person's life.

Those against population screening point out that the diagnosis of hemochromatosis in asymptomatic people may result in job discrimination or rejection for medical or life insurance (or, at the very least, hefty premium increases for these types of insurance). Furthermore, the optimal approach to asymptomatic people discovered to have hemochromatosis by screening is unclear. Some experts believe that less than 1 percent of people with the C282Y mutation will actually develop clinically significant disease. At the present time, population-wide genetic screening is not being conducted. However, it is likely that the screening of high-risk populations (Caucasians of northern European descent) will be standard at some point in the future.

SECONDARY OR ACQUIRED IRON OVERLOAD DISEASES

As discussed earlier in this chapter, iron overload can either be inherited at birth or may be acquired at some point due to a variety of causes. In fact, mere excessive oral ingestion of iron can cause elevated iron studies. Thus, when a person is discovered to have a high iron profile on routine blood tests, a thorough investigation into all of the medicines, vitamins, and supplements (both prescribed and over the counter) that he is taking should be made. Those that contain excess iron should be eliminated from the diet.

There have been occasional reports of people becoming iron overloaded from drinking excessive quantities of beer that had been brewed in cast-iron drums or from consuming substantial quantities of foods cooked in iron cookware. If high iron profiles persist after the elimination of the above-mentioned factors, another cause of high iron levels—such as hereditary hemochromatosis or chronic hepatitis C—should be searched for.

People who have received an excessive number of blood transfusions—say, more than fifty in a lifetime for example—often have elevated iron levels due to iron accumulated from all those transfusions. These people are at risk for the development of iron-related organ damage. A chelation therapy program should be considered if continued transfusions will be needed on a regular basis.

Some people receive iron replacement either orally or by injection after being diagnosed with anemia (a low red blood cell count). Yet anemia can have a multitude of causes—iron deficiency being just one of them. If the anemia is not due to an iron deficiency but to some other cause, such as a vitamin B_{12} deficiency, for example, toxic accumulations of iron can result if iron replacement was given.

Other causes of secondary iron overload include thalassemia major, a genetic defect in red blood cell production; and hemolytic anemia, an accelerated rate of red blood cell destruction.

Excessive Iron and Other Liver Diseases

Iron by itself can have harmful effects on the liver. When excessive iron exists in combination with another liver disorder, there is potential for worsening and/or accelerated liver damage. There are three liver diseases that are associated with high iron levels. They include alcoholic liver disease (see chapter 17), nonalcoholic fatty liver disease (NAFLD) (see chapter 16), and chronic viral hepatitis—especially chronic hepatitis C (see chapter 10). Elevated iron studies occur in about 40 to 50 percent of people with one of these underlying liver disorders. However, since these people do not have hereditary hemochromatosis, their intestines do not absorb an overabundance of iron. Thus, excessive iron deposition in the liver occurs only about 10 percent of the time in this particular group. Furthermore, the degree of iron deposits in the liver is mild compared to that found in people with hemochromatosis.

Why people with these three liver disorders have high iron levels remains an area of speculation and debate among medical researchers. It is believed, but not conclusively proven, that some of these people may be heterozygotes for hemochromatosis (carriers of one mutant gene). If these people are treated with phlebotomy, their LFTs may show some improvement. It has also been suggested that people with chronic hepatitis C who have elevated iron studies may respond better to interferon treatment if they undergo phlebotomy. Therefore, it makes sense for the doctor to obtain hemochromatosis genetic testing on people with these liver diseases who have elevated iron studies.

CONCLUSION

After reading this chapter, you know that iron—though required by the body in small amounts for proper functioning—can be harmful to some people. This includes people with hemochromatosis, other disorders of iron overload, and some chronic liver diseases. Hemochromatosis is another liver disorder where early detection is crucial to halt the progression of the disease. If a person has this disorder, it is highly recommended that their family members be screened.

The next chapter discusses both *benign* (noncancerous) and *malignant* (cancerous) liver tumors and how they are treated.

Nineteen

BENIGN AND MALIGNANT LIVER TUMORS

June, a thirty-year-old receptionist, went to her doctor for evaluation of a fever, cough, and sore throat. The doctor's diagnosis was that June had bronchitis. He gave her a prescription for an antibiotic and took some blood tests. The results of the blood tests were normal with the exception of an elevated GGTP. The doctor noted that in June's medical history questionnaire, she wrote that she'd been on birth control pills since giving birth five years earlier. The doctor advised June to see a radiologist to get a sonogram done to evaluate the cause of her elevated GGTP. The sonogram revealed a large mass on her liver and her doctor advised her to discontinue taking the birth control pills immediately and repeat the sonogram in three months. The repeat sonogram did not reveal any decrease in size of the mass. The doctor sent June for a liver biopsy, the results of which revealed that June's tumor was a hepatic adenoma. The doctor concluded that this benign tumor was caused by June's use of birth control pills. June was referred to a surgeon for the removal of the hepatic adenoma.

For many people, one of the worst fears is that one day a doctor will inform them that they have a *tumor*. However, having a liver tumor is not always a fatal condition. This chapter discusses both benign (not cancerous or fatal) and malignant (cancerous and potentially fatal) liver tumors. It addresses how they are detected, what kind of symptoms they may cause, who is at risk, and what the potential treatments are.

While there are many types of liver tumors, this chapter will detail the most common ones—hemangiomas, hepatic adenomas, focal nodular hyperplasia, metastatic tumors, and hepatocellular carcinoma. It also briefly addresses some conditions, such as focal fatty infiltration, that may be confused with liver tumors.

With the exception of hepatocellular carcinoma, all liver tumors—whether they are benign or malignant—can occur in people regardless of whether there is an underlying liver disease. There are many promising new treatments for malignant tumors. While these treatment options will be discussed briefly, an extensive discussion of them is beyond the scope of this book. People should consult with an oncologist (cancer specialist) for further details regarding these new therapies.

LIVER MASSES

Liver masses are being detected by doctors with increasing frequency. The reason for this is simple. Advances in radiological techniques have given today's doctors access to a wide variety of imaging studies. Thus, radiological studies are regularly being performed in the course of evaluation of medical problems unrelated to the liver, such as nonspecific abdominal pain. A consequence of this frequent use of imaging studies is that liver masses are being discovered by chance. Once a mass on the liver has been detected, it then becomes necessary to conduct further testing in order to determine the exact nature of the mass. Fortunately, most of these masses will be benign (noncancerous).

The liver is a common site of tumors for a variety of reasons. As discussed in chapter 1, the liver has a rich dual blood supply—from the portal vein and from the hepatic artery. These passageways provide a direct route for malignant (cancerous) tumor cells from other organs to navigate into the liver and deposit themselves there. This is known as liver *metastasis*. As you may recall, everything we eat, drink, and breathe—whether it be foods, medicines, or fumes—ultimately passes through the liver to be processed. Therefore, when a person ingests significant amounts of potentially toxic chemicals, such as alcohol or in some cases even oral contraceptives, the liver can potentially suffer adverse consequences. One possible outcome is the formation of a tumor. Furthermore, any diseases with the potential to lead to cirrhosis—including chronic viral hepatitis B or C, hereditary hemochromatosis, or even nonalcoholic fatty liver disease—leave the liver at risk for the formation of a malignant tumor. Before discussing malignant tumors, the following section addresses a variety of benign liver tumors.

THE TYPES OF BENIGN LIVER TUMORS AND THEIR TREATMENTS

There are many types of benign liver tumors. This section will discuss five types: hemangioma, hepatic adenomas, focal nodular hyperplasia (FNH), the solitary liver cyst, and nodular regenerative hyperplasia (NRH). In general, they occur more frequently in women than in men. They are usually discovered by chance during the evaluation of nonrelated symptoms. Liver function tests (LFTs) are usually normal in people with benign liver tumors. In rare circumstances, these benign tumors can become so massive that a person may go to the doctor for abdominal discomfort caused by an enlarged liver. In these uncommon circumstances, results from blood tests occasionally reveal mildly elevated AP or GGTP levels (see chapter 3).

There are no blood tests that specifically indicate that a tumor is in fact benign. Thus the doctor may be uncertain as to whether the tumor is, in fact, benign. While malignant liver tumors may *metastasize* (spread to other organs, most commonly the lungs), benign liver tumors are always confined to the liver. Diagnosing the specific nature of the tumors can generally be done using a variety of radiological techniques (imaging studies) combined with the patient's medical history. When the diagnosis remains uncertain, a liver biopsy is generally performed. Since many of these tumors have an abundance of blood vessels, liver biopsy in some cases carries an increased risk of bleeding. A smaller-than-normal needle, or an aspirate of liver fluid, can be used to decrease the occurrence of this potential complication.

Treatment of benign lesions is generally conservative. Surgery is considered primarily in cases where the tumor is causing significant abdominal pain, or if there is a high risk of rupture of the tumor. Furthermore, surgery should be done if the benign nature of the tumor cannot be confidently established, or if it is felt that the tumor has a risk of progression to a malignancy.

What Is a Hemangioma?

Hemangiomas are the most common benign tumors of the liver. They have no malignant potential and may occur in a person with or without underlying liver disease. The name *hemangioma* derives from the fact that these tumors are filled with *heme* (blood). They resemble the small bright red spots that people commonly get on the skin of their chests and abdomens as they age. These spots, referred to as *senile hemangiomas,* are also benign. Hemangiomas occur in the liver in approximately 7 percent of the population, but some studies have reported ranges of from 1 to 20 percent. About 10 percent of people with a hemangioma will have more than one of them. Some people will also have hemangiomas in other areas of the body such as the skin, lungs, or brain. Hemangiomas are more common in women, but can also be found in men and can occur at any age.

The Symptoms and Signs of a Hemangioma

Typically, an individual who harbors a liver hemangioma will not even be aware of it, as these tumors are usually asymptomatic (without symptoms). Hemangiomas rarely grow. However, when one does in fact grow to a size greater than 4 centimeters, a person may experience abdominal discomfort, usually located in the right upper quadrant of the abdomen. This is attributable to the enlarged liver pushing against other surrounding organs, such as the intestines or the stomach. A person with a hemangioma may also experience periodic pain as the hemangioma grows. This pain is thought to be caused by the formation of blood clots within the vessels of the expanding hemangioma.

An extraordinarily rare but very serious complication that can occur is the rupture of a hemangioma. Rupture can be induced by physical trauma or may be spontaneous. If this occurs, there will be sudden, excruciating abdominal pain and abdominal distention. This is a medical emergency, and immediate surgery will be required.

Diagnosing a Hemangioma

Blood tests are typically normal in people with hemangiomas and therefore are of little to no value in arriving at a diagnosis. Hemangiomas are usually detected by chance during a sonogram performed for the evaluation of an unrelated medical condition. However, a sonogram is not diagnostic, but only suggestive of this type of tumor. Therefore, additional radiological scans are necessary in order to confirm that the tumor in question is in fact a hemangioma. If the sonogram indicates that the mass is larger than 2.5 centimeters in size, a *tagged red blood cell* (RBC) *scan* is ordered. Using this scan, the person's blood is labeled with a radioactive metallic element (known as a tracer), such as technetium. Images of the liver are taken at varying time intervals. Since blood flow through the hemangioma is characteristically slow, if a hemangioma is present, the tracer will accumulate within it after a prolonged amount of time (about two hours), thereby confirming the diagnosis.

If the sonogram indicates that the mass is smaller than 2.5 centimeters in size, an MRI generally can diagnose the mass as being a hemangioma. Repeat imaging studies are generally not necessary for hemangiomas that appear typical on radiologic studies. However, with giant hemangiomas, greater than 10 centimeters, repeat imaging studies should routinely be done after a year to assess for any change of configuration or to determine if there has been any growth.

Liver biopsies are occasionally performed to diagnose a hemangioma, but are not recommended, as they carry an increased risk of bleeding when standard-size needles are used and are sometimes nondiagnostic when smaller needles are used.

Treating a Hemangioma

Treatment of hemangiomas is not necessary, unless they are very large—greater than 10 to 15 centimeters, and/or are causing significant abdominal discomfort. For these people, surgical removal (resection) of the hemangioma should be considered. The only other time that surgery is suggested is if there is uncertainty that the tumor in question is, in fact, a hemangioma. Other options, such as radiation therapy and the use of steroids, have not been very successful and are not recommended. In rare cases, such as when multiple, large, symptomatic hemangiomas are present, liver transplantation may be the only option. There are no pills, either prescription or over the counter, that will cause a hemangioma to resolve.

Reducing the Chances That a Hemangioma Will Grow

Some researchers believe that excess estrogen can cause hemangiomas to grow. In fact, growth of hemangiomas has been observed in some women during pregnancy and in others while taking birth control pills. Furthermore, these people may be at increased risk for rupture. Although the effect of estrogen on hemangiomas is not conclusive, it is advisable for people with hemangiomas to stay off birth control pills and all other forms of estrogen replacement.

What Is a Hepatic Adenoma?

A *hepatic adenoma* is a rare tumor found on the liver. It is made of hepatocytes (liver cells) that have abnormally multiplied numerous times, forming a benign mass. In contrast to hemangiomas, hepatic adenomas occur infrequently. These tumors were very uncommon in the United States prior to the widespread use of oral contraceptives, which began in the 1960s and 1970s. The typical person discovered to have this tumor is a woman in her thirties who had used birth control pills at some time in her life—usually for longer than five years. However, some tumors are discovered in women who took birth control pills for as little as six months, and some tumors are found in women up to ten years after they have discontinued using birth control pills. It is thought that the estrogen in birth control pills may be the cause of hepatic adenomas. However, since most of these pills presently contain a lower amount of estrogen than they did in the past, hepatic adenomas are becoming more uncommon. Occasionally, this type of tumor has been found in women who have never used birth control pills and in men—especially in those men who have used androgens or anabolic steroids. About one-quarter of people will have more than one hepatic adenoma.

The Symptoms and Signs of a Hepatic Adenoma

In contrast to the asymptomatic nature of hemangiomas, about 50 percent of people with adenomas have abdominal pain or feel an abdominal mass in the right upper quadrant, and the other 50 percent have no symptoms. Approximately 20 percent of people with a hepatic adenoma have no symptoms until the adenoma ruptures, which is marked by the sudden onset of excruciating abdominal pain. This is a serious situation that can result in massive hemorrhage and must be treated with emergency surgery.

Diagnosing a Hepatic Adenoma

About 10 to 20 percent of people will be discovered to have a hepatic adenoma by chance when imaging studies of the abdomen are obtained for an unrelated problem or complaint. In other cases, an abdominal mass may be found during a routine physical exam. Still others are detected at the time of abdominal surgery for an unrelated reason. Sonograms, CT scans, and MRIs can all be utilized to detect a hepatic adenoma. However, these imaging studies are merely suggestive of the diagnosis. Therefore, a liver biopsy is necessary to confirm the presence of a hepatic adenoma.

Treating a Hepatic Adenoma

Treatment entails the discontinuation of any estrogen-containing medications, such as birth control pills. While this tumor is typically benign, there is a small, yet significant, potential for it to progress to liver cancer. Therefore, if this tumor does not regress after birth control pills are discontinued, surgical removal of the tumor is recommended. Furthermore, surgery may be recommended after an assessment has been made as to the tumor's risk of rupturing. In people opting not to undergo surgery, regular follow-up scanning is crucial in order to monitor and detect tumor growth.

Special Precautions to Take for Those with a Hepatic Adenoma

As hormonal imbalances during pregnancy may trigger the hepatic adenoma to grow and rupture, pregnancy is not recommended. However, once the adenoma has been surgically removed, pregnancy should be safe. People with hepatic adenomas should avoid taking birth control pills, any form of estrogen supplementation, and anabolic steroids-androgens.

What Is Focal Nodular Hyperplasia (FNH)?

Focal nodular hyperplasia (FNH) is a benign liver tumor made of liver cells that have multiplied numerous times around a malformed or abnormally formed hepatic artery. It is more common among women than men. While estrogens probably do not actually cause the development of FNH, the hormonal effects of birth control pills and pregnancy may cause an existing tumor to grow.

The Symptoms and Signs of Focal Nodular Hyperplasia

Most people have no symptoms, but in cases where the tumor is very large, some people experience abdominal pain or notice a mass that can be felt through their skin. Unlike hemangiomas and hepatic adenomas, rupture and hemorrhage are unlikely, and progression to liver cancer has never been reported.

Diagnosing Focal Nodular Hyperplasia

As with the other benign tumors, most people are found to have FNH by imaging studies performed during the evaluation of unrelated complaints. These tumors have a characteristic appearance that an experienced radiologist can detect on a sonogram, CT scan, or MRI. Liver biopsy is infrequently necessary, as results are usually not diagnostic. A hepatic arteriogram—an X ray of an artery after the injection of dye—is often needed to make a definitive diagnosis. If the diagnosis still remains in question, surgical removal of the lesion is undertaken to make a definitive diagnosis.

Treating Focal Nodular Hyperplasia

Since this tumor has little risk of complications, surgery is not indicated unless the person is having symptoms, such as abdominal pain, or if repeat imaging studies document an increase in size. Since hormonal imbalances can cause the tumor to grow, birth control pills should be discontinued and future pregnancies should be avoided. Occasionally, the doctor cannot definitively determine that the tumor is benign. When the diagnosis is in doubt, surgical removal of the tumor is indicated. When surgical removal is undertaken, it usually corrects the condition.

What Is a Solitary Liver Cyst?

A cyst is an enclosed sac or cavity containing either air, fluid, or semisolid material. They are a relatively common finding in the liver and are usually solitary. Liver cysts are usually benign. Occasionally they are present at birth, but they are not inherited. They are most frequently found in the right lobe of the liver and are more common in women than in men.

The Symptoms and Signs of a Liver Cyst

Most liver cysts are asymptomatic. Thus, they are most commonly detected during the evaluation of unrelated problems. Right-sided abdominal pain or abdominal distention may occur when cysts exceed 5 centimeters in size. In rare cases a cyst may bleed, become infected, or become cancerous. If one of these complications occurs, a fever, abdominal pain, or elevated liver enzymes will typically be present. If a repeat radiologic imaging study reveals growth or change in the size of the cyst, close follow-up will be necessary, and needle aspiration or biopsy of the cyst should be considered. Cancer is diagnosed by aspiration of fluid from the cyst using a needle guided by a radiologic imaging study.

Diagnosing a Liver Cyst

Liver cysts are usually diagnosed by radiologic imaging studies, such as sonogram, CT scan, or MRI. These tests are typically performed during evaluation of an unrelated problem and, thus, the cyst is diagnosed incidentally. The benign nature of the cyst can usually be determined by its radiographic features.

Treating a Liver Cyst

Asymptomatic cysts do not need any treatment. Symptomatic cysts may be treated by sonogram or CT-guided percutaneous (through the skin) cyst aspiration. In this procedure, known as ablation therapy, a solution such as alcohol or the antibiotic doxycycline is injected into the cyst, causing it to shrink, thus ablating or destroying the cyst and eliminating symptoms. Cysts may recur after ablation approximately 5 to 15 percent of the time. If ablation is not successful or available, the cyst can be ablated surgically—either laparoscopically or by an open surgical technique.

What Is Nodular Regenerative Hyperplasia (NRH)?

Nodular regenerative hyperplasia (NRH) is a condition in which normal liver tissue is totally replaced by nodules of regenerating liver cells. This condition is usually found in people over the age of fifty and is usually associated with other factors and conditions such as the use of anabolic steroids, the use of some chemotherapy medications, toxic oil exposure, rheumatoid arthritis, amyloidosis (a disease characterized by the deposition of the protein amyloid in various organs of the body), polyarteritis nodosa (a disease characterized by inflammation and scarring of small arteries), and bone marrow or liver transplantation. It is believed that these associated factors and/or conditions may contribute to the formation of NRH. Most experts believe NRH to be a benign condition. However, there have been occasional reports of liver cancer developing in people with NRH.

The Symptoms and Signs of NRH

In many cases, NRH is an incidental finding in patients with symptoms and signs of the associated condition—for example, joint aches in people with rheumatoid arthritis. Among people with NRH, liver function tests (LFTs) are typically normal or slightly elevated but are nondiagnostic. Although believed to be a benign condition, some people have had serious complications. These complications have occurred in people with particularly severe cases affecting the entire liver—a condition that resembles cirrhosis. Thus, occasionally this condition progresses to portal hypertension with variceal bleeding, ascites, and even liver failure requiring a liver transplant (see chapter 6).

Diagnosing NRH

NRH is difficult to diagnose. Radiologic imaging procedures such as sonogram or CAT scan are usually not diagnostic. Furthermore, a standard liver biopsy typically cannot detect this abnormality. In order to confirm a suspected diagnosis of NRH, a large piece of liver must be obtained through a laparoscopic or surgical liver biopsy.

Treating NRH

The treatment of NRH depends upon the patient's symptoms. Most people have no symptoms and require no specific therapy. People who have progressed to portal hypertension may need liver transplantation.

OTHER LIVER ABNORMALITIES THAT MAY BE CONFUSED WITH A PRIMARY LIVER TUMOR

There are three other types of liver tumors that need to be discussed. These are focal fatty infiltration, pseudotumor, and metastatic liver tumors.

Focal fatty infiltration of the liver is a totally benign condition. It consists of fat deposits in the liver concentrated in one area. This gives the appearance of a mass. It can be due to a variety of causes, such as obesity, diabetes, or alcoholic liver disease. It usually resolves when the underlying disease is corrected, such as with weight reduction in overweight people.

A *pseudotumor* is a fake tumor. It is medically known as macroregenerative nodules or adenomatous hyperplasia. It consists of cirrhotic nodules that give the appearance of a mass. These pseudotumors, which are found in about 25 percent of people with cirrhosis, rarely become cancerous.

A *metastatic liver tumor* is a cancer that originally started in an organ other than the liver (known as the *primary organ*) and then spread to the liver. In the United States, metastatic tumors are the most common malignancies that occur in the liver. Thus, when some doctors inform their patients that they have liver cancer, most of the time the doctors are actually referring to metastatic tumors, as opposed to primary liver cancer. Cancers originating in the colon, stomach, esophagus, pancreas, gallbladder, breast, kidney, uterus, and lungs commonly metastasize (spread) to the liver. In fact, approximately one-third of all cancers have the potential to spread to the liver.

WHAT IS HEPATOCELLULAR CARCINOMA?

A *primary malignant liver tumor* is a cancer that originates in the liver. The most common primary liver cancer in the world is known as hepatocellular carcinoma, also known as HCC or hepatoma. HCC is one of the most common cancers in the world, accounting for 6 percent of all cancers worldwide. Approximately 500,000 to 1 million cases of HCC occur each year. This makes HCC the fifth most common malignancy in men, and the ninth most common in women. Its greatest frequency occurs in Southeast Asia and Africa. Although its rate of occurrence has been rising over the past twenty years in the United States, it is still uncommon, accounting for only 0.5 to 2 percent of all cancers. The cause of this rise has been linked to the prevalence of chronic hepatitis C in the United States.

The characteristics of this cancer vary with geographic location. For example, in areas of the world where HCC is prevalent, such as in Asia and Africa, people are generally afflicted at an early age and often have a sudden onset of illness. In the United States, where this type of tumor is not as common, age of onset is generally at a later age and the tumor usually progresses slowly and silently. In general, men appear to be affected more frequently than women. In fact, in parts of the world where HCC is common, men are affected as much as eight times as frequently as women.

The following is a discussion of what causes HCC, what the associated symptoms and signs are, how a person is diagnosed, what the long-term prognosis is, and what some of the treatment options are for both operable and inoperable tumors.

THE CAUSES OF HCC

There is no simple explanation for why some people develop HCC and others do not. Most likely, there are multiple factors involved. The most significant known factor is the presence of cirrhosis due to any cause. Other factors may include genetic potential, hormonal influences, advancing age, state of general health and nutrition, lifestyle habits (especially alcohol abuse), and exposure to viruses and chemicals. While some of these factors are merely speculated to attribute to the development of HCC, other associations are definitively known. These specific factors are discussed below.

Cirrhosis

It is well established that there is a correlation between the presence of cirrhosis and the development of HCC. In fact, cirrhosis is present in approximately 60 to

90 percent of people with HCC. Furthermore, autopsy studies show that up to 28 percent of people with cirrhosis at the time of death also had HCC that went unrecognized during their lifetimes. In parts of the world where HCC is not very common, such as in the United States, cirrhosis is present in the vast majority of people with HCC. In contrast, in areas such as Mozambique, Africa, where 20 out of 100,000 people each year are afflicted with HCC, the association with cirrhosis, while common, is not as extensive This is probably due to the increased incidence in Africa of chronic hepatitis B, in which HCC may occur without cirrhosis, and the frequent consumption of foods contaminated with the liver toxic fungus-aflatoxin (see page 301). Regardless of the geographic location, it does appear that repeated liver damage, independent of the cause of damage, can predispose the liver to abnormal cell growth, thereby resulting in HCC.

The risk of developing HCC in people with cirrhosis is between 1 and 6 percent per year. The risk of developing HCC differs somewhat depending upon the cause of cirrhosis. For example, people with chronic hepatitis B have a high risk of developing HCC in their lifetimes—up to two hundred times the risk that the general population has. In contrast, the risk of HCC in a person with primary biliary cirrhosis, although present, is very low. For more information on cirrhosis, see chapter 6.

Chronic Viral Hepatitis

People with either chronic hepatitis B (HBV) or hepatitis C (HCV) have an increased risk of developing HCC. However, since the genetic makeup of these viruses differs—DNA for HBV, and RNA for HCV—the mechanism of causing HCC also differs. The next few paragraphs discuss the relationship between these viruses and the development of HCC. See part 2 for a complete discussion of viral hepatitis, which includes chapters on each of the above-mentioned hepatitis viruses.

HBV

There is a strong correlation between chronic hepatitis B and the development of HCC. Overall, HBV is responsible for approximately 75 percent of all HCCs. In fact, in countries with a high incidence of HCC, between 60 and 90 percent of people are found to have chronic hepatitis B. As previously noted, chronic hepatitis B infection can increase a person's risk of developing HCC up to two hundred times! Furthermore, HCC can occur in people with chronic hepatitis B even in the absence of cirrhosis. This may be partly due to an unidentified gene (HBx gene) that may make a person prone to developing HCC. Also, since hepatitis B is a DNA virus, it may actually incorporate its DNA into the DNA of the liver cells of the person it has infected. The mixing of genetic material from the hepatitis B virus and the patient may promote gene mutations leading to HCC even without underlying cirrhosis. The risk for an HBsAg carrier of developing HCC ranges from 0.06 percent to 6.6 percent each year. The risk increases with the severity of liver disease and the activity of the virus. Thus, those with cirrhosis and/or positive HBV DNA have the highest risk of developing HCC. Other risk factors for developing HCC include older age (greater than forty), male sex, and a family history of HCC.

While progression of disease is more rapid in people with both hepatitis B and hepatitis D, it is not clear whether these people who are doubly infected have a greater risk of developing liver cancer than those infected with HBV alone. In fact, some researchers believe that HDV may actually suppress the replication of HBV as some studies have noted a reduced incidence of liver cancer in those who are doubly infected. Other researchers believe that if people infected with both HBV and HDV do not rapidly progress to liver failure then the risk of developing HCC may be quite high. More research needs to be done in this area before definitive conclusions about the interaction between these viruses can be drawn.

People doubly infected with both the HBV and the HCV do carry an increased risk of HCC. People with chronic hepatitis B who drink excessive amounts of alcohol have been found to develop HCC, on average, more than ten years earlier than those people who do not drink alcohol excessively. Therefore, people with chronic hepatitis B should avoid all alcohol as it can hasten progression to HCC.

It takes approximately twenty to thirty years for HCC to form in a person with chronic hepatitis B. Thus, people infected with the hepatitis B virus (HBV) at birth can develop HCC as early as twenty years of age, whereas people infected with HBV in adulthood tend to develop HCC in their sixties or seventies. The annual risk of developing HCC for people with chronic hepatitis B has been estimated to be between 0.5 and 3 percent.

HCV

A strong correlation exists between chronic hepatitis C and the development of HCC. In contrast to hepatitis B, cirrhosis is present in all cases of hepatitis C–associated HCC. This is presumably because HCV is an RNA virus and therefore cannot incorporate itself into the DNA of the person it has infected. There is increasing evidence that certain undefined HCV proteins may also contribute to the formation of HCC. People with hepatitis C who drink alcohol excessively appear to have a greater risk of developing HCC. This underscores the importance of total abstinence from alcohol in people with chronic hepatitis C.

As stated above, it appears that coinfection with both HBV and HCV greatly increases a person's chance of developing HCC. Therefore, obtaining the hepatitis B vaccination is crucial for people with hepatitis C who are not already infected with hepatitis B. (See chapter 24 for more information on vaccinations.) It usually takes more than thirty years from the time a person becomes infected with HCV for HCC to develop. Once cirrhosis has developed, it is estimated that there is a 1 to 6 percent chance each year for HCC to develop. It has been demonstrated that treatment with the drug interferon prior to the development of HCC actually lowers the incidence of HCC in some people with chronic hepatitis C. In fact, interferon treatment was found to be associated with a decreased risk of HCC even if the virus was not eradicated during therapy. This underscores the importance of early recognition and aggressive treatment of chronic hepatitis C in the early stages of the disease, prior to the development of HCC.

Iron

As you learned in chapter 18, iron is toxic to the liver. Iron can potentially cause gene mutations that may lead to HCC. Hemochromatosis is a genetically acquired liver disease of iron overload. While by itself hemochromatosis does not cause HCC, once it has progressed to cirrhosis, there is up to a 200-fold increase in the risk of developing HCC as compared with the general population. Phlebotomy helps prevent progression of the disease. And, if started prior to the onset of cirrhosis, phlebotomy can help prevent the development of HCC in people with hemochromatosis. However, once cirrhosis has developed, the risk of developing HCC exists. This is true even if a person with cirrhosis has undergone successful phlebotomy. Once again, this demonstrates the importance of early recognition and treatment of liver disease.

Chronic Liver Diseases

Autoimmune hepatitis, primary biliary cirrhosis, and nonalcoholic fatty liver disease are three other chronic liver diseases—discussed in chapters 14, 15, and 16, respectively—that can lead to cirrhosis and thus to HCC. However, the incidence of HCC in these diseases is very low compared with the incidence of HCC in other chronic liver diseases, such as chronic hepatitis B, chronic hepatitis C, and hemochromatosis.

Lifestyle Factors—Alcohol Consumption and Cigarette Smoking

It is a well-known fact that alcohol can be toxic to the liver. In fact, most people associate the word *cirrhosis* with alcohol. Alcohol liver disease (ALD) is perhaps the most common cause of cirrhosis in the United States and most cases of HCC in the United States are found in people with alcoholic cirrhosis. However, most research has shown that alcohol itself is not actually a direct cause of HCC. Rather, it is when alcohol causes liver damage and cirrhosis that HCC can develop. In people with either chronic hepatitis B or chronic hepatitis C, alcohol accelerates the course of the disease, leading to cirrhosis and HCC at an earlier age compared with people who do not drink alcohol. Thus, alcohol, in effect, acts as a *cocarcinogen*—a substance that, when combined with another carcinogenic factor, hastens the progression to cancer.

It is estimated that approximately 15 percent of people with alcoholic cirrhosis will develop HCC in their lifetimes. This percentage applies even to people who stopped drinking after they developed alcoholic cirrhosis. However, people with alcoholic cirrhosis who stop drinking live, on average, ten years longer than people with alcoholic cirrhosis who continue to drink. It is most likely that this increased survival time provides these people with an extra ten years in which to develop HCC. The close connection between alcoholic cirrhosis and HCC was underscored by an autopsy study performed on people who had alcoholic cirrhosis. Researchers discovered HCC in 55 percent of livers examined. A final note on this subject: People with any liver disease would be wise to abstain from alcohol due to the potentially toxic impact of alcohol on the liver.

The role of cigarettes in the development of HCC is not clear. However, some studies suggest that cigarette smoking may be a risk factor leading to HCC in some people with liver disease—especially those without evidence of chronic hepatitis B. Since cigarette smoking has been proven to be detrimental to health in so many ways, anyone who has liver disease is advised to not smoke cigarettes. This advice applies to all tobacco products.

Aflatoxin

Aspergillus flavus is a fungus (mold) that produces a toxic by-product known as aflatoxin. Aflatoxin has been shown to be hepatotoxic and to have the potential of leading to HCC. Foods stored in hot, humid conditions for prolonged periods of time are prone to mold and thus aflatoxin contamination. In certain parts of Africa, the incidence of HCC can be directly correlated with the amount of aflatoxin-contaminated food consumed. In parts of Africa and Asia, this fungus commonly poisons foods such as peanuts, soybeans, corn, and rice. Researchers have speculated that aflatoxin leads to liver cancer by causing a genetic mutation (mutation of the p53 gene). It is believed that aflatoxins may increase the toxic effect that hepatitis viruses have on liver cancer production; that is, it may act as a cocarcinogen. Aflatoxin contamination of foods is rare in the United States; therefore, aflatoxin is not considered to be a significant cause of liver cancer in the United States.

Drugs—Anabolic Steroids and Oral Contraceptives

Some people use anabolic steroids (muscle-building hormones) for medical reasons. Others use them to increase their competitive edge in sports. Men and women who take anabolic steroids for prolonged periods of time are at increased risk for the development of HCC. Therefore, unless there is a medical reason to use anabolic steroids, their use should be avoided.

Women who take oral contraceptives for a period of greater than eight years have a slightly increased risk of developing HCC. As noted on page 293, hepatic adenoma, which is associated with oral contraceptive use, has a small risk of developing into HCC.

Diabetes

Many researchers believe that diabetes may be a risk factor for HCC. This may be linked to elevated insulin levels in the blood (hyperinsulinemia) that occurs in people with diabetes. It is believed that insulin activates certain factors that can cause gene mutations that lead to cancer. There is also increasing evidence that people with NASH (nonalcoholic steatohepatitis, chapter 16), many of whom have either diabetes and/or hyperinsulinemia, are at increased risk for progression to HCC. Finally, many people with type 2 diabetes are obese, and some researchers believe that obesity may be a risk factor for the development of HCC.

Gender and Race

Men are two to four times more likely to develop HCC than women. This is partly attributed to the increased incidence of viral hepatitis and alcoholic cirrhosis in men. Hormonal factors—androgens—likely contribute to this increased incidence, but this association has not as yet been proven.

Within the United States, there are great differences among ethnic groups as to the incidence of HCC. Asians, Hispanics, and Native Americans are diagnosed with HCC almost three times more frequently than African Americans, who are diagnosed almost three times more frequently than Caucasians. These racial differences in HCC are most likely due to variations in time of acquisition of the liver disease, life style differences, and different incidences of HCV, HBV, and alcoholic cirrhosis among different ethnic groups. A specific ethnicity per se does not actually cause HCC.

Age

Gene damage and gene mutations may lead to HCC. As people age, there is an accumulation over time of gene damage due to a variety of factors. HCC is more frequently discovered as people age. In fact, it is rarely found in people under the age of forty. A major exception to this is in areas of the world where HBV is endemic (e.g., sub-Saharan Africa and China). In these people, HCC may occur as young as twenty years old.

THE SYMPTOMS AND SIGNS OF HCC

As previously noted, geography has considerable relevance to HCC. This relevance pertains to the rate of occurrence of HCC, as well as the array of symptoms associated with HCC. In areas with a low rate of occurrence of HCC, such as the United States, people with chronic liver disease or cirrhosis are more likely to be aware of their conditions and to be under a doctor's care. In these people, HCC usually progresses slowly and silently, and symptoms experienced, if any, are those that pertain to cirrhosis. These people are usually detected to have HCC at a point when the tumor is quite tiny. Consequently, these people usually have no tumor-related symptoms at the time. This early detection of HCC is due to the fact that in the United States—as in many other developed countries—people with cirrhosis are commonly screened and monitored on a regular basis.

However, some individuals are first detected to have HCC when there has been an abrupt deterioration of an otherwise stable chronic liver disease course. Symptoms of HCC in these people can include abdominal pain, weight loss, fatigue, or manifestations of decompensated cirrhosis, such as encephalopathy. The liver is usually enlarged, rock hard, and nodular. Jaundice is present in some people, but is usually mild. Signs suggestive of cirrhosis may be present, or there may be obvious signs of decompensated cirrhosis, such as ascites (accumulation of fluid in the abdomen).

In contrast, in less developed areas of the world, such as sub-Saharan Africa, which has a high incidence of HCC, HCC is usually an aggressive disease with a rapid downhill course. These people are usually younger than those in geographic areas of low incidence and are often not aware that they have a chronic liver disease. These people often complain of sudden abdominal distention and tenderness, and a physical exam commonly reveals a mass in the right upper abdominal region. The doctor may hear a bruit over the liver during an exam. A *hepatic bruit* is a harsh, abnormal noise that can be heard through a stethoscope when it is placed over the liver. This is suggestive of a vascular tumor (a tumor that is chockful of blood vessels, such as HCC). Often, the initial complaint in these people is excruciating abdominal pain. Typically, the cause of this pain is that the tumor has ruptured. This is a medical emergency requiring immediate surgery. Low-grade intermittent fevers may also be present.

Some people will have symptoms of HCC that are exhibited in other organs of the body. This is due to secretion of substances, such as hormones, by the tumor to other parts of the body through the bloodstream. HCC-related symptoms when manifested in other parts of the body are known as *paraneoplastic syndromes*. Paraneoplastic manifestations occur as one of the first symptoms of HCC in about 5 percent of people, although this percentage is higher for people in areas of high incidence of HCC. There are many types of paraneoplastic manifestations of HCC, but the two most common are a low glucose level (known as hypoglycemia) and a high cholesterol level (known as hypercholesterolemia). Less common manifestations include a high calcium level (known as hypercalcemia), an elevated red blood cell count (known as polycythemia), high blood pressure, signs of feminization in men (such as gynecomastia), and watery diarrhea.

DIAGNOSING HCC

A person may be diagnosed with HCC through a combination of blood work, imaging studies, and liver biopsy. The following is a discussion of each of these diagnostic methods.

Blood Tests

In its earliest, most treatable stages, HCC can be very difficult to detect. Laboratory blood tests such as those discussed in chapter 3 may reveal few clues beyond an elevated AP or GGTP. Other blood test abnormalities, such as elevated liver enzymes or a decreased platelet count, are not due to HCC but to the underlying liver disease, such as hepatitis or cirrhosis, respectively. Most of these tests are nonspecific and will give only vague hints that something more serious is wrong. Immediate suspicion for HCC should be raised when a person with a relatively stable course of liver disease abruptly develops a significant rise of liver function tests (LFTs). As emphasized throughout this book, the liver is a master of camouflage. Thus, a large tumor can be present in the liver despite minimal blood test abnormalities and a lack of symptoms. In fact, it is possible for more than half of one's liver to be replaced by a tumor without causing significant blood test abnormalities or symptoms.

The only diagnostic test to detect HCC is a blood test known as *alpha-fetoprotein (AFP)*. This test is one of the *tumor markers* (a blood test indicative of, but not diagnostic of, cancer). Normal adult level is less than 20 nanograms per milliliter (ng/ml). If the level in a person's blood is over 400 ng/ml, then it is pretty safe to say that liver cancer is present. Levels under 400 ng/ml are a little more confusing. This is due to the fact that AFP levels can also be elevated as a result of many other conditions (see bulleted list below), especially any conditions in which there may be liver damage, such as cirrhosis or acute hepatitis. These other conditions rarely cause one's levels to exceed 100 ng/ml. Recent studies have shown that AFP is less effective as a predictor of HCC in African Americans with hepatitis C than in other racial groups. Therefore, other methods of screening African-American patients with HCV, such as a yearly MRI, should be considered.

Causes of an elevated AFP other than HCC include:

- Hepatitis—both acute and chronic

- Cirrhosis

- Liver metastases

- Pregnancy

- Cystic fibrosis

- Gastric cancer

- Pancreatic cancer

A rapidly rising AFP level, say from 60 ng/ml to 230 ng/ml within a few months—even if levels do not reach 400 ng/ml—is also suggestive of HCC. This abrupt increase signals the need to commence an intensive search for the tumor. It has been shown that initial AFP levels above 100 ng/ml in a person with chronic liver disease may foreshadow the development of HCC within the next five years. These people should be closely observed for tumor development. The degree of elevation of AFP is usually related to the size of the tumor—the larger the tumor, the higher the value. Thus, with very small lesions, AFP is often barely elevated.

After successful treatment of HCC, the level of AFP should normalize. It should rise again if there is a recurrence of the tumor. It can be seen that the AFP blood test is useful as a marker for the recurrence, as well as the initial detection of HCC. However, a person should not be lulled into a sense of total security if his AFP level is normal. Only about 67 percent of HCCs secrete AFP. This means that 33 percent of HCCs occur in people whose AFP are normal. Therefore, while this marker is very useful, it does have limitations.

Des-gamma-carboxyprothrombin (DCP), an abnormal form of prothrombin (a protein produced by the liver involved in blood clotting), is found to be elevated in 60 to 90 percent of people with HCC. DCP is positive even in some people with HCC whose AFP level is normal. However, DCP is rarely positive when HCC is less than 3 centimeters in size. The accuracy of this blood test is presently being evaluated through research. If the statistical significance of DCP is confirmed, combined AFP and DCP blood tests will greatly improve the ability of physicians to detect HCC.

Imaging Studies

One or more imaging studies (discussed in chapter 3) are usually performed on people suspected of having HCC. The first is usually a sonogram. Tumors less than 2 centimeters in size (and possibly less than 1 centimeter in size) can be detected by this imaging study. Sonograms are the study most commonly recommended for HCC screening.

CT scan is often the next study obtained. A contrast dye is used to enhance the tumor, thus giving improved accuracy of diagnosis. A substance known as *lipoidal,* an iodinized poppy-seed oil contrast dye, is injected into the hepatic artery. This substance is promptly cleared from the rest of the liver but remains in the HCC, where it identifies abnormal tumor cells. HCC can be detected by a repeated CT scan performed about two weeks thereafter. Lipoidal creates an obvious contrast between normal tissue and the tumor. Tumors as small as 0.2 to 0.3 centimeters can be identified using lipoidal-enhanced CT scans.

MRI is also being used with increasing frequency to detect liver masses. It has an accuracy that is comparable to that of an enhanced CT scan. An enhancing substance such as gadolinium is used, as it improves diagnostic accuracy for some tumors by creating an identifiable contrast between normal tissue and a tumor.

Hepatic angiography is also used to aid in the detection of an HCC. It is the most invasive and expensive of all the imaging techniques, and it is used primarily to determine operability. In this technique, a catheter is placed into the hepatic artery, and contrast-enhancing dye is introduced into the vessels that feed the tumor. A tumor is more *vascular* (contains an abundance of vessels) than the surrounding liver tissue, and vessels present in the tumor can be directly seen, thereby enabling the doctor to successfully locate the tumor.

Liver Biopsy

In cases where a tumor has been detected but the diagnosis is still in question, a liver biopsy is sometimes performed. The biopsy is usually performed by sonogram or CT scan guidance. Due to the fact that liver tumors are very vascular, the risk of bleeding increases. Also, there is a small risk of spreading the tumor along the track of the needle. Therefore, the use of a smaller-than-normal size needle is generally recommended. However, the tissue sample extracted using a small needle is often too small. Therefore, many times diagnostic uncertainties still cannot be resolved. Thus, for people with liver tumors, the role of liver biopsy is somewhat controversial. For a complete discussion of liver biopsies, see chapter 5.

SCREENING AND SURVEILLANCE FOR HCC

Screening and surveillance is done in order to detect HCC at an early enough stage so that surgery can either successfully remove the tumor in its entirety and thereby cure the condition or significantly improve the person's chances for long-term survival. The importance of screening people who are at risk for liver cancer cannot be overemphasized. The chances of successful treatment are far greater when a tumor is detected in its earliest stages, as opposed to an advanced stage, where it may have already spread to other areas of the body. Anyone with cirrhosis from any cause and people with chronic hepatitis B (HBsAg positive) with or without cirrhosis are at risk of developing HCC. These people should be screened regularly for HCC. In this way, if a tumor forms, it is more likely to be detected in its earliest stages when it is most amenable to treatment.

While the exact method and interval of screening are subject to differing opinions, as a general rule, screening is advisable approximately every six months. This is based on the fact that the time it takes for HCC to double in size ranges from one to nineteen months with a median time of six months. Screening is simple, quick, relatively inexpensive, and painless. It generally consists of a sonogram and the AFP blood test and should be done at least once every six months. Diligent surveillance will detect approximately 25 to 65 percent of tumors at a size of 2 centimeters or smaller. Since, as previously noted, up to 37 percent of people with HCC will have normal levels of AFP, it is important to use both screening methods for anyone who is at risk of HCC.

THE LONG-TERM PROGNOSIS FOR THOSE WITH HCC

When a small tumor (less than 5 centimeters) is detected by screening and surveillance techniques, there is a chance that it can be successfully removed in its entirety through surgery. Once the HCC has grown to greater than 5 centimeters, it is probably not curable, as it most likely will have already spread to other areas of the body (metastasized)—most commonly nearby lymph nodes and the lungs. For these people, some form of therapy (discussed on the following pages) should be initiated. Without therapy, only 1 percent of these people will survive two years from the time HCC is detected.

THE POTENTIAL TREATMENT OPTIONS FOR HCC

For people with HCC, prolonged survival is possible, but, in general, long-term prognosis is somewhat poor. The most common treatment options for HCC include surgical resection, liver transplantation, and the injection of alcohol directly into the tumor. Other options include tumor embolization, chemotherapy, hormonal manipulation, radiotherapy, and immunotherapy. Sometimes, a combination of these therapies will maximize results. All of these options will be discussed in more detail below.

Options differ greatly for those tumors that are surgically correctable (that is, single tumors and those less than 5 centimeters in size) as compared with tumors that are not amenable to surgery (that is, tumors at multiple sites in the liver and those that are greater than 5 centimeters in size or that have metastasized to other organs). The size of the tumor, the number of tumors present in the liver, and the status of the underlying liver disease are the important variables looked at when deciding which therapy would provide the best long-term results in each particular case.

Surgical Resection

Surgical *resection* (the removal of the tumor through surgery) is often the first option considered for people with HCC. In the absence of cirrhosis, up to 80 percent of a person's liver can be removed, and the remainder will "regenerate" to its former full size, as discussed in chapter 1. Surgical resection, performed on people who meet specific criteria, can potentially cure a person of HCC. The best candidate for surgical resection is a person with a solitary tumor less than 5 centimeters in size in a liver without cirrhosis. The tumor should also be isolated just to the liver and not have spread to other sites such as the lungs. Those who have an increased likelihood of positive results include people who are in otherwise good health and people younger than fifty years old. Unfortunately, only about 5 percent of all HCC diagnosed in the United States fall into these categories. Approximately half of those who undergo surgery will still be alive at least five years after surgery. The major disadvantage of surgical resection is that there remains a high risk of tumor recurrence because new tumors may develop in the remaining portion of the liver. And, if cirrhosis was initially present, overall liver function is not improved.

Liver Transplantation

As noted above, only a small percentage of people with liver cancer have surgically resectable tumors at the time they are diagnosed. The remaining people must consider liver transplantation. Liver transplantation has the potential for removing from the body not only the tumor, but also any underlying cirrhosis. Thus, in people with a single HCC less than 5 centimeters in size or in people with less than three HCC all less than three centimeters in size, liver transplantation is a good treatment modality. In such cases, the five-year survival time is 75 percent. Unfortunately, the waiting period for a liver transplant can make this option less effective. However, the newly implemented system for determining liver organ distribution—*Model for End-stage Liver Disease (MELD)*—gives a higher priority to people with HCC, thereby lessening their waiting time. *Living donor transplantation,* in which part of the liver from a suitable donor (such as a relative or other person with the same blood type) is transplanted into the patient, is a particularly good option as it eliminates this delay. Some of the therapies used for inoperable tumors (see below) may be used as an interim therapy for people awaiting a liver transplant. The topic of liver transplantation is discussed in further detail in chapter 22.

Therapy for Inoperable Tumors

Due to the clandestine nature of liver disease, many tumors are already in advanced stages by the time they are recognized and, as such, are not amenable to any form of surgery. Some people are not candidates for surgery due to advanced age or poor general health. For these people, options include percutaneous alcohol injection, embolization and chemoembolization, chemotherapy, radiation therapy, hormonal therapy, cryosurgery, and gene therapy. The following is a discussion of these options.

Percutaneous Alcohol Injection (PEI)

This therapy consists of a small needle being inserted percutaneously (through the skin) into the liver, much in the same manner as a liver biopsy is performed. The exact location of the tumor is pinpointed using a sonogram. Alcohol is then injected directly into the tumor through the needle. The alcohol acts to kill the cancer cells. The most common complaints concerning this procedure include mild pain and low fever, but otherwise it is well tolerated. People who do best with this treatment are those who have a tumor smaller than 5 centimeters, those who have less than three tumors in the liver, and those who do not have advanced cirrhosis. In fact, up to 90 percent of small, solitary tumors less than 3 centimeters in size can be successfully killed using this method. Up to 70 percent of people whose tumors are eliminated are alive four years later. People with larger tumors or advanced cirrhosis do not have as high a success rate, and the incidence of recurrence of the tumor in these people is high, even when the original tumor was successfully killed using this method. For these people, other options are offered. These alternatives include combining PEI with chemoembolization (see below), the use of solutions other than alcohol (such as hot saline or acetic acid) for injection into the tumor, and even the placement of a microwave electrode directly into the tumor. The success rate, incidence of recurrence, and number of years of prolonged life applicable to each of these therapies are currently being reviewed by researchers. Although definitive numbers have not been established, some preliminary studies involving these treatments have shown positive results.

Tumor Embolization and Chemoembolization

When a cholesterol plaque becomes lodged in an artery that leads to the heart, blood flow to the heart stops. This blockage of blood flow causes part of the heart muscle to die. This is commonly referred to as a heart attack, or *myocardial ischemia*. Extrapolating this principle, if the hepatic artery (the artery that leads to the liver) is clogged, liver cancer cells may die. This deliberate clogging process is known as *embolization*. Substances that are used to block blood flow to liver cancer cells include gelatin-sponges (Gelfoam) and metallic coils. In many cases, anticancer drugs such as doxorubicin or cisplatin are introduced through the hepatic artery at the same time as Gelfoam or other substances. This is known as *chemoembolization*. This provides an increased concentration of the chemotherapy directly into the tumor with less of the side effects of typical chemotherapy. While this treatment method does appear to reduce tumor growth, especially when lipiodal solution is added to the regimen, long-term survival is only slightly improved.

Other Options

Chemotherapy, using agents such as 5-fluorouracil, doxorubicin, or mitomycin, whether introduced as a single agent or in combination with each other, has not been found to significantly prolong survival.

Radiation therapy is used primarily to reduce pain associated with the tumor. Promising research is being conducted on *proton irradiation* and *intraarterial irradiation,* discussions of which are beyond the scope of this book.

Hormonal therapy using substances that inhibit both male and female hormones has been attempted. *Antiandrogens* (male-hormone inhibitors) have had poor results. *Antiestrogens* (female-hormone inhibitors), such as tamoxifen, have shown promising results in some, but not all, studies. Research continues to be conducted in this interesting area.

Interferons are proteins made naturally in the body. They play an important role in regulating the immune system. It has been shown that they have both antiviral and antitumor properties. One group of researchers has demonstrated that the administration of interferon can prolong survival in people with inoperable HCC. Additional research will need to be done in this area before definite conclusions can be established. Interferon was discussed in more detail in chapters 11, 12, and 13.

The freezing of liver tumor cells, also known as *cryosurgery,* is another technique being studied. Cryosurgery consists of destroying the tumor and surrounding liver tissue by injecting subzero liquid nitrogen into it. One drawback to this therapy is that it requires surgery. Another promising treatment involves the burning of liver tumor cells. This is known as *thermal ablation* and consists of transferring energy, in the form of radiofrequency waves, directly to tumor cells. One advantage to this technique is that no surgery is needed. Delivery of this thermal energy is via a needle inserted directly into the tumor under sonogram or CT-scan guidance. In this manner, liver tumor cells are killed by literally being "fried" to death. Both of these therapies take advantage of the fact that cancer cells are sensitive to temperature extremes.

Preliminary studies in Japan with *polyprenoic acid,* a form of vitamin A, appear promising. Also, vitamin K in combination with other forms of conventional treatment may improve survival by preventing tumor extension into the portal vein.

Gene therapy, while still in experimental stages, is a promising new type of treatment for combating cancers. HCC seems to be well suited to this treatment method, as some scientists believe that HCC involves a mutant gene—the p53 gene mutation. It is hoped that if the defective p53 gene can be replaced with a healthy copy of the p53 gene, the cancer process might be halted or even reversed.

Angiogenesis inhibitors are undergoing intensive research in mice. *Angiogenesis* is a term that means the development of new blood vessels. Just like all the organs in the body, cancers need a blood supply in order to live and grow. Angiogenesis inhibitors aim to block the signals that cancer cells release in order to entice new blood vessels. If this signaling process is blocked, tumor cells would die, as their blood supplies would be cut off. Thalidomide is an agent that has antiangiogenic properties. This medication was initially used to treat morning sickness in pregnant women. However, thalidomide was withdrawn from the market around 1961 due to its potential to cause severe birth defects—missing digits, arms and legs—in children whose mothers consumed it during pregnancy. Due to its antiangiogenic capabilities, thalidomide is now being used in experimental studies as a treatment for HCC. Preliminary results are encouraging.

CONCLUSION

This chapter underscores how important it is for all people with liver disease to be under the care of a knowledgeable liver specialist. With regular screening and monitoring, if a malignancy has formed, it can be detected in its earliest, most treatable stage. With rapidly advancing new treatment regimens and the implementation of preventive measures, we should be experiencing a substantial decrease in the incidence of HCC in years to come. This chapter also discussed how HCC manifests so differently in different parts of the world. We have seen from this chapter that there are numerous benign masses of the liver. It is important to remember this fact, because if a mass is detected on the liver, there is no need to automatically assume a fatal outcome.

This concludes part 3 of the book. In part 4, treatment options and lifestyle changes will be discussed. Part 4 will also provide an in-depth look at liver transplantation.

Part Four

Treatment Options and Lifestyle Changes

Twenty

TREATMENT OF COMMON SYMPTOMS AND COMPLICATIONS

Since liver disease may occur without symptoms, it has the potential to go undetected for many years. During this time, a person may unknowingly progress to cirrhosis. There are, however, a significant number of people with liver disease who do have symptoms. Symptoms of liver disease may include fatigue, itching, and abdominal pain and can be relatively mild or can be so severe as to be debilitating. Sometimes it is specifically these symptoms that first bring a person to the attention of her doctor. As you've learned in previous chapters, the severity of symptoms does not always correlate with the severity of the liver disease. In other people, serious complications of liver disease—including ascites and encephalopathy—initially cause them to seek medical attention. When these serious complications occur, it indicates a severe liver disorder. In any case, symptoms and complications of liver disease tend to be similar no matter which liver disease a person has.

Getting medical treatment is the most important step a person with liver disease can take to improve her health. However, treatment is only complete when the symptoms and complications of liver disease are treated as well as the liver disease itself. This chapter discusses the treatment of some of the most common symptoms and complications that pertain to liver disease. Treatment options for some of the complications associated with chronic liver disease are also addressed.

TREATMENT OF SYMPTOMS

Some of the symptoms that commonly occur in people with liver disease were discussed in chapter 2. Here you will read about the treatments of these symptoms. Read on to learn about some medical treatments and some helpful ways to treat fatigue, insomnia and other sleep disturbances, psychiatric disorders, itching, headaches, and abdominal pain and distention. Many of these symptoms are due to the side effects of the drug interferon (used to treat hepatitis B and C). The specific topic of interferon-related side effects and their treatment is discussed in detail in chapter 11.

Treatment of Fatigue

One of the most common, relentless, and debilitating symptoms experienced by people with liver disease is fatigue. The symptom of fatigue is universal to liver disease. Some people do not experience fatigue until several years after they have been diagnosed with liver disease. In others, fatigue is the primary reason that they seek medical attention. Fatigue does not correlate with either the duration or the severity of the disease, so it may be as debilitating to a person in the early stages of liver disease as it is in a person with advanced cirrhosis. Fatigue is particularly common in people with chronic hepatitis C as well as among women.

Successfully treating fatigue can be a challenge. In attempting to combat fatigue, all of the possible causes of a person's fatigue should be looked into. Some causes are easily managed. Some occur commonly in people with liver disease. The potential causes of and/or contributors to fatigue include the following:

- thyroid disease (may be primary cause of or contribute to fatigue)

- anemia (may be primary cause of or contribute to fatigue)

- disorders of other organs, including the heart (for example, congestive heart failure) or the brain (for example, brain tumors)

- nutritional deficiencies (for example, a lack of iron or a lack of protein)

- disturbances in fluid and electrolyte balance (for example, a low sodium level)

- depression

- some medications and drugs (a doctor should review all prescription and over-the-counter medications that a patient is taking; if possible, those that cause fatigue should be discontinued)

- excessive use of caffeine

- excessive use of alcohol

- emotional stress

- lack of exercise

- lack of sleep

- overwork

If fatigue continues to persist after ruling out or correcting any of the above factors, there are some lifestyle changes that may be helpful. For example, eating a healthy, low-fat, well-balanced diet; quitting smoking; refraining from alcohol consumption; and exercising daily are all lifestyle changes that can ameliorate fatigue. Also it is recommended to drink plenty of water and limit caffeine-containing beverages to one or two servings per day. Never consume large, heavy meals. Four to six small meals throughout the day will keep energy levels high and will minimize fatigue. It goes without saying, but bears repeating anyway: People with liver disease should avoid drinking alcohol. Alcohol can worsen any liver disease and is a cause of fatigue as well. It's also a good idea when necessary to begin a healthy weight-reducing diet to eliminate any excess weight. (Never lose more than one to two pounds per week.) See chapter 23 for more information on exercise and nutrition.

The demands of a hectic job or harried home life may need to be reduced. Overwhelming stress may cause fatigue even in a person who is not suffering from liver disease. Excessive stress, including emotional stress, is often the cause of fatigue in people with liver disease. Therefore, friends and family should attempt to reduce the normal load of obligations and expectations that they may normally have had of the person.

In some cases, it may be necessary for a person with liver disease to incorporate naps into her daily schedule. If possible, a thirty- to forty-five-minute daytime nap should be taken daily. This can help rejuvenate a person with liver disease. Often, a doctor's letter to the patient's employer or supervisor may be needed. A person with fatigue should feel free to ask her doctor for such a note. If a daytime nap is impossible, try to do some midday exercises. When sitting at a desk job all day, for example, blood tends to move away from the head and muscles. This results in both mental and physical fatigue. It is important to get your blood circulating throughout your entire body. Try to get up and walk around or simply do some stretching exercises. Even a little exercise will help get you concentrating and motivated again.

Remember, fatigue cannot be cured by a pill! Be especially wary of any products that boast "improved energy levels" on their labels. Because the liver is in charge of breaking down all supplements and medications, more harm than good may result from taking such products. Also, be aware that taking excessive amounts of vitamins and minerals in an attempt to combat fatigue—especially vitamin A, niacin, and iron—can lead to a worsening of liver disease. This will be discussed in more detail in chapter 23. It is essential that a person with liver disease consult a liver specialist prior to taking any supplements or products that promise to cure fatigue.

Ondansetron (Zofran) is a medication used in the treatment of nausea and vomiting associated with cancer chemotherapy. There have been anecdotal reports on the use of Zofran (4 mg twice a day) in the management of fatigue associated with liver disease. Since some people with liver disease also suffer from nausea (especially those taking interferon and ribavirin treatment for chronic hepatitis C), Zofran may be worth a try. Other medications have been found to be helpful in treating fatigue associated with other diseases such as HIV, melanoma, and chronic fatigue syndrome. These medications include bupropion (Wellbutrin), methylphenidate (Ritalin), and modafinil (Provigil). A preliminary study on a small group of patients with hepatitis C showed that Ritalin significantly improved interferon-induced fatigue. Provigil is a medication approved for the treatment of narcolepsy—a neurological disorder marked by uncontrollable attacks of daytime sleepiness. Anecdotal evidence suggests that Provigil at a dose of 200 mg per day may be a useful adjunct in the treatment of fatigue associated with liver disease. More studies need to be conducted on patients with liver disease before any of the above-mentioned medications can be routinely recommended for use in the management of fatigue.

Treatment of Insomnia and Other Sleep Disturbances

The average person requires between seven and eight hours of sleep per night. However, some people require as much as ten hours and others require only four. No matter what your personal requirement, the main objective is to feel rejuvenated upon awakening. People with liver disease often suffer from sleep disturbances. In fact, approximately 35 to 50 percent of people with cirrhosis report having sleep-related difficulties. Some people have trouble falling asleep and others have difficulty staying asleep. Many people complain of being tired all day and awake all night. Others complain of erratic sleeping habits characterized by days of excessive sleep (a condition known as *hypersomnia*) alternating with days of lack of sleep (a condition known as *insomnia*). Still others state that they experience delays of their usual bedtimes and wake-up times. For most people suffering from these sleep disorders, the sleep they do get is not refreshing.

Sleep disturbances may cause decreased concentration, poor coordination, excessive fatigue, anxiety, and depression. It may affect personal relationships, work performance, and physical appearance. These symptoms and consequences of sleep disorders are magnified in people with liver disease as they may already be suffering from one or more of the aforementioned symptoms.

The cause of sleep disorders in people with liver disease is unclear, but most likely it relates to alterations in the body's production of *melatonin*—a hormone that is produced by the pineal gland and is involved in the sleep cycle. Sometimes sleep disturbances stem from medications used for the treatment of liver disease. For example, interferon, ribavirin, prednisone, and propanolol all may cause insomnia. Pruritus (itching) can sometimes cause a sleeping disorder. People suffering from intense itching (discussed on page 319) may find themselves awake half the night scratching. People on interferon therapy for chronic hepatitis may be drinking up to a gallon a day of water to diminish the side effect of dehydration and therefore they may be awakening throughout the night to go to the bathroom. Discontinuation of water or fluid intake two to three hours prior to retiring along with urinating before bedtime may alleviate this problem. Caffeine, nicotine, and alcohol consumption may disturb sleep habits. Abstaining from these substances will likely assist in the quest for a good night's sleep. Note that sleep disturbances may also be a sign of impending encephalopathy (see page 328).

Treatment of sleep disorders associated with liver disease consists of both behavioral modification and medical management. Unwind from the day's tensions for about an hour before lying down. Take a warm shower or bath and consider using soothing aromatic lotions to enhance relaxation. Try drinking warm milk or a tranquilizing herbal tea such as chamomile. Milk contains the chemical tryptophan, which causes drowsiness. Try to avoid watching late-night thrillers or scary movies as well as late-night news, as these shows may cause undue stress. Soft music may enhance your ability to relax. If you are fortunate enough to own a dog or a cat, try petting or brushing your pet prior to bedtime. The soft purr of a cat enhances relaxation and calms the nerves, making it easier for one to fall asleep. Do not eat three hours prior to bedtime. Certain foods, as well as a heavy meal in general, can cause reflux symptoms (heartburn and nausea), thereby inhibiting a good night's sleep. Make sure your bed and bedroom are comfortable. The room temperature of your bedroom, as well as the texture of your bedsheets, can affect your night's sleep. People should use their beds only for sleeping and never for other activities, such as reading, watching television, or eating. These activities should be performed in other areas of the home. If a person is unable to fall asleep within twenty minutes of retiring, she should get out of bed and read a book or perform some other relaxing activity in another room. Lights should be kept low and the television should be kept off. Only after becoming tired should she return to bed. Also, people should make an effort to arrange their schedules so that they wake up at the same time each day, regardless of the amount of time spent sleeping during the night. This type of consistency can help reduce fatigue. Although long naps of two to three hours during the day are not recommended for people with sleep disturbances, a twenty- to thirty-minute nap in the early afternoon, if it can be arranged, may have an energizing effect.

Under no circumstances should alcohol be used as a sleeping aid. Also, as most prescription and over-the-counter sleeping pills are broken down by the liver, they should be avoided unless their use (in low doses and for short periods) is authorized by a liver specialist. People with liver damage are at increased risk for prolonged sedative effects if these medications are used at their generally prescribed dosages. Avoid herbal medications such as kava and valerian as sleep aids. These herbs can cause serious liver damage, even in people without underlying liver disease. In people who already have liver disease, they may worsen the disease and may even lead to liver failure and death.

Although used primarily for the treatment of depression, selective serotonin reuptake inhibitors (SSRIs)—Paxil, Celexa, Zoloft, Wellbutrin, and Lexapro—are generally safe for most people with liver disease and may help treat insomnia. These medications, with the exception of Lexapro, must be taken on a daily basis for a period of two to eight weeks to become effective. Lexapro may become effective within a week of its initial daily use. SSRIs are discussed in detail in the next section of this chapter on psychological/psychiatric disorders.

Extra-strength Tylenol PM may be used in moderation as a sleeping aid. This over-the-counter medication contains 500 mg of acetaminophen, which functions as a pain medication and helps relieve aches, pains, and headaches (associated with interferon), as well as 25 mg of diphenhydramine (Benadryl), which promotes drowsiness. Melatonin, taken in dosages of 1 to 2 mg half an hour before bedtime, may be helpful. Keep in mind that melatonin supplements are not regulated by the FDA, and the amount of active ingredient contained in each pill may vary depending on the brand. Ambien (manufactured by Searle), a prescription sleeping aid, may be used on occasion. However, if Ambien is used nightly, its effectiveness will typically diminish after a few weeks. Furthermore, if used every night for more than two weeks, a dependence upon this medication may occur. It should be noted that Ambien has been associated with memory problems, a side effect that interferon therapy may worsen. Therefore, one should use Ambien on a limited basis only and under the strict guidance of a doctor.

Treatment of Psychological/Psychiatric Disorders

Any chronic illness may cause a person to become anxious and depressed. This is especially true of chronic liver disease. In fact, it has been noted that approximately 20 percent of adults with severe psychiatric disorders have hepatitis C as well. And between 11 and 30 percent of people with hepatitis C suffer from depression. Many of the medications used to treat liver disease can cause psychological symptoms. Furthermore, many of these medications can worsen an already existing psychiatric disorder. Interferon has been associated with depression, irritability, confusion, emotional instability, insomnia, and lack of concentration. One or more of these symptoms occurs in approximately 57 percent of people who undergo interferon therapy. Prednisone, used after liver transplantation and to treat autoimmune hepatitis, has been associated with mood swings, personality changes, depression, and irritability.

People who do not have severe psychiatric problems but who are prone to depression, anxiety, and/or emotional instability may benefit from taking antidepressant or antianxiety medications prior to starting interferon or prednisone therapy. In fact, most people will benefit from going on antidepressant or antianxiety medication prior to starting interferon therapy. People who already suffer from severe depression, especially those with suicidal thoughts, those who've made suicide attempts, or those with a serious psychiatric disorder, should postpone interferon therapy until their underlying psychiatric problems have either stabilized or abated. Most important, a person should not be reluctant or feel ashamed to seek support from a psychological counselor or psychiatrist. Obtaining as much additional help as possible is generally a good idea.

All drugs are metabolized, at least to some extent, through the liver. While people with a chronic liver disease should avoid any nonessential medications, this may be outweighed, in some cases, by the greater benefit of treatment with antidepressant or antianxiety medications. As discussed above, the safest antidepressants are the selective serotonin reuptake inhibitors (SSRIs). All SSRIs appear to be equally effective in the treatment of depression and anxiety. Although comparative studies on the different SSRIs in people with liver disease have not been done, some distinctions have been noted. Pretreatment of patients with Paxil has been found to be quite effective in preventing severe depression in patients with melanoma treated with high dosages of interferon. Wellbutrin may have less sexual side effects than other SSRIs. Lexapro's antidepressant/antianxiety action takes effect sooner than the other SSRIs. For people being treated with either interferon or prednisone, if depression, anxiety, or any other psychiatric problem becomes severe, a reduction in the dose of these medications may be necessary. These medications typically decrease anxiety levels, but additional antianxiety medications, such as buspirone (Buspar) or alprazolam (Xanax), are sometimes needed. Use of Xanax should be limited due to its potential for addiction and/or liver toxicity. People who already have a psychiatric condition or who experience side effects while on interferon or prednisone should be managed jointly by a liver specialist and a psychiatrist. For those desiring an alternative approach, the herb St. John's wort (*Hypericum perforatum*) has been considered by some. It should be noted that studies conducted so far have shown that St. John's wort does not provide any benefit in cases of moderate to severe depression. (See chapter 21 for more information on herbs.)

A doctor should investigate all possible causes of a patient's psychiatric symptoms, as certain symptoms may be readily remedied. For example, thyroid disorders (symptoms of which may mimic psychiatric disorders) are often associated with certain liver diseases and their treatments. Thyroid disorders are usually correctable with medications and, once treated, the associated psychiatric symptoms typically abate. Certain types of anemia may cause psychiatric symptoms, which may be readily correctable with proper treatment. Moreover, excessive alcohol use has been associated with hallucinations and abnormal thoughts and behavior. This may be remedied by cessation of alcohol use and by hospitalization. Also, the beginning stages of encephalopathy (the treatment of which is discussed on page 328), which is associated with cirrhosis, may be the cause of altered mental status or psychotic behavior. Finally, negative lifestyle factors—including excessive stress, lack of sleep, lack of exercise, and poor dietary habits such as excessive caffeine consumption or inadequate water intake—may lead to or contribute to psychological or psychiatric symptoms. Therefore, certain lifestyle changes may have a corrective effect on certain psychiatric symptoms.

Treatment of Itching (Pruritus)

Pruritus is a localized or generalized intense sensation of itching that necessitates the need to scratch. The cause of pruritus associated with liver disease is unknown. It is most often found in people with cholestatic liver diseases, such as primary biliary cirrhosis (PBC), or in cases in which cholestasis complicates any liver disease, as can occur in people with advanced cirrhosis who have jaundice.

Pruritus occurs in approximately 80 percent of people with PBC and in approximately 20 to 50 percent of people with jaundice. It can also occur as a side effect of medication used to treat liver disease, such as ribavirin for hepatitis C. It is usually at its worst at night and often is most severe on the palms and soles. The intensity of this symptom varies from mild itching, which does not interfere with a person's life, to *intractable* (incapable of being relieved) itching, which may severely interfere with normal daily activities. Pruritus can become so severe that it can lead to sleep deprivation and suicidal thoughts. In fact, intractable pruritus is sometimes so bad that liver transplantation may be the only way to relieve it. The severity of itching does not always correlate with the degree of abnormality of liver function tests—alkaline phosphatase, gamma glutymyl transpeptidase, or bilirubin.

The treatment of pruritus can be difficult and is often unsatisfactory. Scratching does not commonly relieve pruritus. In fact, some people with pruritus, having found their fingernails to be insufficient, have attempted to scratch themselves using sharp objects, such as forks, knives, and hair brushes. This should be avoided as it can lead to chronic skin irritation, scarring, and infections. Treatment of infected skin involves the use of antibiotics and meticulous cleaning of wounds. It is important for people suffering with pruritus to wear loose-fitting clothes made of soft, smooth material and to keep their skin as moisturized as possible. During hot and humid weather, these people are advised to stay indoors in air-conditioned places.

The medication that has been most successful for treating pruritus is *cholestyramine* (Questran). Cholestyramine is known as a bile-acid binder (also known medically as an anion-exchange resin). It captures bile acids and eliminates them from the body via the stools. This generally results in relief from itching. It is recommended to take one packet of cholestyramine immediately before as well as one immediately after breakfast. This will enable a person to maximize the elimination of bile (which has accumulated from not eating overnight) from the gallbladder. If further doses are needed, they should be taken with meals. As cholestyramine may inhibit the absorption of other medications, it is crucial that any other medications be taken at least two but preferably four hours before or after taking cholestyramine. Cholestyramine usually begins working within a few days but needs to be taken daily for maximum effectiveness. Dosages range from 4 to 16 grams per day. Colestipol (Colestid) is another bile-acid binder that is used to treat itching. Chronic use of cholestyramine may lead to malabsorption of vitamins, especially the fat-soluble vitamins A, D, E, and K, and thus necessitate supplementation.

Antihistamines, such as diphenhydramine hydrochloride (Benadryl) or loratadine (Claritin), may help reduce itching but usually need to be taken in conjunction with cholestyramine. When taken alone, the relief of itching it provides is most likely due to its sedative effects. As people with PBC complicated by Sjögren's syndrome already suffer from a dry mouth, antihistamines should be avoided in these people since they can worsen this symptom.

Phenobarbital is a *barbiturate* (a central nervous system depressant) that has—in rare instances—been successfully used to treat pruritus. It also has sedative properties, which may account for its anti-itching effect. People should be particularly careful to avoid consuming alcohol when taking phenobarbital, as alcohol (another central nervous system depressant) will enhance the sedative effects of phenobarbital. This has the potential to lead to coma.

Rifampin is an antibiotic that has been shown to alleviate itching in some people with cholestasis. Dosages range from 150 mg two to three times per day. It usually takes about one month for rifampin to start working. Since rifampin can be toxic to the liver, its use must be very closely monitored.

Opiate antagonists are medications capable of blocking the effects of narcotics. Naloxone, naltrexone, and nalmefene are examples of opiate antagonists that have been used in the treatment of pruritus. Naloxone works only if given intravenously. It may provide benefit where the itching is so severe that it is considered a medical emergency and/or in people with intense itching who are awaiting liver transplantation. Its use in the management of chronic itching is not practical, due to the necessity of intravenous administration. Nalmefene and naltrexone may be administered orally, and some studies have shown that they can significantly reduce pruritus. Nalmefene is awaiting FDA approval in the United States, and naltrexone is potentially hepatotoxic. Therefore, neither of these drugs can be recommended at the present time.

Methotrexate, a chemotherapy medication, has been reported to decrease scratching activity, but more study is needed to confirm this. Techniques such as *plasmapheresis* (removal of plasma without the removal of other cells—that is, red blood cells—from the body), *charcoal hemoperfusion* (a form of blood cleansing), and ultraviolet light (without sunblock) have been experimentally used to treat pruritus, although none of these techniques has been shown to be consistently effective. Numerous other medications have been tried or are under study, including serotonin antagonists (ondansetron [Zofran]) administered intravenously, codeine (a narcotic pain reliever), S-Adenosy-L-Methionine (SAMe; an anticholestatic substance), the anesthestic propofol, and the enzyme-inducer flumecinol. However, until further studies have been performed, none of these options can be recommended for use in the treatment of pruritus. Ultimately, liver transplantation is indicated when pruritus becomes unbearable.

Some patients find relief using gentle anti-itching soaps and lotions made for sensitive skin such as Aveeno, Cetaphil soap, L'Occitane, or other brands containing an oatmeal base. Also, over-the-counter topical hydrocortisone cream or Benadryl lotion may be helpful. People experiencing itching are advised to avoid perfumed soaps and lotions. Hot baths and showers have been noted to exacerbate itching and should be avoided. Instead, take lukewarm baths and showers. It is advisable to wear loose-fitting, all-cotton clothes. Finally, make sure you are adequately hydrated—drink up to one gallon of bottled water each day.

Treatment of Headaches

Headaches are common among the general population, and those with liver disease are no exception. In fact, it is estimated that 15 to 20 percent of women and

6 percent of men without liver disease suffer with migraines. This number is probably higher in people with liver disease due to the side effects of some of the medications (such as interferon) used to treat the disease or from immunosuppressive agents (such as cyclosporine or tacrolimus), used after a liver transplant.

Medication-induced headaches may be eased by reducing the dose of the medication. If this is not an option, sumatriptan (Imitrex) and zolmitriptan (Zomig) are very helpful in the treatment of migraine-type headaches. However, the dosages of these medications may need to be lowered in people with cirrhosis. Some people obtain relief from headaches with beta-blockers (such as propanolol [Inderal]), which have the added benefit of reducing portal pressure in people with portal hypertension (discussed under "Treatment of Bleeding Varices" on page 326). Acetaminophen (Tylenol), taken in moderation (two to four tablets per day), with or without codeine, may help alleviate headaches, especially if one stays well hydrated by drinking at least twelve 8-ounce glasses of water per day. Riboflavin (vitamin B$_2$) at a dose of 400 mg daily may be helpful in decreasing the incidence and reducing the frequency of headaches. Acupuncture may also be considered, but more studies need to be conducted on this alternative form of therapy before it can be recommended.

Lifestyle changes, stress-reduction techniques, plenty of rest, regular exercise, and avoidance of all alcohol can help reduce the frequency and severity of headaches. It is important not to consume an excessive amount of caffeine. People who are used to drinking more than three to four cups of caffeinated beverages daily need to reduce caffeine use slowly in order to prevent caffeine-withdrawal headaches. Bright lights and noisy environments should be avoided. Other causes of headaches, such as dental problems (e.g., TMJ [temporomandibular joint syndrome]), allergies, sinus infections, and eye problems need to be considered if symptoms continue despite the above management. High blood pressure is also a common cause of headaches. Therefore, people experiencing frequent headaches should have their blood pressure routinely monitored. Finally, persistent severe headaches need to be evaluated with an MRI (a type of imaging study) and perhaps with other tests as well.

Treatment of Abdominal Pain and Distention

Abdominal pain and/or pain over the liver (right upper quadrant pain) in a person with liver disease may have many causes. Therefore, this type of pain should not automatically be attributed to a liver disorder: Other causes should be investigated. In fact, abdominal and right upper quadrant pain is rarely due to chronic liver disease. Right upper quadrant pain, when due to the liver, occurs most commonly in the acute stages of liver disease or during a flare-up of a chronic liver disease. In these circumstances, the cause of this pain is due to acute inflammation, irritation, and distention of the liver. By comparison, the liver is rarely tender in people with chronic liver disease. Yet many people with chronic liver disease state that although they do not actually experience pain, they do feel a vague sense of "fullness," or an "awareness," of the liver. The cause for this is unclear.

Gallstones, as the name suggests, are stones that form in the gallbladder. Approximately 20 million Americans have gallstones. Gallstones often occur in people with liver disease—especially those with primary biliary cirrhosis (PBC)—or those with cirrhosis due to any liver disease. Other risk factors for gallstones include female gender, obesity, a family history of gallstones, multiple pregnancies, rapid weight loss, and biliary-tract narrowing (known as *biliary strictures*). The typical pain from gallstones is a right upper quadrant discomfort that usually lasts from a half hour to six hours and then abates. Pain tends to be severe and usually recurs. Diagnosis of gallstones is typically made by obtaining an abdominal sonogram. People with symptomatic gallstones require surgical removal of the entire gallbladder, not just the gallstones. This is known as a *cholecystectomy* and is usually performed using a laparoscope (a type of endoscope inserted through a small incision in the abdominal wall). This is known as a laparoscopic cholescystectomy. Ursodeoxycholic acid (Actigal, URSO, ursodiol) has been used in the past to dissolve some small gallstones. But in such cases, recurrence commonly occurs, and surgery is eventually required. Therefore, this medication cannot be recommended as a treatment for gallstones. Gallstones can sometimes fall out of the gallbladder and the bile ducts (the passageways connecting the liver and the gallbladder), which carry bile into the intestines. Blockage of a bile duct is a serious complication, resulting in jaundice, excruciating pain, and infection. Thus, if one is suffering from abdominal pain due to gallstones, surgery is typically recommended. Prevention of gallstones is difficult if a person is prone to forming them. However, avoidance of rapid weight loss and maintaining a low-fat diet with lots of vegetables may help.

People with chronic liver disease from any cause are at risk for the development of liver cancer, which may also cause pain in the right upper quadrant. Diagnosis and treatment of liver cancer are discussed in chapter 19.

Stomach disorders are also common among the American population and among people with liver disease as well. *Peptic ulcer disease (PUD)* and *gastritis* (inflammation of the stomach lining) may be the cause of abdominal pain in people with liver disease. An *upper endoscopy* (a procedure wherein a flexible tube with a light at the end is inserted down the esophagus into the stomach and then into the first part of the small intestine) is typically performed in order to diagnose these stomach disorders. During an upper endoscopy, a biopsy is typically performed for *Helicobacter pylori,* a bacteria that may cause gastritis and ulcers. These stomach ailments are readily treatable with medications, known as proton-pump inhibitors (Nexium, Prevacid, Protonix, and Aciphex), either alone or in combination with antibiotics, depending upon the precise diagnosis.

Intestinal pain caused by irritable bowel syndrome (IBS) must also be considered as a cause of abdominal or right upper quadrant pain. The right side of the large intestine lies in close proximity to the liver, and the transverse colon lies in the middle of the abdomen (see figure 1.1 on page 9). Therefore, spasms of the intestines, a symptom that characterizes IBS, are often mistakenly attributed to the liver by the person experiencing the symptom. IBS is a benign digestive disorder, which most commonly occurs among young women but can also occur in men and older women. The symptoms of IBS, such as abdominal pain and cramping, bloating, and excessive gas, are often successfully treated with *anticholinergic* medications (such as clindinium [Librax] and hyoscyamine [Donnatal]) in combination with dietary restrictions and stress reduction.

A colonoscopy (a flexible tube with a light at the end used to visualize the large intestine) may need to be performed in situations in which abdominal pain does not abate and remains unexplained. Other more serious disorders of the intestines that may cause abdominal and right upper quadrant pain may be discovered during a colonoscopy, such as Crohn's disease (an inflammatory disease that may affect the small and/or large intestine) or colon cancer. In fact, as a general recommendation, it is important for everyone over the age of fifty to obtain a colonoscopy.

Other causes of abdominal and right upper quadrant pain that should be investigated in people with liver disease include scar tissue from prior abdominal surgery, known as *adhesions,* and inflammation of the pancreas, a condition known as *pancreatitis.* Pancreatitis may occur with increased frequency in people who drink excessive alcohol and in those with primary biliary cirrhosis. There is a possible association between interferon therapy used for the treatment of chronic hepatitis C and pancreatitis. While the studies reporting this association are anecdotal, for people on interferon therapy, pancreatitis should be considered as a possible cause of abdominal pain.

If a person experiences abdominal pain along with distention and swelling of the abdomen, *ascites* must be considered as a cause. Ascites is associated with cirrhosis and is discussed below. However, abdominal distention occurring in people with liver disease may be due to ailments other than ascites. Abdominal distention can result if the digestive tract fills with gas. When this happens, a person may experience the sensation of being bloated. This type of abdominal distention may be due to impaired or inadequate absorption (known as malabsorption) or digestion (known as maldigestion) of certain foods (see chapter 23 for more information). This is a controllable condition and may be treated by the avoidance of specific foods, such as dairy or wheat (*gluten*) products. Fatty liver is another condition that can lead to abdominal distention and liver abnormalities. In people whose fatty liver stems from being overweight, a distended abdomen may occur due to excessive adipose (fatty) tissue. This condition, which was discussed in chapter 16, is often reversible with weight reduction.

TREATMENT OF COMPLICATIONS

Complications associated with cirrhosis were covered in chapter 6. The following section discusses the treatment of four complications of chronic liver disease: ascites, bleeding varices, encephalopathy (all three of which can occur in people with cirrhosis and portal hypertension), and osteoporosis, which often occurs in people with chronic liver disease (most of whom have cirrhosis and portal hypertension but some of whom don't).

Treatment of Ascites

Ascites is characterized by massive accumulation of fluid in the abdominal cavity. This results in abdominal swelling and distention. Treatment of ascites will not improve the functioning of the liver, nor will it improve one's prognosis. Thus, once ascites has developed, liver transplantation should be considered. Nevertheless, treatment of ascites is important. First, it improves the quality of life of the cirrhotic patient. Second, spontaneous bacterial peritonitis (SBP), a life-threatening infection of ascitic fluid, will not occur if ascites is not present.

Treatment of ascites includes a low-sodium diet, with sodium intake limited to approximately 500 to 1,000 mg of sodium per day. Fluid restriction to about one liter of fluid per day is important in people whose blood sodium level is 120 mmol/l and under. Low-sodium diets are discussed in detail in chapter 23. Treatment via sodium and fluid restriction alone will adequately decrease ascites in only about 20 percent of people. Therefore, diuretics (water pills) are usually combined with dietary restrictions in an effort to maximize results. The most commonly used diuretics are furosemide (Lasix) and spironolactone (Aldactone). Optimal diuretic therapy consists of 160 mg per day of Lasix and 400 mg per day of Aldactone. This type of therapy works well in approximately 90 percent of people.

Diuretic therapy may be associated with a number of side effects and complications and therefore it is important to be closely monitored by an experienced doctor while on therapy. In general, to minimize complications, the goal of weight loss should be set at one pound per day if leg swelling (edema) is absent, and two pounds per day if edema is present. Side effects of diuretic therapy include dehydration (with associated kidney dysfunction), low sodium levels, high or low potassium levels, and leg cramps. These side effects should be managed by discontinuing medication until complications resolve or by adjusting the dosage of diuretic medication and fluid intake. Encephalopathy (see page 328) may be precipitated by this therapy. Thus, any disorientation as well as any behavioral changes need to be immediately reported to the doctor. Spironolactone often causes tender, enlarged breasts, a painful condition known as *gynecomastia*. This is due to the antiandrogenic activity of spironolactone. When gynecomastia occurs, a decrease in the dose (or possibly even discontinuation) of spironolactone may be required. Tamoxifen is an estrogen antagonist typically used in the treatment of breast cancer. At a dose of 20 mg twice a day, it has been demonstrated to control the painful gynecomastia associated with spironolactone. However, tamoxifen has also been associated with liver abnormalities, including a fatty liver, and therefore must be used with extreme caution.

When the maximum doses of diuretic therapy fail, a person is known as having *refractory ascites*. This occurs approximately 10 percent of the time. Before it is determined that refractory ascites exists, it is important to make sure that dietary restrictions are being adhered to and that nonsteroidal anti-inflammatories (NSAIDs) such as aspirin, Motrin, Advil, and/or Celebrex are not being taken. In addition to being quite dangerous for people with cirrhosis, NSAIDs diminish the effectiveness of diuretics (see chapter 24 for more about NSAIDs). Refractory ascites can be managed by physically removing the fluid via a process known as a *paracentesis*. A paracentesis involves the removal of large amounts of fluid through a needle inserted into the abdomen. Bleeding is a rare complication of this procedure. As such, the possibility of bleeding is not grounds for avoiding the procedure. A paracentesis should be performed on all patients with ascites at the time ascites first develops in order to examine the fluid for possible infection—a condition known as *spontaneous bacterial peritonitis (SBP)*—or for evidence of liver cancer or other cancers (such as ovarian). People with SBP commonly have a fever and abdominal pain, although these symptoms are sometimes absent. SBP requires hospitalization and treatment with intravenous antibiotics.

If the ascitic fluid is not infected, four to six liters of it can be safely removed at one time. A paracentesis should be performed at two-week intervals. However, if paracentesis procedures are repeatedly required over time in order to prevent fluid reaccumulation, a *transjugular intrahepatic portosystemic shunt (TIPS)* should be considered. TIPS is a procedure that entails creating a *shunt* (an alternative passageway) in the liver between the portal and hepatic veins. Creating this shunt has the effect of decreasing the portal pressure and diminishing the amount of ascitic fluid. Originally, TIPS procedures were performed strictly to control bleeding from esophageal and gastric varices (discussed below). Yet TIPS is now considered to be very useful in the control of refractory ascites.

The TIPS procedure is performed by a radiologist. The patient is given only a local anesthetic and a mild sedative. Neither a surgical operation nor general anesthesia is required. The radiologist inserts a needle into the jugular vein in the neck, passes the needle into the hepatic vein, and advances the needle into the portal vein. This creates a passageway (shunt) for a catheter to be left in place between the hepatic and portal veins. One complication of TIPS is encephalopathy. It occurs in approximately 25 percent of people who undergo this procedure. Another complication is the potential for occlusion (blockage) of the shunt, thereby necessitating its replacement. While TIPS makes ascites much more manageable, this procedure has no effect on liver function, the progression of disease, or the patient's survival. Furthermore, people with refractory ascites have less than a 50 percent chance of living more than one year. Therefore, people with refractory ascites inevitably need a liver transplant (see chapter 22 for more information).

Treatment of Bleeding Varices (Bleeding Blood Vessels)

The most serious complication of cirrhosis is bleeding esophageal varices. This complication occurs when the blood pressure in these blood vessels becomes too high, a condition known as portal hypertension. This causes the blood vessels to dilate to such a degree that they literally explode. When this happens, profuse, life-threatening bleeding results. In fact, it is estimated that between 30 and 50 percent of people could die within one to two months of their first episode of bleeding varices. Approximately one-third of people with cirrhosis have esophageal varices. Fortunately, bleeding only occurs in one-third of these people. And with appropriate preventive medical care, this number can be cut in half.

As noted in chapter 6, an upper endoscopy is required for both diagnosis and treatment of bleeding esophageal varices. Most liver-disease experts recommend that an upper endoscopy be performed every two to three years on patients with cirrhosis in order to determine the presence of esophageal varices and the risk of bleeding. Once varices are found, patients should be placed on a medication to reduce the pressure in the esophagus, which will significantly decrease the risk of bleeding from esophageal varices and improve survival. This type of therapy that acts to prevent a disease (in this case, hemorrhage) is known as *prophylactic therapy*. The most frequently used drug to reduce portal pressure is the beta-blocker propanolol (Inderal). The optimum dose of Inderal is determined by the pulse rate. Dosages range between 10 and 80 mg per day. The goal is to achieve a pulse rate of approximately 55 beats per minute while resting. Sometimes another medication, isosorbide mononitrate (Isordil) in doses up to 20 mg twice a day is added to propanolol in an effort to further decrease portal pressure. However, this medication should not be used by itself as a prophylaxis of variceal bleeding. Patients should continue Inderal lifelong. If stopped prematurely, the risk of variceal hemorrhage returns.

Prophylactic therapy will not help patients who are already actively bleeding. Active bleeding is a medical emergency requiring hospitalization, preferably in an intensive care unit. In this scenario, doctors can stop the bleeding during an endoscopy by injecting a clotting agent directly into the dilated blood vessel (also known as a *varix*). This procedure is known as esophageal and/or gastric *sclerotherapy*. Alternatively, the doctor can stop the bleeding during an endoscopy by strangling the bleeding varix with a miniature rubber band. This procedure is known as esophageal and/or gastric variceal band ligation. Ligation is the preferred method to stop acute variceal bleeding, as less complications arise with this form of therapy, and recurrent bleeding occurs less often. Recurrent bleeding from varices takes place within six weeks of the initial episode in approximately two-thirds of people. Sclerotherapy, or preferably band ligation, should be performed every ten to fourteen days until the varices have been totally destroyed. This usually takes three to four rounds of therapy. Patients should also be placed on a beta-blocker, such as propanolol (Inderal), possibly in combination with isosorbide (Isordil), as these medications further reduce the risk of recurrent bleeding and ultimately prolong survival. Isordil, however, should not be used without Inderal for the control of recurrent bleeding.

Endoscopic ligation and/or banding can stop bleeding 90 percent of the time. If these methods fail to stop recurrent bleeding, a man-made shunt should be considered. *Portal-systemic shunts (PSS)* were the first types of shunts used to control variceal bleeding. This procedure entails surgically joining the portal vein to the inferior vena cava. PSS is performed by a surgeon, and the patient must undergo general anesthesia. Although this technique can successfully control variceal hemorrhage, a secondary consequence is that blood flow is diverted away from the liver. Thus, the liver actually becomes starved for blood. This may lead to an increased incidence of encephalopathy and accelerated progression of the patient's underlying liver disorder. Another type of surgical shunt is known as the *distal splenorenal shunt (DSRS)*. The DSRS procedure involves joining the splenic and kidney veins together. In this manner, blood flow to the liver is preserved, as blood is able to flow to the liver through the portal vein. As such, the incidence of encephalopathy and the rate of progression of liver disease are less among people undergoing DSRS than among those undergoing PSS. TIPS, as discussed above, creates a shunt connecting the hepatic and portal veins, thereby decreasing pressure in the esophagus and decreasing the risk of bleeding. TIPS does not require surgery or general anesthesia. While any of the above-mentioned man-made shunts may successfully control variceal bleeding, they do not prolong survival. In fact, the chance of surviving an additional month is slim. Therefore, people with variceal bleeding, like those with refractory ascites, ultimately need a liver transplant (see chapter 22).

Treatment of Encephalopathy

Encephalopathy is an altered or impaired mental status that occurs in people with cirrhosis and typically leads to coma. Treatment should begin with eliminating the factor that started the encephalopathy. Factors that can cause encephalopathy include the following:

- excessive use of *diuretics* (water pills), known as *overdiuresis*

- use of pain medications, sleeping pills, or tranquilizers

- excess consumption of animal protein

- infection

- constipation

- bleeding in the digestive tract (for example, bleeding esophageal varices)

- blood transfusion

- electrolyte imbalances (for example, low potassium level, a condition known as *hypokalemia*)

- dehydration (for example, fluid restriction, excessive diarrhea, overdiuresis)

- kidney dysfunction

- portal-systemic shunts (PSS)

- excessive alcohol consumption

- liver cancer

Treatment includes the discontinuation and avoidance of all sedatives, tranquilizers, and pain medications; discontinuation or reduction in the dosage of all diuretics; treatment of infection (particularly SBP); elimination of constipation; control of gastrointestinal bleeding; and reduction in amount, or total elimination of, animal protein from the diet. Some liver experts believe that strict vegetarian diets can help improve encephalopathy.

Further management involves oral administration of an antibiotic, most commonly *neomycin* (4 to 6 grams per day). Since bacteria that naturally live in the intestines produce ammonia, and since ammonia has been linked to encephalopathy, treatment with neomycin (which reduces bacteria) should improve encephalopathy. Neomycin should not be used in people who have renal (kidney) failure, as it can be toxic to the kidneys. Metronidazole (Flagyl) at a dose of 800 mg per day taken for a period of one week may be used as an alternative to neomycin. People found to have *Helicobacter pylori* in their stomachs must be treated with antibiotics and a proton-pump inhibitor such as Prevacid. Since this bacteria produces *urease* (an enzyme needed to produce ammonia), it may have a role in precipitating encephalopathy. Lactulose is a very sweet, synthetic sugar that acts as a powerful laxative. It acidifies the stool and thereby traps ammonia and drags it out of the body along with other fecal material. Therefore, lactulose can be quite useful in the management of encephalopathy. Kristolose (manufactured by Cumberland Pharmaceuticals) is a crystalline form of lactulose. It is not as sweet tasting and syrupy in texture as lactulose and is thus more palatable to some people than lactulose. The dose for either lactulose or kristolose ranges from 30 to 60 grams per day. The goal is for the patient to have two to four loose bowel movements per day. Once the initial bout of encephalopathy has been overcome, maintenance with lactulose should continue with a goal of one to two loose bowel movements per day.

Zinc levels should be checked and supplemented if found to be deficient, as zinc deficiency may be a contributing factor to encephalopathy. Thiamine deficiency should also be considered, and supplements should be routinely administered if the patient has a known history of alcoholic liver disease. Administration of branched-chain amino acids (leucine, isoleucine, and valine) may have some benefit; however, evidence supporting this is inconclusive. Two other drugs, flumazenil and bromocriptine, may be useful in the treatment of encephalopathy, although further study is needed to confirm this. Fortunately, if the precipitating factor is promptly corrected and if treatment with lactulose is expeditiously started, encephalopathy, in most cases, will be reversed—at least on a temporary basis.

Liver dialysis should be considered if encephalopathy does not improve despite the use of conventional medical treatments. Liver dialysis is analogous to kidney dialysis. A catheter is inserted into a vein in the patient. Some blood is removed through the catheter and is passed through the liver dialysis unit. In liver dialysis, toxins such as ammonia, which may cause encephalopathy, are removed from the patient's blood. Then the newly cleaned blood is returned to the patient through the same catheter. It takes about four to six hours to clear the blood of potential toxins that may cause encephalopathy. The HemoTherapies Unit is currently the only FDA-approved liver dialysis device in the United States. Many other devices are in the process of being developed. In any case, people with encephalopathy should be evaluated for a liver transplant.

Treatment of Osteoporosis

Osteoporosis is a condition marked by decreased bone mass and decreased bone density. This leads to a weakening of bones, thereby increasing the risk of bone fractures. People with any chronic liver disease are at increased risk for the development of osteoporosis due to any or all of the following: a lack of activity resulting from excessive fatigue; poor nutritional habits; reduced muscle mass; disturbances in hormonal levels (a condition known as *hypogonadism*); and medications used to treat certain liver diseases, such as prednisone for autoimmune hepatitis or after a liver transplant, and interferon and ribavirin combination therapy for chronic hepatitis C. People with cholestatic liver diseases such as primary biliary cirrhosis are at a particularly high risk for osteoporosis.

Osteoporosis can be quite painful and debilitating. Furthermore, there often are no warning signs of osteoporosis until a fracture occurs. Since osteoporosis can be so incapacitating, prevention of this complication of liver disease is crucial. Therefore, as postmenopausal women are already at high risk for bone fractures, they should try to avoid long-term treatment with prednisone or use the lowest dose possible, as this medication can worsen osteoporosis. This applies especially to those postmenopausal women discovered to have autoimmune hepatitis and those who have undergone a liver transplant. Prior to liver transplantation, it is especially important to take all steps possible to avert osteoporosis, as liver transplant recipients, regardless of age and menopause status, inevitably lose bone mass during the three- to six-month period following transplantation. Furthermore, the presence of osteoporosis prior to transplantation is predictive of the occurrence of fractures after the transplant.

All people with advanced chronic liver disease, especially women over the age of fifty, should undergo bone-mineral-density testing in order to determine whether they have osteoporosis. This test is performed by a radiologist and should be repeated once every three to five years. Blood tests, by themselves, are an insufficient means of measuring bone density and calcium requirements. If bone density is found to be low, it is strongly advised that the patient start on medication, such as Fosamax (alendronate sodium), aimed at inhibiting bone loss, in addition to taking a calcium and vitamin D supplement. In fact, people who are at a particularly high risk for osteoporosis (women with primary biliary cirrhosis, for example) should start taking Fosamax before the development of bone loss. See below for a further discussion of Fosamax and other biphosphonates.

There are some steps that people with liver disease can take to reduce the likelihood of osteoporosis. People should supplement their diets with calcium (1,000 to 2,000 mg per day) and vitamin D (400 to 800 IU per day). Also, an exercise routine, including weight-bearing exercises, must be incorporated into one's lifestyle. Weight-bearing exercises not only increase muscle size, but they increase underlying bone mass, thus decreasing the likelihood of osteoporosis. These issues are discussed in more detail in chapter 23. Smoking, alcohol, and excessive caffeine should be avoided. Since the incidence and severity of osteoporosis correlate with the dose and duration of prednisone therapy, people should attempt to taper off this medication as soon after transplantation as possible. Most transplant centers have begun to routinely decrease the dose of prednisone soon after transplant, and some transplant centers discontinue prednisone use altogether one year after transplant.

Estrogen-hormonal therapy has been demonstrated to increase bone mass. However, oral estrogen replacement should generally be avoided in people with liver disease, as it may cause additional liver problems, such as worsening of cholestasis. Furthermore, estrogen supplementation may cause certain benign liver tumors, such as hemangiomas and/or hepatic adenomas to enlarge (see chapter 19). Estrogen patches are generally a safer choice. Implantable estrogen, a recent development, is probably safe, but long-term studies as to its effect on liver disease have not been done. Soy estrogen, originally thought to be a safe alternative, should be avoided, as recent reports have suggested that it may cause drug-induced hepatitis.

Biphosphonates are phosphate derivatives that bind to the surface of the bone, thereby blocking bone removal and decreasing bone loss. Currently, there are three biphosphonates—alendronate (Fosamax), etidronate (Didronal), and risedronate (Actonel)—that have been approved by the FDA for the prevention and treatment of osteoporosis. These medications have been shown to increase bone mass, prevent bone loss, and decrease the incidence of bone fractures. Fosamax and Actonal have the advantage of a once-a-week administration, as opposed to the alternative of daily administration. Biphosphonates should be taken on an empty stomach, along with at least eight ounces of water. The patient should swallow the tablet while in an upright position and not lie down for thirty minutes after taking this drug. Calcium should not be taken at the same time. People with liver disease, especially those with cholestatic liver disease, may benefit from starting biphosphonate therapy before they develop osteoporosis. Any person who already has osteoporosis should begin biphosphonate therapy promptly. These medications may also be protective if used after liver transplantation. However, people with esophageal varices should probably avoid these medications because of the drug's capability to cause ulcers in the esophagus, which may precipitate esophageal variceal hemorrhage.

Calcitonin (Miacalcin) is a hormone produced by the thyroid gland (a gland in the neck) that decreases the release of calcium from the bones. Calcitonin has been shown to reduce the incidence of bone fractures and bone loss in post-menopausal women with osteoporosis. Synthetic calcitonin, known as miacalcin, is FDA approved for the treatment of osteoporosis. When sprayed into the nose, miacalcin is quickly absorbed into the bloodstream. It may also be taken as a sub-cutaneous injection. Miacalcin has also been shown to decrease bone pain associated with bone fractures caused by osteoporosis. In addition, it appears to be quite beneficial in preventing bone loss after liver transplantation. Thus, miacalcin can be an effective alternative for people who do not wish to or are unable to take biphosphonates.

Men with chronic liver disease are also at risk for osteoporosis and the resulting bone fractures and bone loss. This is primarily due to decreasing hormonal levels, known as hypogonadism. Men with cirrhosis often have decreased testosterone levels, and because testosterone is metabolized into estrogen, this results in a decreased level of estrogen in the blood. Testosterone levels further decrease with advancing age. And testosterone levels may be decreased by licorice ingestion, which is used by some individuals in the treatment of hepatitis. Few studies have been done on the safety and efficacy of testosterone replacement in hypogonadal men with liver disease. Since testosterone may be dangerous for the liver, and since it certainly is dangerous for men with prostate cancer, testosterone replacement therapy cannot be recommended at the present time.

CONCLUSION

Often the symptoms and/or complications of chronic liver disease discussed in this chapter are what prompt people to see their doctors, thereby leading to the diagnosis of liver disease. Treating the symptoms and complications of liver disease and cirrhosis can be as challenging as treating the underlying liver disorder. In fact, it is specifically the unresponsiveness of some symptoms and complications to therapy that typically leads a person to liver transplantation (which will be discussed in chapter 22). While appropriate and effective treatment of the symptoms and complications of liver disease is not the same thing as a cure, it is a crucial step toward improving a person's well-being. People with chronic liver disease who experience severe symptoms, such as fatigue, often seek out herbs and other alternatives to the conventional medical therapies discussed in this chapter. Therefore, the next chapter will discuss herbs and alternative therapies for liver disease, and will address issues related to their safety and effectiveness.

Twenty-one

HERBS AND OTHER
ALTERNATIVE THERAPIES

Recent surveys have indicated that Americans now make more visits to healthcare professionals who specialize in alternative medicine than to doctors who practice conventional medicine. *Alternative medicine* is any therapy used to treat an illness that is not within the realm of conventional and/or accepted medical therapies. People with liver disease are no exception to this trend. For example, most people with chronic hepatitis C have tried (or have at least inquired about) the herb milk thistle. Well, why not? It is now commonplace to find an entire aisle at the local drugstore or even the supermarket devoted to herbal remedies, some of which claim to help protect liver cells and help support liver function. Dozens of publications and books proclaim the proficiency of herbs for the treatment of medical conditions including hepatitis, cirrhosis, and other liver diseases. Some of these books have even made it to the *New York Times* best-seller list. On the Internet, numerous websites proclaim the effectiveness of herbs for treating liver disease. However, as you will learn, there is much more information to consider.

Some alternative therapies may be helpful if used properly under the guidance of a knowledgeable licensed healthcare professional and may be beneficial when used as part of a total treatment regimen in conjunction with conventional medical therapies. Some medical insurance companies have started to cover the cost of visits to practitioners of alternative therapies. Many well-respected institutions and organizations, including the National Institutes of Health, have conducted seminars on complementary and alternative medicine, and funding for research in this area has greatly increased in recent years. It appears that the worlds of conventional and alternative medicine may be moving in the direction of integration. In fact, there is a burgeoning field of medicine known as *integrative medicine,* which seeks to treat disease using a combination of conventional and alternative methods. However, be aware that some alternative therapies are simply a waste of time and money and can even be outright harmful and may cause complications that can result in liver failure. This is why it is important for people with liver disease to obtain a clear understanding of both the pros and cons of using herbs and alternative therapies.

This chapter will help you do just that. It discusses herbal remedies and some other alternative therapies for chronic liver disease and hepatitis. It provides a guide to help you distinguish among empty promises, helpful therapies, and those treatments that are flat-out dangerous. What constitutes an alternative treatment, as well as what an herb is, is defined within this chapter. Also, the Dietary Supplement and Education Act of 1994 (DSHEA) and its implications are discussed. This chapter also explains how to research information concerning the efficacy and side effects of some of the most popular herbs being used in the treatment of liver disease. Milk thistle (silymarin) and other herbs that claim to benefit the liver, as well as herbs that have the potential to harm the liver, are discussed in detail. In addition, alternative therapies other than herbs are discussed. Finally, conclusions on the safety and efficacy of various alternative remedies are provided, and recommendations for the use of alternative therapies are spelled out.

TAKING A CLOSER LOOK AT HERBS

Herbs are plants or plant parts that are used for healing purposes. These herbs, which generally have a bitter taste, are known as *medicinal herbs.* They are distinct from *culinary herbs,* which are tasty and used to season food. There has been a surge in the popularity of herbal remedies, as many people are desperately searching for alternatives to conventional synthetic medications. In fact, herbal products are estimated to be a multibillion-dollar-a-year industry whose revenue has increased dramatically in recent years and continues to increase with each year. It's easy to understand why herbal remedies are becoming such a popular alternative to Western medicine. With each new advance, medical science seems ever more intimidating. The latest technological breakthroughs often alienate as much as they ameliorate. Herbs, on the other hand, are a much friendlier commodity— as comfortably familiar as the kitchen spice rack. They can be purchased over the counter (without a prescription) in drugstores, supermarkets, health-food stores, by mail order, and over the Internet.

There are several things that people with liver disease in particular need to know about herbal medicines and how they differ from standard pharmaceuticals. The following information provides the facts—both good and bad.

A Brief History of Herbal Medicine

Herbs have been used throughout history by every culture to treat virtually every type of ailment—from the common cold to cancer, and yes, of course, liver disease. They have been consumed as teas, slices of root, and in modern times, pill or capsule form. The first written records describing treatment of disease with herbal remedies date back to about 1500 B.C. and are inscribed by the ancient Egyptians on papyrus. In China, the basis of traditional Chinese medicine was first recorded in the Materia Medica, which was written about two thousand years ago. In fact, traditional herbal remedies continue to form the backbone of modern Chinese medicine. Many institutions in China are devoted to the controlled study of medicinal herbs, and the Chinese Ministry of Public Health oversees the administration of new herbal products. Traditional Japanese medicine, known as *kampo,* is based on herbs. In 1988, laws were established in Japan to regulate the manufacture and quality of kampo medicine and to ensure compliance with the Japanese government's regulations for quality control in the manufacture of drugs. In Germany, where herbal remedies are commonly used by people and often recommended by doctors, Commission E oversees the safety of these preparations and requires that certain standards of purity be met. And the European Parliament is in the process of enacting legislation to ensure that all herbal products demonstrate efficacy and safety.

In the United States, much of our knowledge about herbs comes from the Native Americans, who had numerous uses for the plants that grew in abundance around them. Until the 1940s, medical textbooks often made reference to the medicinal uses of berries, bark, leaves, and roots. However, with the fantastic advances of modern technology during the twentieth century, these more natural remedies took a backseat to the scientifically developed synthetic medicines of today. Note, however, that approximately 10 to 20 percent of today's prescription drugs contain at least one active ingredient derived from plants or herbs. For example, digitalis, a popular drug used to treat certain heart conditions, is derived from the leaves of the herb foxglove. Salicin, which is used to make aspirin, was originally extracted from the bark of willow trees (now it is made synthetically). And some cough drops contain menthol, lemon, eucalyptus, or mint—all derived from herbs.

The Reasons Why Some People Are Turning to Herbal Medicine

There are many reasons why people with liver disease are turning to herbal remedies for answers. First, many people equate herbs with being safe because they are natural. Remember, however, that natural does not mean harmless. In fact, some herbs, which will be discussed on page 348, can be harmful to the liver. Second, some people who fail to respond to accepted medical treatments become disillusioned with conventional medicine and begin to look for alternatives. Third, many people with liver disease feel fine and may find it difficult to consider taking a medication that has the potential to make them feel ill—especially if they believe that herbal preparations can make them feel even better. Finally, while all herbs aren't inexpensive, they may still be cheaper than prescription medications over the course of long-term treatment. This is particularly true for people without medical coverage.

How to Evaluate the Research on Herbal Medicine

Walking through the aisles of a healthfood store or supermarket, you are likely to see many everyday products, such as green tea, licorice, artichokes, dandelion root, peppers, and turmeric, claiming to be beneficial in the treatment of liver disease. Obviously, one should and must research an herb more thoroughly before taking it with the expectation that it will help the liver. Simply reading the label on a supplement bottle, reading the description in an herbal remedy book, or asking the owner of the healthfood store if a particular herb will help the liver may not be enough. There are many steps a person can take on her own to determine if the herbal product that she is considering taking is, in fact, effective.

Many libraries, as well as the Internet, have access to MEDLINE (an electronic database maintained by the National Library of Medicine), which contains thousands of medical research papers. From MEDLINE you can get copies of original scientific articles cited in magazines, books, or journals. This will provide you with information as to what doses the investigators used and under what conditions they were used. Also, it is advisable to consult the *Physicians' Desk Reference (PDR) for Herbal Medicines.* This book provides a wealth of important information on herbs. It provides indications for an herb's use, including whether the indication is considered controversial; some of the known side effects of the herb; and some possible interactions with other drugs. Anyone contemplating the use of an herbal preparation is urged to purchase this book. Thanks to this book, people now have a good starting place for researching a particular herb or dietary supplement. In addition to the *PDR for Herbal Medicines,* the Office of Dietary Supplements (ODS) at the National Institutes of Health (NIH) has an up-to-date comprehensive website containing a database of scientific publications related to dietary supplements. And, in 1998, the Commission E Monographs was translated into English—*The Complete German Commission E Monographs: Therapeutic Guide to Herbal Medicines.* This book describes which herbs have been approved or rejected in Germany for medicinal uses, the recommended dosages and uses of approximately 250 specific herbs, and the contraindications, possible adverse reactions, and drug interactions that may occur with specific herbs.

As a general rule, there isn't as much scientific research on herbal remedies as there is on conventional therapies. Much of what does exist is usually based on a small number of test subjects who have taken the herb in question for a short duration. Still, it's worthwhile finding out exactly what sort of information exists. With the increased interest in herbal products, there are bound to be more and better-controlled scientific studies in the future. In fact, randomized controlled trials have begun to be conducted in the United States on the efficacy of certain herbs. Unfortunately, results so far have been disappointing. For example, studies on the herb St. John's wort, which is commonly used to treat depression, concluded that this herb did not have significant efficacy. Studies done on ginkgo, an herb purported to improve memory, have concluded that it does not provide significant benefits to memory. Studies done on milk thistle (silymarin) have concluded that this herb does not provide any benefit to people with the liver disease primary biliary cirrhosis (PBC).

In order to evaluate a research study, a few guidelines must be kept in mind. First and foremost, no single study can be considered to truly prove anything. Find out if the results have been reproduced in other laboratories or by other researchers. Next, try to determine the study's credibility: Has it been published in a well-respected medical journal, or has it only been self-published—as in a book or pamphlet that does not require any type of review? Look closely at the details of any study you are trying to evaluate. Did the investigators actually compare two groups of subjects (a control group and an experimental group), or had they simply performed an observational study, which involves looking at what happened to people taking the product in question? If they used a control group, how did they ensure that the two groups were indeed comparable in every way before the study began? Is there a possibility that the control group was actually sicker than the experimental group? What criteria did they use to include people in their study? Have they made sure that there weren't other disorders or other medications that confounded their results? How long did the study last, and what happened after the treatment was stopped?

After examining the methods that were used to conduct the experiment, look at the conclusions. Are they warranted by the evidence? Have the investigators taken into account the *placebo effect* (an improvement in response to treatment with a placebo, not the substance being tested)? Be particularly wary of research that does not include possible alternative explanations for its findings.

If a person can't find any useful information from independent sources on the efficacy of the particular herbal remedy in question, then it may be time to ask some tough questions, including: Do I want to be a guinea pig for an untested product? How do I know if the product is safe if I become pregnant? What guarantees do I have that the compound won't promote cancer, trigger ulcers, or contribute to liver failure? How do I know what dose I should use and how often? If the person still decides to take the compound, she should be sure to tell her doctor, so that the doctor can be on the lookout for any potential side effects or drug interactions.

What We Don't Know About Herbal Medicine

While the amount of information and research concerning herbs is increasing, there are still two important matters that have not been clearly defined as to herbs. First, due to the lack of controlled research on herbal remedies, the exact extent of drug-herb interaction is not entirely known. Thus, an herb that a person may be taking in an attempt to prevent liver damage may have a negative interaction with the medication that she is taking to control high blood pressure. For example, licorice—proclaimed to be beneficial in the treatment of viral hepatitis—might cause fluid retention and worsen high blood pressure. Furthermore, licorice may cause a decrease of libido in men, which is a potential side effect of interferon therapy, in addition to being a side effect of many antidepressants that are often used during interferon therapy for hepatitis C. Many herbs may increase or decrease the action of conventional medicines. For example, the herb cannabis sativa (marijuana) has been demonstrated to diminish the effectiveness of interferon and to suppress the immune system. Though potential adverse drug-herb interactions can be looked up in the *PDR for Herbal Medicines,* this list may be incomplete. An example of such an interaction includes the death of a woman who was taking St. John's wort at the time she underwent anesthesia with the drug Demerol. Due to an adverse drug-herb interaction, this patient experienced fatal cardiac arrest. This also resulted in the filing of a large lawsuit against the herb manufacturer.

Furthermore, the noted side effects of an herb, in general, may be incomplete. This is due to the fact that it can be very difficult to trace side effects to a particular herb. It may take weeks, months, or even years for problems to show up. By that point, people don't always remember that they have taken an herbal remedy, or they have become so accustomed to a particular side effect that they dismiss it. Complicating matters even further, many natural remedies contain dozens of active ingredients depending on exactly how they were prepared by the manufacturer. The composition of these ingredients may vary greatly (even among bottles of the same type of herb). Finally, there are no regulatory laws mandating that the manufacturer or distributor of an herbal preparation report possible adverse reactions of the herb to the FDA or other government agency (see "The Dietary Supplement Health and Education Act of 1994" on page 339). In all likelihood, all the possible drug-herb interactions and other side effects associated with a given herb are not listed in the *PDR for Herbal Medicines.* This is made clear by reports that appear on a regular basis alerting the public to the danger of an herb that was once thought to be safe. Usually the herb in question has caused some unsuspecting consumer to suffer severe, or even fatal, side effects, including cancer, kidney failure, and liver failure, thereby necessitating the removal of the herb from the market or at least stronger warning labels on the bottle. Examples of such herbs include kava and ephedra.

Second, there is a lack of standardization among herbal products. It is important to be aware that not all parts of the herb contain the active ingredient proclaimed to produce the beneficial effect. For example, one study compared ten different brands of the herb ginseng and found that the active ingredient ginsenoside varied drastically among different brands, although all were essentially similar in their descriptions of ingredients contained in the bottle. In fact, some pills or capsules contained almost none of the active ingredient. A different study found that up to one-quarter of the products on health-food store shelves did not contain any of the listed ingredients.

Due to the absence of regulation, it is possible that a totally different herb can be substituted for the one on the label. Furthermore, there have been reports that some herbs have been spiked with steroids, painkillers, tranquilizers, thyroid extracts, or other substances to improve their effectiveness. Toxic metals (including lead and arsenic) and even powerful heart stimulants (such as digitalis), the blood thinner warfarin, and the diabetic medication glyburide have been discovered mixed in with herbal preparations. And some herbs have been found to contain dangerous microorganisms, such as staphylococcus aureus, *Escherichia coli* (E. coli), salmonella, and shigella, each of which can make a person quite ill. Of course, the product labels did not mention the addition of any of these adulterants, and all labels claimed to contain only "natural" ingredients. So how can someone determine whether the contents listed on the label of an herbal product accurately reflect its contents? First, it is important to determine whether the company manufacturing the herbal product is a well-known, legitimate company with a good track record of providing consumers with safe and effective products. Second, a person can request a "certificate of analysis" from the manufacturer concerning a particular herbal product. This ensures that the ingredients listed on the label have been analyzed by a laboratory and are accurately represented on the label. Or a sample of the herbal product can be sent to an herbalist, a nutritionist, or a compound pharmacist, all of whom are capable of performing an analysis of the ingredients contained in the herb. Lastly, a *compound pharmacist*—a pharmacist who prepares, mixes, assembles, packages, and labels medications from scratch—can prepare an herb in its active form.

THE DIETARY SUPPLEMENT HEALTH AND EDUCATION ACT OF 1994

For a synthetic drug to become available by prescription, it must undergo rigorous premarket scrutiny by the United States Food and Drug Administration (FDA). Similarly, foods must meet manufacturing standards before they are deemed safe to eat. Herbal remedies have always presented a problem for the FDA. Should they be classified as food or drug? Until 1994, the FDA pretty much resolved this dilemma by treating herbal products as food additives. The manufacturers refrained (for the most part) from making any medical claims about their products. And if the FDA felt that an herbal product was unsafe, it could pull the product from the market and subject it to further testing.

In 1993, the FDA decided that herbal manufacturers would soon have to provide more scientific data about their products because more and more people were taking them. This decision was met with opposition. Members of Congress were bombarded with complaints from health-food store owners, herbal medicine manufacturers, and the supplement-taking public.

The outcome of this upheaval was the Dietary Supplement Health and Education Act of 1994 (DSHEA). This legislation essentially declared that any herb, vitamin, mineral, or other botanical product (other than tobacco) that was marketed as a dietary supplement was exempt from regulation by the FDA. The maker must simply provide "reasonable assurance" that no ingredient "presents a significant or unreasonable risk of illness or injury." Herb manufacturers still couldn't claim that their products prevented, treated, or cured disease, but they were allowed to make one claim that they had never before been allowed to make: They could advertise that their products "supported the structure or function" of various organs in the body. But in order to make such a claim, they had to include on the label the following disclaimer: "This statement has not been evaluated by the Food and Drug Administration. This product is not intended to diagnose, treat, cure, or prevent any disease."

While there are still some rules about what can go on product labels, the FDA has no jurisdiction over what is written in books, said on videos, or written on the Internet. As a result, claims about cures and the treatment and prevention of disease have proliferated. It is now totally up to the consumer to evaluate the validity of these claims.

How DSHEA Affects Consumers

Due to this law, no proof of safety or effectiveness of an herbal product needs to be submitted to any governmental regulatory agency before becoming available to the public. This means that side effects and toxic reactions caused by herbs or herbal products may get discovered only after they have happened to consumers who have purchased the products. Moreover, there is no regulatory process mandating that adverse reactions to herbs be reported to the public or to any governmental entity. For example, the manufacturer of Metabolife, the popular herbal weight-loss remedy that contains the potentially lethal combination of ephedra and caffeine, withheld from the public more than 14,000 adverse reactions, including 80 fatal or near-fatal incidents, that were reported to them by consumers of their product. However, under DSHEA the manufacturer had a legal right to do so. Therefore, the toxicity associated with herbal remedies is most likely greatly underestimated. (In contrast, serious adverse reactions to prescription drugs must be made public, and typically the drug is promptly pulled from the market.) The Congressional Research Service reports that according to their analysis, many people believe that "any product that appears in pill form has been reviewed for safety by the FDA." Thus, many people who use herbal remedies incorrectly assume that these products are regulated by the FDA for safety and efficacy.

How DSHEA Affects the Labeling of Herbs

Although claims that an herbal product prevents, treats, or cures disease are not permitted to appear on a product label, claims can be made about the effect of the remedy on an organ's structure or function. For instance, the label on a bottle of milk thistle can claim that the product "may support the liver" or "may inhibit factors responsible for liver damage," but it cannot state that it cures or prevents liver disease. However, though a label cannot make such blunt claims, other advertising venues are not prohibited from making them. This leads to confusion over exactly what claims manufacturers are making about their products. Also, since

The Dietary Supplement Safety Act of 2003 (DSSA)

As this book was being written, Congress was considering legislation that would amend DSHEA. Introduced in Congress in March 2003, the Dietary Supplement Safety Act of 2003 (DSSA) would require manufacturers and distributors of dietary supplements to report serious adverse consequences to the secretary of health and human services. Under the proposed DSSA, a supplement manufacturer would have to prove its product is safe before it could be marketed. Whether this proposed legislation will eventually become law is unknown. As well, it is unknown what specific provisions might be included in the law in its final form. In any event, the fact that such legislation is being debated in Congress suggests that stricter government regulation of the supplement industry is likely in the near future. Certainly, a welcome development for the consumer would be the enactment of laws mandating extensive and conspicuous warning labels on all supplement products. Also welcome would be the creation of a government-run Internet website providing detailed information (including name of manufacturer and distributor) on adverse consequences experienced by consumers of supplements.

the labeling of herbs is unregulated, it may often lack crucial information—such as the exact ingredients and the amount and potency of the ingredients. Some herbal remedies contain only one ingredient, whereas other remedies contain a mixture of ingredients. Consumers should research the quality and efficacy of any herbs or herbal products that they intend to use and shouldn't rely solely on the manufacturers' claims.

MILK THISTLE—THE MOST WIDELY USED HERB FOR LIVER DISEASE

Milk thistle (also known as silymarin and its scientific name, *Silybum marianum*) is a tall plant characterized by sharp spines that resemble artichokes and leaves that are riddled with distinctive white veins. It was originally discovered growing in the Kashmir region bordering India and Pakistan. It can now be found all over the temperate world, growing in dry and rocky soil. Its stems and leaves secrete a milky substance when crushed. The following sections contain important information regarding this popular herb. It is important to be aware that some preparations of milk thistle may contain iron; therefore, milk thistle should be avoided by people with liver diseases associated with iron overload such as hemochromatosis and some cases of chronic hepatitis C.

The History of Milk Thistle

As with so many other herbs, the medicinal claims for milk thistle have an ancient history. Originally believed to help nursing mothers produce milk, milk thistle became more well known over time for its effects on the liver. This can be traced back to ancient Roman times when Pliny the Elder (A.D. 23–79) referred to the milky juice of this plant as being excellent for "carrying off bile." John Gerard, a sixteenth-century British herbalist, recommended milk thistle for "expelling melancholy," a symptom attributed to liver disease during that era. In Germany during the nineteenth century, doctors commonly treated jaundice and other liver diseases with an extract from milk thistle seeds. The scientific study of herbs continued to be concentrated in Europe, and in 1949 German researchers found that milk thistle appeared to protect the livers of animals exposed to high doses of carbon tetrachloride, a potent liver toxin.

In 1968, it was found that the active ingredient in milk thistle is located in the seed and that it consists of three components—silybin, silydianin, and silychristin. These components are now collectively referred to as "the flavonoid silymarin." Silymarin is currently used in Europe to treat all types of liver disorders. In the United States, due to the lack of FDA regulation, the actual percentage of biologically active silymarin in a given preparation of milk thistle is unknown.

The Benefits Claimed for Milk Thistle

The following claims have been made about milk thistle:

- milk thistle may reverse liver damage in alcoholics

- milk thistle may reverse liver injury in patients with chronic hepatitis

- milk thistle may slow the advancement of cirrhosis

- milk thistle may improve the long-term survival rate among cirrhotic patients

Herbalists claim that milk thistle achieves the above in three different ways: First, milk thistle is said to strengthen the outer protective membrane of liver cells so that they are better at deflecting toxins. Second, milk thistle is said to shield the liver from free radicals, which are potentially dangerous, yet inevitable, by-products of some of the body's basic metabolic functions. And finally, milk thistle is said to stimulate the production of new liver cells to replace old damaged ones. This section will examine some of the evidence that forms the basis for each of these alleged properties of milk thistle.

Ability to Inhibit Factors Responsible for Liver Damage
by Strengthening the Outer Membrane of Liver Cells

This characteristic of milk thistle would prevent the entrance of potentially toxic substances into the liver. This property can be demonstrated if a person decides to go on a wild mushroom–picking expedition and accidentally eats the deadly fungus deathcap. These mushrooms are found in North America and Europe and are part of the Amanita phalloides family of mushrooms. They are known for containing deadly toxins known as phallotoxins that are famous for causing liver failure or even death when consumed—thus the nickname "deathcap fungus." Unfortunately, a person would have to be a *mycophagist* (an expert mushroom picker) to tell the difference between a deathcap and other tasty amanita mushrooms that are edible and nontoxic. It doesn't take much for a poisonous mushroom to destroy the liver. Within about eight hours of ingestion, diarrhea, stomach pains, nausea, and vomiting will occur. About a week later, LFTs will elevate and total liver failure, along with encephalopathy and death, is not too far off. That's where milk thistle comes in. Milk thistle has been shown to compete effectively with these mushroom toxins to occupy the same site on the liver cell membrane. If ingested in time, milk thistle may block the entrance of these mushroom toxins into the liver and prevent damage from occurring. Or, if taken soon after ingestion, milk thistle may actually displace the toxins from their sites and thereby stop any further damage.

It must be emphasized that most of the evidence of the liver-protective properties of milk thistle stems from experimental animal studies. For example, laboratory animals were experimentally poisoned with Amanita phalloides. The animals given milk thistle at five hours and twenty-four hours after poisoning displayed little evidence of liver damage and had normal levels of liver enzymes. Animals that did not receive milk thistle either died of liver damage or had elevated liver enzymes. Case reports of humans who ingested poisonous mushrooms revealed marked improvement of liver-related abnormalities and a successful outcome when treated with milk thistle. However, these results must be interpreted with caution. These are isolated incidences, consisting of only three people. Moreover, other treatments, such as antibiotics and steroids, were also administered along with the milk thistle. Therefore, whether the benefits achieved were due to milk thistle or other therapies is unclear.

As you can see from the above, there is some very suggestive, though not conclusive, evidence in favor of milk thistle's ability to help protect the liver from acute mushroom poisoning. Many people would consider the data to be good enough to warrant trying milk thistle along with other medical treatments, especially in the event of such an emergency. But don't forget that most people who have been poisoned by mushrooms are otherwise in good health. Their liver cells have not been damaged. They have not lived for years with a scarred liver. So even if milk thistle is one day proven to be the standard antidote for some kinds of mushroom poisoning, it doesn't necessarily mean that it will protect people with other forms of liver disease.

Protects Liver Cells from Free-Radical Damage

Free radicals are highly reactive molecules that the body creates as a natural consequence of just being alive. The number of free radicals produced often skyrockets under the influence of such factors as a high-fat diet, smoking, and exposure to the sun or excess radiation. Free radicals may result in severe damage of cells and tissues in the body. Most free radicals in the body consist of toxic oxygen molecules. Oxygen in its toxic state can oxidize molecules in the body, corroding them, similar to the formation of rust—which is simply oxidized iron. Since the body can't live without these rogue chemicals, it also produces antioxidants that gobble up any free radicals they can find and render them harmless. Probably one of the hardest-working antioxidants produced by the liver is an enzyme called *glutathione peroxidase,* which protects the liver from free-radical damage. In fact, one of the ways that alcohol and liver toxins damage the liver is by interfering with the body's ability to create glutathione. A few tissue studies have suggested that milk thistle can boost the level of glutathione in liver cells, thus affording protection to the liver from these toxins. Commonly known antioxidants include vitamins A, C, and E. Milk thistle claims to possess ten times more antioxidant power on the liver than vitamin E.

Iron is a major catalyst of free-radical reactions and can be a potent toxin to the liver. Iron overload diseases are associated with liver damage and cirrhosis. Iron-induced oxidation of cellular membranes is known as lipid peroxidation. Lipid peroxidation by-products, such as hydrogen peroxide, are believed to be the mediators of the toxic effects of iron on the liver. This is thought to be an important mechanism leading to iron toxicity. Milk thistle is believed to possess antioxidant activity and specifically scavenge hydroxyl and peroxyl radicals. Experimental studies done on rats who were fed high iron diets showed lack of iron-induced liver toxicity when administered milk thistle. Comparative studies will need to be done before conclusions can be made for humans. Additional experimental studies on animals given liver toxins, such as carbon tetrachloride (CCL4), alcohol, or acetaminophen, and on small groups of humans exposed to toluene and xylene vapors, showed similar protective effects of milk thistle. However, one study attempting to demonstrate the protective effect of milk thistle on acetaminophen-induced liver damage not only failed to show protection, but it actually demonstrated that milk thistle can cause liver-cell death.

The largest human studies with the longest follow-up time and that best demonstrate the beneficial effects of milk thistle on the liver have been conducted on people with alcoholic liver disease. Some of these studies have suggested that mortality in people with alcoholic cirrhosis may be reduced by treatment with milk thistle when compared to a group of people with similar alcohol-induced, disease-related characteristics who were not treated with milk thistle. However, many flaws can be found in these studies. For example, upon closer examination of one study, it was noted that patients in the nontreated group were slightly sicker and had on average higher bilirubin levels and a more advanced stage of liver disease compared with people in the group treated with milk thistle. Some studies done on people with alcoholic cirrhosis have demonstrated a normalization of liver enzymes after one month of treatment with milk thistle. However, other large studies in which people with alcoholic liver disease were treated with milk thistle have shown no benefits to either liver enzymes or mortality.

Stimulates Production of New Liver Cells to Replace Old Damaged Ones

In experimental studies (not performed on human subjects), milk thistle was demonstrated to increase the production of ribonucleic acid (RNA). Since RNA is one of the building blocks of life, the production of protein was thereby increased and therefore, theoretically, stimulating the production of new liver cells to replace destroyed liver cells. Once again, it must be emphasized that it has never been demonstrated that this property of milk thistle applies to humans.

Summary of What Milk Thistle May Do

From the above evidence it appears that milk thistle is very helpful in cases of acute mushroom poisoning. It may be helpful for people with alcoholic liver disease or liver disease caused by certain drugs. However, milk thistle does not appear to have any antiviral properties. Thus, although it may decrease liver enzyme elevations, it cannot eradicate the hepatitis C or B viruses from the body, nor can it lessen the amount or toxicity of these viruses in the body.

The Most Effective Way to Take Milk Thistle

If a person decides that she wants to try milk thistle, how should she take it in order to maximize its proclaimed effects on the liver? Well, since milk thistle does not easily dissolve in water, its purported benefits cannot be reaped by drinking it as a tea or by eating the leaves. The best way to take milk thistle is either in capsule form, especially from concentrate, or in a form that combines it with other substances—such as beta-cyclodextrin or phosphatidylcholine (silipide)—that render milk thistle more soluble in water. In this way, milk thistle becomes more bioavailable to the body, and its effects are maximized. The concentration of silymarin is highest in the seeds of the plant, although it is also found in the fruit and leaves.

With milk thistle, as with all herbal remedies, there is no standard recommended dose or length of time to take the herb in order to best achieve its purported benefits. Recommendations made on labels and in herbal publications vary from as low as 70 mg twice per day to as high as 420 mg three times per day. Recommendations for duration of use range from one month to as long as nine months. There are no standard recommendations as to the best time of day to take the herb or whether to take it with food as opposed to on an empty stomach. *The PDR for Herbal Medicines* recommends 200 to 400 mg of silymarin daily, but contains no additional recommendations regarding its use.

The Side Effects of Milk Thistle

Most reports on milk thistle claim that there is a total lack of side effects when taking this herb. However, on close review of the literature, the following side effects were noted: headache, irritability, nausea, minor gastrointestinal upset, and, most commonly, diarrhea. These side effects are similar to those commonly encountered in connection with the use of interferon (the FDA-approved treatment for hepatitis B and C). One experimental study, which has not been duplicated, demonstrated that liver cell damage occurred as a result of exposing liver cells to milk thistle. The long-term side effects of milk thistle usage are not known.

OTHER HERBS USED FOR HEPATITIS AND LIVER DISEASE

This section discusses six of the most common herbs used in the treatment of liver disease—licorice, green tea, dandelion, artichoke, turmeric, and black peppers and long peppers. Read on to learn about some of the facts that people with liver disease need to know before deciding to take these herbs.

Licorice

The word *licorice* tends to conjure up an image of chewy black or red candy. However, licorice (*Glycyrrhiza glabra*) is also a powerful herb that has been proclaimed to help the liver. The active ingredients of licorice come from its roots and are believed by some to be due to glycyrrhizic acid, which also accounts for licorice's sweet taste. This acid functions similarly to the body's own naturally occurring hormone *aldosterone,* which regulates salt and water in the body. Thus, side effects of licorice may include high blood pressure, water retention, and potassium depletion. It is important to avoid licorice during pregnancy. Also, people who have glaucoma, heart disease, or high blood pressure should avoid licorice.

Licorice has been shown in some experimental studies to stimulate production of the body's natural supply of interferon. This may account for its popularity in Japan, where it is sometimes used in the treatment of chronic viral hepatitis. When used intravenously, licorice has been demonstrated to lower liver enzymes. However, these results have not been confirmed, and some studies have concluded that licorice provides no beneficial effects on the liver in humans. Furthermore, it has been noted that if licorice is taken for more than one week, there is an increased risk of serious side effects, such as high blood pressure or dangerously low potassium levels. Sustained beneficial effects from licorice use have not been clearly demonstrated. The *PDR for Herbal Medicines* states that licorice is *contraindicated* (use is inadvisable) in people with chronic hepatitis, cholestatic liver disease, and cirrhosis. Licorice may contain iron and should therefore be avoided by people with iron overload diseases, such as hemochromatosis and sometimes chronic hepatitis C. Licorice may interact adversely with the steroid drug prednisone. Prednisone is used in the treatment of autoimmune hepatitis (AIH) and after liver transplantation as an immunosuppressant. Licorice may cause levels of this steroid to become dangerously elevated, thereby resulting in low potassium levels as well as salt and water retention. Licorice can also counteract the effects of the water pill (diuretic) spironolactone, used in the treatment of ascites. Finally, licorice has been shown to decrease testosterone levels. Thus, men suffering from decreased libido, which can occur in people with cirrhosis, as a side effect of interferon therapy (for hepatitis C), and as a side effect of many antidepressant medications (such as Celexa), should avoid taking licorice.

Green Tea

Green tea (*Camellia sinensis*), popular in Asia, contains a high dose of catechin, a plant chemical. By comparison, black tea, which is popular in the United States, has undergone the process of fermentation, resulting in a lower concentration of catechin. Catechin is a flavonoid with antioxidant properties that has the ability to stabilize cell membranes. Therefore, the proclaimed liver-protective properties of catechin are similar to those that are claimed for milk thistle.

Experimentally induced liver damage in rats and liver cell cultures has demonstrated the protective effects on the liver afforded by catechin. However, most human studies have failed to show similar results. Side effects noted in one study involving humans included fever, hemolysis (breakdown of red blood cells), and urticaria (an allergic rash). Dosages used in humans were 20 to 40 mg/kg daily as opposed to 200 mg/kg daily used in rats. It has been suggested that higher dosages should be used on humans in order to reap the herb's benefit of liver protection. However, the side effects that accompany higher dosages render such an approach impractical.

Dandelion

Anecdotally, it has been claimed that dandelion (*Taraxacum officinale*) possesses liver-healing properties. In fact, dandelion has been purported to enhance bile flow and to improve both hepatitis and jaundice. However, actual studies involving dandelion are difficult to locate. Dandelion has an extremely high vitamin A content, higher than that of carrots. Since high levels of vitamin A can lead to serious liver damage (which will be discussed in chapter 23), it is not advisable to use any herbal preparation that contains dandelion. (Please note: Dandelion may contain iron and therefore should be avoided by people with iron overload diseases.)

Artichoke

The active ingredient of artichoke is found in the leaves and is known as *caffeylquinic acid* or *cynara*. The alleged properties of artichoke are similar to those alleged for milk thistle. Studies using artichoke on people with liver disease are difficult to locate.

Turmeric

Turmeric (*Curcuma domestica*) is the main ingredient in Indian curry powder. For thousands of years, this herb has been used by India's practitioners of traditional Ayurvedic medicine as a cure for liver disease. The herb's active component is

the yellow pigment *curcumin.* This herb is proclaimed to have antioxidant properties. In experimental animal studies, it has been shown to inhibit liver damage
from aflatoxin and other liver toxins. It might, therefore, be concluded that the
Indian population has a lower incidence of liver disease than the rest of the
world, but this has not been demonstrated.

Black Peppers and Long Peppers

Piperine is the active ingredient of black peppers (*Piper nigrum*) and long peppers (*Piper longum*), which are among the most commonly used spices. In cases
of experimentally induced liver disease in mice, piperine has been shown to reduce the damaging effects of toxins on the liver. These studies explained this
beneficial effect on the liver by asserting that piperine had the ability to prevent
depletion of glutathione, the liver's own protective antioxidant. There are no
known studies comparing the occurrence of liver disease in people who consume
these peppers with those who don't.

HERBS THAT MAY HARM THE LIVER

As mentioned previously, the mere fact that herbs are natural does not mean that
they are harmless. In fact, there have been many reports of people suffering serious health problems or even dying as a result of their use of herbal remedies.
Since everything that enters the mouth is metabolized through the liver, the liver
is a prime target for the toxic effects of some herbs. People with normal-
functioning livers and no history of prior liver disease have suffered adverse consequences to the liver as a result of taking certain herbs. Obviously, the potential
for adverse consequences in people with liver disease is greatly increased. Remember, it is the liver's job to rid the body of potentially harmful substances. A
liver that is already damaged will have to work overtime to clear a toxic herb
from the body. Quite obviously, it is inadvisable to subject a poorly functioning
liver to this type of stress. A doctor, unaware that a patient with liver disease has
taken herbal remedies, or unaware of the hepatotoxic effects of certain herbal
remedies, may attribute any worsening of the patient's condition to the natural
course of the liver disease.

    The following is a brief discussion of some of the herbs that have been de-
termined to be dangerous to the liver along with an extensive list of herbs that
have been linked to hepatitis, liver damage, and liver failure. Although not
proven, it appears that women are more susceptible to herbal-induced liver disease than men. Also, some significant drug-herb interactions specifically relevant
to people with liver disease are discussed.

    In general, a key point to keep in mind is that any herb containing *pyrrolizidine
alkaloids* is potentially hepatotoxic. Hepatotoxicity due to pyrrolizidine-containing
herbs can result from either small amounts ingested over long periods of time or
from large amounts ingested over a short period of time. Pyrrolizidine alkaloids

have been found in approximately 350 different plant species. The most toxic of these have been noted to be from the *senecio, heliotropium, crotalaria,* and *symphytium* species. Pyrrolizidine poisoning is common in Africa and Jamaica, two areas of the world where herbal teas containing this substance are consumed as folk remedies for a number of ailments. The pyrrolizidine alkaloids have been associated with a severe type of liver disorder known as *veno-occlusive disease.* In this disease, the hepatic vein becomes clogged, blocking off the blood supply to the liver. This can result in abdominal pain, vomiting, ascites, hepatomegaly, edema, cirrhosis, liver failure, and even death due to extensive liver damage.

The most well-established example of a liver-toxic pyrrolizidine alkaloid–containing herb is comfrey (*Symphytum officinale*). Comfrey has been used to relieve joint and stomach aches and is commercially available as a tea or in tablet or capsule form in the United States. Many herbal preparations that contain a mixture of herbs include comfrey, but due to the lack of labeling regulations of herbal products, comfrey may or may not be listed as an ingredient on these products.

Germander, an herb marketed as safe and natural, was at one time widely used in France as a weight-loss remedy. Since 1992, this herb has been banned from the French market because it was discovered to be the cause of twenty-six cases of severe hepatitis. Additional cases of hepatitis due to germander were also reported in Canada. It is thought that the diterpenoid content of germander is the culprit causing hepatotoxicity.

Chaparral, an herb proclaimed to be an aging retardant, has been reported to cause jaundice, fulminant hepatitis, and liver damage. In one reported case, the damage was so extensive that the patient required a liver transplant. Jin Bu Huan, typically used as an herbal sedative, has been reported to cause acute hepatitis. Some herbs may be dangerous to ingest while pregnant. In fact, death of a newborn baby was reported in a woman who consumed a hepatotoxic herbal preparation during pregnancy.

The above are just a few examples of herbs that have led to liver damage, which is often permanent and occasionally fatal, though sometimes reversible. The following is a list of herbs that are known to have caused liver problems. Although this is long, it cannot be considered complete due to unreported data. Herbs that have been associated with liver disease include the following:

- black cohosh

- buckthorn (*Rhamnus cathartica*)

- callilepsis laureola (*Impila*)

- cascara sagrada

- celandine (also known as greater celandine) (*Chelidonium majus*)

- chaparral (also known as creosote bush or greasewood) (*Larrea taridentata*)

- comfrey and other herbs containing pyrrolizidine alkaloids (heliotropium, senecio, crotalaria, symphytum)

- coxidan (Danthron 1,8-hydroxyanthroquinone and dioctyl calcium sulfosuccinate)

- germander (*Teucrium chamaedrys*)

- green tea leaf

- groundsel (*Senecio vulgaris*)

- impila root

- Jin Bu Huan

- kava (also known as kava kava or *Piper methysticum*)

- kombucha

- lobelia (*Lobelia inflata*)

- ma huang (ephedra)

- mate (also known as paraquay tea) (*Ilex paraguariensis*)

- mistletoe (*Viscum album*)

- nutmeg (*Myristica fragrans*)

- pau d'arco (*La pachol*)

- pennyroyal (*Mentha pulegium*)

- pokeweed (*Phytolacca americana*)

- ragwort (*Senecio jacoboea*)

- sarsaparilla (*Smilax species*)

- sassafras (*Sassafras albidum*)

- saw palmetto (the main ingredient of the herbal preparation known as "Prostata")

- senna (*Cassia acutifolia*)

- skullcap (*Scutellaria laterifolia*)

- soy phytoestrogen

- sweet clover (*Melilotus officinalis*)

- tansy (*Tanacetum vulgare*)

- t'u-san-chi

- valerian (*Valeriana offinalis*)

- woodruff (*Galium odoratum*)

- certain Chinese herbal formulas, typically a complex mixture of a variety of different herbs

- herbal preparations containing the recreational drug "ecstasy" (3,4-Methylene-dioxymetamphetamine)

It is also important to be aware that there are many known drug-herb inter-actions of potential significance to a person with liver disease. For example, gar-lic, gingko, dong quai danshen, devil's claw, and papaya extract (papain) all may increase the tendency to bleed. Thus, people with liver disease undergoing a sur-gical procedure or any invasive procedure, such as a liver biopsy, should be aware of this potential effect. Furthermore, people with esophageal varices may also be at increased risk for hemorrhage when taking these herbs. People who have had a liver transplant should avoid the herb St.-John's-wort. This herb may cause cy-closporine levels (a medication used after transplantation to prevent rejection of the new liver) to decrease, thereby putting one at risk for rejection of the trans-planted liver. As discussed, licorice may reduce prednisone levels, thus putting a transplant recipient at risk for rejection of the transplanted liver.

OTHER ALTERNATIVE TREATMENTS FOR LIVER DISEASE

It is important for people to explore all of the options that are available to treat hepatitis and liver disease. However, it is also important that they not allow them-selves to be fooled into trying therapies that clearly do not work or that may ex-acerbate their liver conditions. Conventional medical therapies have proved their ability to save the lives of many people with liver disease. It is important to keep this point in mind when considering alternative treatments as a substitute for the time-tested conventional therapies. This section discusses some alternative ther-apies other than herbs that people with hepatitis or other liver diseases may be tempted to try.

Ozone Therapy

Most people are somewhat familiar with the ozone layer. This protective layer in the atmosphere is responsible for absorbing toxic forms of radiation emitted from the sun. Without this protective layer, all forms of life on earth would die. Proponents of ozone therapy theorize that because ozone is, in essence, saving our lives, administering it directly into the body can cure a whole host of diseases, in-cluding cancer, AIDS, and hepatitis. Advocates of ozone therapy contend that viruses (such as the hepatitis B and C viruses) and other microorganisms that are responsible for causing disease survive and actually flourish in a low-oxygen environment. Consequently, they believe that if an oxygen-rich environment (such as ozone, which is made of three oxygen molecules) is substituted for the oxygen-poor environment of the body (oxygen is comprised of two oxygen molecules) that viruses, such as the hepatitis viruses, would die. To date, no study has confirmed this hypothesis. In fact, there have been a few reported cases of people who acquired hepatitis C (and also HIV) as a result of poorly sterilized ozone-therapy equipment. Finally, if ozone can actually kill viral cells, it would also have the potential to kill healthy human cells. Therefore, ozone therapy for people with hepatitis or other liver diseases cannot be recommended at this time.

Alpha-lipoic Acid Therapy

Alpha-lipoic acid, also known as thioctic acid, is a *coenzyme* (an enzyme helper) manufactured by the body that functions as an antioxidant. It also helps cells in the body to produce energy. Alpha-lipoic acid has been proclaimed to be a substance that can protect the liver from toxins. In fact, it is approved in Germany to treat liver disease. In people with acute liver poisoning (such as from toxic mushrooms or an acetaminophen overdose), alpha-lipoic acid (administered intravenously) may protect the liver when administered soon after such poisoning. It probably functions similar to the herb milk thistle. However, these findings are based on anecdotal reports. In people with chronic liver disease, there is no conclusive evidence that alpha-lipoic acid protects the liver, slows progression of disease, reverses cirrhosis, or eradicates chronic hepatitis B or C. Therefore, until further research establishes the efficacy of this coenzyme, it cannot be recommended to people with chronic liver disease. If taken, it is important not to exceed 1,200 mg intravenously per day or 100 mg orally per day.

Thymosin Therapy

The thymus is a gland located in the neck that secretes hormones (*thymosin, thymopoietin,* and *serum thymic factor*) involved in the regulation of the immune system. These hormones may stimulate the body's production of interferon. People with low levels of these hormones are often susceptible to infection. Thus, some researchers have suggested that people with hepatitis B and C possibly can benefit from the administration of thymus gland hormones, either by mouth (Complete Thymic Formula manufactured by Preventive Therapeutics, Inc.) or by injection (Thymosin-alfa1[Zadaxin] manufactured by SciClone Pharmaceuticals).

A study conducted on people with chronic hepatitis C who did not respond to or who could not tolerate interferon failed to show any benefits from taking Complete Thymic Formula (an over-the-counter supplement containing thymosin, thymopoietin, thymic humoral factors, herbs, vitamins, minerals, and enzymes).

Studies investigating the benefits of injectable thymosin (Thymosin-alfa1

[Zadaxin]) did not appear to help people with chronic hepatitis C. However, when Zadaxin was used in combination with interferon, some people with hepatitis C experienced a sustained eradication of the virus. Furthermore, preliminary studies on the use of Zadaxin in combination with pegylated interferon alpha-2a (PEGASYS) for people with chronic hepatitis C who failed to respond to previous interferon/ribavirin combination therapy look promising. These results are discussed in chapter 13.

Zadaxin used alone or in combination with interferon also appears to be beneficial in treating patients with chronic hepatitis B. These studies are discussed in chapter 12.

Metabolic Therapies

Metabolic therapies are based on the belief that harmful substances that accumulate in the body are the cause of disease. These therapies vary but often include a combination of high-dose vitamins, dietary restrictions, and coffee enemas. For people with liver disease, metabolic therapies can be especially harmful. Metabolic therapy diets usually include high doses of carrot juice. Carrot juice, consumed in excess, may lead to elevated levels of vitamin A, a vitamin that can potentially cause liver damage if taken in extreme amounts. Coffee enemas are purported to stimulate the secretion of bile and eliminate poisons from the liver as well as to remove them from the body. However, excessive use of enemas may lead to a serious dehydration problem, dangerous electrolyte imbalances, and a loss of muscle tone in the colon, all of which may result in chronic constipation. Furthermore, this form of treatment has not been proven to be beneficial for people with liver disease and should be avoided.

Megadose Vitamin Therapy

Some practitioners of alternative medicine believe that megadoses of vitamins (in the case of hepatitis, megadoses of vitamin C) can cure disease. This belief is unsubstantiated. Furthermore, megadose vitamin therapy is potentially harmful. Since vitamin C promotes the absorption of iron, toxic levels of iron may accumulate in the liver, leading to additional damage. Also, as discussed in chapter 23, megadoses of vitamin A can lead to severe liver damage. Therefore, megadose vitamin therapy is not recommended.

Other Alternative Therapies

There are numerous (too numerous to describe in this book) alternative therapies that, although they have no proven merit, have been touted as beneficial to the liver. These therapies include placing hot and cold castor oil packs on the skin over the area of the liver (supposedly to draw poisons out of the body) and using medicinal mushrooms, such as reishi, which can be deadly if confused with the liver-toxic mushroom amanita. Any alternative therapy that a person may be considering should first be discussed with her liver specialist.

Supportive Therapy

Supportive therapy from friends, loved ones, religious groups, and other organizations is an important part of getting better, no matter what liver disease a person has. Some people find that joining a local support group is also helpful. In fact, it has been medically proven that psychological and moral support can help people get better faster and can help them live longer lives. So, while supportive therapy is technically not a form of alternative therapy, it should be considered an important adjunctive therapy for all people with liver disease.

RECOMMENDATIONS CONCERNING THE USE OF ALTERNATIVE THERAPIES

The role of alternative therapies for the treatment of people with liver disease and hepatitis remains inconclusive. Many studies performed to date have been based on animal subjects, and most of the clinical trials conducted on humans lasted only a short period of time (approximately one to two months in many studies) and involved small numbers of people. Many studies with encouraging results unfortunately used generalized terms such as *liver disease* or *hepatitis*. So, which liver diseases actually improved as a result of the alternative therapy utilized in the study is unclear. Therefore, any benefits to the liver achieved with an alternative therapy may not be equally applicable to all liver diseases. Furthermore, follow-up observation time was too short to attribute any long-term benefit to most alternative therapies studied.

While a decrease in liver enzymes was demonstrated in many people treated with a given alternative therapy (such as people with hepatitis C treated with milk thistle), the therapy's effect on other parameters (such as HCV RNA viral loads in the case of people with hepatitis C treated with milk thistle) was typically not addressed. Furthermore, whether liver enzyme normalization was sustained once the alternative therapy was discontinued was also not addressed in all studies. Finally, the effect of the alternative therapy on inflammation and/or scarring (as per liver biopsy samples before and after therapy) was not addressed in any alternative therapy study. So, taking these issues into consideration, the following list contains some guidelines that a person interested in exploring alternative therapies for liver disease and hepatitis should follow:

- If a person decides to try an alternative treatment regimen, her liver specialist should be informed of this prior to its commencement. This will allow the doctor to monitor the results of the alternative therapy through blood tests and physical exams. Furthermore, the doctor will be able to observe the patient with an eye toward possible adverse effects or drug interactions. The patient should keep a diary of symptoms, side effects, and laboratory reports. This is necessary in order to assess the degree of improvement and to track adverse reactions.

- The patient should be jointly managed by the conventional medical doctor and the alternative healthcare practitioner. This will help minimize any conflicting therapies and will facilitate prompt recognition of an adverse reaction due to therapy.

- Licensure laws and practice guidelines for alternative healthcare practitioners vary from state to state. It is important for a person to review the credentials of the alternative healthcare provider she is considering seeing. Some helpful information concerning questions to ask a prospective doctor can be found in chapter 4.

- Any alternative therapy that the patient intends to use should be fully researched by both the patient and the conventional medical doctor prior to commencement of therapy. There are numerous reference books and resources available to a person desiring to investigate or find the most knowledgeable alternative-medicine practitioners.

- If an herb is being used, start with the lowest dose recommended. Do not exceed usage for over six months' time or for longer than any of the study periods. Also, since most studies on the benefits of milk thistle observed positive results within one month, it is probably advisable to discontinue its use if benefits are not experienced within this time period. The same holds true for any herbal preparation.

- Do not use herbal mixtures. These contain a variety of herbs and often miscellaneous other ingredients. Due to the multiplicity of uncontrolled substances found in herbal mixtures, there is a likelihood of ingesting substances that may be harmful to your liver.

- If at any time side effects are experienced, or if a woman discovers that she is pregnant, the alternative therapy should be discontinued immediately. Under such circumstances, the patient should promptly inform her doctor of her pregnancy or side effects experienced.

- It is important to keep in mind that any form of alternative therapy, no matter how harmless, no matter how safe, may still have the effect of endangering a person if its use delays the commencement of a proven therapy. No matter how effective an alternative therapy claims to be, it should never be substituted for proven medical therapies. It is essential that all people discuss the full range of conventional options with their doctors before starting alternative remedies.

- The validity of some alternative therapies for people with liver disease or hepatitis may ultimately be established through controlled medical studies. Standardized double-blinded, placebo-controlled studies must be conducted before any alternative therapy can be recommended for use in the treatment of liver disease. Research in this area is ongoing but needs to be conducted in large numbers of people in a reproducible manner.

CONCLUSION

Disillusionment with conventional medicine (especially in light of the less-than-optimal success rate in the treatment of chronic hepatitis C) has led many people with hepatitis and other liver diseases to seek out alternative treatments—the majority of which do not have sufficient research backing them. The surge of interest in the area of alternative medicine will undoubtedly spark some rigorously conducted research protocols that will hopefully determine exactly what and how much benefit an alternative therapy has on the liver. Such studies should be aimed at clearly defining those groups of people who can benefit from herbal remedies and/or other alternative treatments. Furthermore, these studies should provide guidance on whether to administer such remedies alone or in combination with more conventional treatments. Medical therapy for liver disease may eventually see a mutually beneficial partnership between conventional and alternative therapy. Certainly this appears to be the outlook for the future.

When all therapies, whether conventional, alternative, or a combination of the two, fail to help a person suffering from complications of liver disease, liver transplantation is the only viable option. The next chapter discusses this procedure.

Twenty-two

LIVER TRANSPLANTATION

ortunately, most people with chronic liver disease will never need a liver transplant. So why read this chapter? Well, all people who have chronic liver disease are at risk (which varies, depending upon a multitude of factors) for the complications associated with chronic liver disease. These include cirrhosis, liver failure, liver cancer, and intolerable symptoms, such as severe itching and fatigue. If one or more of these complications occurs, a person may become a candidate for a liver transplant. Therefore, all people with chronic liver disease and their family members can benefit by reading this chapter to increase their understanding of liver transplantation. Furthermore, it is important for people to be aware that liver transplantation is an accepted standard treatment option for those with liver failure and that it is a life-saving operation with a high success rate.

Only people who have the greatest likelihood of survival should undergo a liver transplant; therefore, this chapter will differentiate the good candidates for transplantation from the poor candidates. This chapter also discusses the evaluation process that leads to a person becoming listed for a liver transplant. Both general and specific (based on individual liver disorders) indications for transplantation will be reviewed. The biggest problem in the field of liver transplantation is that there is an ever-increasing scarcity of available livers for donation. This issue, as well as some potential solutions to this problem, will be discussed in this chapter. This chapter will conclude with a review of post-transplant medications, post-transplant complications, and what to expect after a liver transplant.

THE HISTORY AND SUCCESS RATE OF LIVER TRANSPLANTS

The first successful human-to-human liver transplant was performed by Dr. Thomas Starzl in 1968. (The first attempt at liver transplantation occurred in 1963 but was unsuccessful.) Liver transplantation is now a routinely successful operation. The high success rate is due to the many advances that have occurred

since the early days of transplantation, when less than 30 percent of transplant recipients survived beyond one year. Currently, approximately 85 to 90 percent of
people will survive at least one year, and approximately 75 to 85 percent of people will survive at least five years after receiving a new liver. Not only can people live a long life after a liver transplant (one person has been living with a
transplanted liver for over thirty-two years!), but the quality of life is typically
excellent. Most people can return to their regular jobs and daily routines without
limitations.

There are approximately 125 transplant centers in the United States, and
more than 5,000 liver transplants are performed in this country each year. As of
August 29, 2003, 17,696 people were on the liver transplant waiting list.

DETERMINING WHO NEEDS A LIVER TRANSPLANT

Having chronic liver disease or even cirrhosis does not automatically give rise to
a need for a liver transplant. Nor does it qualify a person for a liver transplant.
Yet, in cases where a transplant is warranted, a person does not want to wait until it is too late to be evaluated for a transplant. On the other hand, it is not necessary that everybody with chronic liver disease be evaluated for a liver transplant
as soon as a liver problem is discovered. So, is there some kind of special gauge
hidden on the body that only an experienced liver specialist can see that tells her
when it is time to send her patient for a transplant evaluation? Well, not exactly.
However, there are some specific criteria that are used to make this decision. Indications for a transplant that are specific to the cause of liver disease will be addressed on page 361. The following section is a discussion of some general
indications for liver transplant independent of the type of liver disease.

GENERAL INDICATIONS FOR LIVER TRANSPLANT

A person is referred for a liver transplant when it is estimated that she will not
live more than two years without a new liver. Accordingly, evidence of decompensated cirrhosis (such as ascites, variceal bleeding, or encephalopathy) is an
indication for liver transplantation. Any manifestation of liver failure, whether
due to acute or chronic liver disease (such as persistent jaundice or coagulopathy)
is an indication for liver transplantation. People who have developed liver cancer
due to chronic liver disease should also be evaluated for a transplant. Liver disease patients with symptoms such as relentless fatigue or intractable itching so
intolerable that they significantly diminish the quality of life may also be candidates for a liver transplant evaluation. Finally, a person who had a liver transplant
in which the newly transplanted liver is not functioning may be a candidate for
transplantation. While it is essential that a patient be evaluated by a liver transplant center, once one of the above-mentioned conditions has developed, medical
treatment should be the first line of therapy and should be undertaken to stabilize
the patient until a new liver is available.

THOSE WHO ARE POOR CANDIDATES
FOR LIVER TRANSPLANTATION

A liver transplant is a very serious undertaking for everyone involved—the transplant surgeon, the transplant team, the patient, and the patient's loved ones. It is of utmost importance that the decision to go ahead with a liver transplant takes into account the likelihood of a successful outcome. There is a shortage of donor livers available for transplantation, and this is a problem that continues to worsen. Because of the improved success rate of liver transplantation, the number of transplants being undertaken keeps increasing, thereby increasing the need for more livers.

Certain conditions disqualify a person from undergoing a liver transplant because a successful outcome is unlikely. These conditions are known as *absolute contraindications*. They include:

- AIDS

- cancer presently existing in an organ other than the liver

- metastatic cancer of the liver (advanced liver cancer that has spread to another organ)

- alcoholic liver disease coupled with failure to abstain from alcohol for the last six months

- severe active infection

- active substance abuse (for example, alcohol or heroin)

- irreversible brain dysfunction

- advanced heart or lung disease

Many other conditions are less than optimal for a liver transplant, but do not rule out the possibility. These conditions are known as *relative contraindications*. They include:

- age (approximately sixty-five years old or older)

- previous cancer in an organ other than the liver (a two-year or longer waiting period is required between completion of cancer treatment and the time of liver transplantation; this is because there is a high likelihood of cancer recurrence if a person is treated with transplant immunosuppression drugs within this two-year period)

- kidney failure

- HIV positivity (typically as part of a research protocol)

- morbid obesity

- malnutrition

- prior portal systemic shunts (see page 327)

- a blood clot in the portal vein, known as *portal vein thrombosis*

- psychosocial assessment indicating an inability to adhere to post-liver transplant medication regimen and instructions

- lack of social support

EVALUATING A PATIENT FOR A LIVER TRANSPLANT

Once the doctor has determined that a patient should be evaluated for a liver transplant, many diagnostic tests will need to be performed. First, the patient must meet with and be evaluated by the entire liver transplantation team. This team generally consists of a transplant surgeon, liver specialist, psychiatrist, and social worker. Other specialists, such as a cardiologist (heart doctor) or a pulmonologist (lung doctor), may need to be consulted as well. The opinions of each of these people are factored into the final decision as to the patient's suitability for a liver transplant. And the extent of additional testing required will hinge upon the evaluation of these healthcare professionals. Such testing may include special imaging studies of the liver such as MRI, heart exams such as an echocardiogram and a stress test, a chest X ray and pulmonary function tests, a purified protein derivative (PPD) skin test to test for tuberculosis exposure, a colonoscopy if over fifty years old, an upper endoscopy to evaluate for esophageal varices, a dental evaluation, and further blood tests. Finally, financial issues are considered.

Since the evaluation process can seem scary and overwhelming, it's always a good idea for the patient to bring a family member, loved one, or close friend along to the appointment. Not only will this person serve as emotional support, but she will assist in recalling and sorting through all the details of the day and can help arrange future testing.

Once the transplant team determines that a person is a candidate for a liver transplant, she is placed on a waiting list. Prior to 2002, transplant candidates were wait-listed based on the United Network for Organ Sharing (UNOS) status-ranking system. Rankings were based on the points accumulated when assessed for severity of liver disease. The more points accumulated, the higher the status on the transplant list. Patients were also listed according to time spent on the list, their blood type, and donor size requirements—height, weight, chest circumference, and liver volume. In 1998, the Department of Health and Human Services decreed that organs should be allocated on the basis of medical urgency and that the amount of time spent on the liver transplant waiting list should no longer be a factor in determining who should get a liver. The new scoring system eliminated transplant list waiting time and hospital status as factors for determining who should get a liver. As of 2002, liver allocation is based on the MELD score.

MODEL FOR END-STAGE LIVER DISEASE: THE MELD SCORE

It was felt by some experts that the former system of liver allocation often did not prioritize patients based on their severity of liver disease. It used criteria such as geographical region, time spent on the waiting list, and some subjective medical criteria (assessments that were subject to the evaluating doctor's opinion) to determine placement on the waiting list, which some experts believed should not be taken into consideration. Furthermore, the public became disenchanted with the old method of liver transplant allocation after reading reports of celebrities and sports figures leapfrogging ahead of thousands of regular people (many of whom were on the verge of death) on the transplant waiting list. The shortcomings of the old system led to the institution, as of February 27, 2002, of a new methodology for allocating livers for transplantation.

The new system, known as the Model for End-Stage Liver Disease (MELD) score, leaves no room for subjective criteria, favoritism, or hospital-shopping, as it is based on a mathematical equation. The equation seeks to calculate a patient's likelihood of dying within three months from their liver disease. In other words, under the MELD scoring system, the sickest patient gets the liver transplant. Three blood tests—the bilirubin; the prothrombin time (PT), measured as international normalized ratio (INR); and the creatinine (a measure of kidney function)—are used to determine this value. The MELD score is calculated using the following equation:

$$3.8 \times \log(e) \text{ (bilirubin mg/dl)} + 11.2 \times \log(e) \text{ (INR)} + 9.6 \log(e) \text{ (creatinine mg/dl)}$$

Don't let this equation scare you. There are many Internet websites that have automatic calculators. All you have to do is plug in your bilirubin, INR, and creatinine. One such website is the UNOS website: www.unos.org. Scores range from 6 to 40. A score of 6 indicates the least ill patient, and a score of 40 indicates the sickest patient. The MELD score is re-configured many times while the patient is on the transplant waiting list. MELD scores go up and down depending upon the patient's health.

Patients with a diagnosis of liver cancer will be assigned a MELD score based on how advanced the cancer is. This staging system is known as the TNM. *T* stands for the extent of the tumor, *N* stands for the presence or absence of lymph nodes, and *M* stands for the presence or absence of metastasis (tumor spread to another organ such as the lung in the case of liver cancer).

TRANSPLANTATION FOR SPECIFIC LIVER DISEASES

Regardless of the cause of chronic liver disease, when all medical therapies have failed or if complications from cirrhosis have developed, liver transplantation must be considered. The general indications for liver transplantation were discussed on page 358. This section discusses liver transplantation for specific liver diseases, all of which were discussed in detail in either part 2 or 3.

Hepatitis A

People with hepatitis A (discussed in chapter 8) do not progress to chronic liver disease. Therefore, the usual indications for liver transplantation (discussed on page 358) do not apply to people with hepatitis A. However, in very rare instances (about one hundred cases per year), people with hepatitis A develop a particularly severe form of acute hepatitis known as fulminant hepatitis A, which was discussed in chapters 7 and 8. These people become extremely ill, developing severe jaundice, encephalopathy, and coagulopathy. Liver failure develops abruptly—usually within eight weeks from the onset of symptoms or within two weeks from the onset of jaundice. Everyone with fulminant hepatitis A needs immediate hospitalization in an intensive care unit and prompt referral for a liver transplant. People who receive liver transplants due to fulminant liver failure have approximately a 70 percent chance of surviving one year, a much lower rate than for people who receive a liver transplant due to complications of cirrhosis.

Hepatitis B

Each year in the United States, approximately 5,000 people die from liver failure due to hepatitis B (discussed in chapter 9). Therefore, liver transplantation can be a potentially life-saving option for people with complications due to hepatitis B. Until recently, people who received transplants due to hepatitis B–related liver failure fared poorly as compared to transplant recipients with other liver diseases. Prior to the development of current preventive therapies, the chance that the hepatitis B virus (HBV) would reinfect the newly transplanted liver was approximately 80 percent. And in people who had high levels of HBV DNA prior to transplantation, reinfection was almost universal. Some of these people developed severe acute hepatitis B after transplantation, which led to immediate retransplantation. Others developed rapidly progressive liver damage leading to liver failure and/or death. In fact, cirrhosis had been seen to occur in people reinfected with HBV after transplantation in as little as one year! Whereas the five-year survival rate after transplantation is approximately 80 to 85 percent for all other liver diseases, until recently, the five-year survival rate for people who received a liver transplant due to hepatitis B was only 48 percent. (Presently the five-year survival rate for hepatitis B transplant recipients is comparable to that for all other liver diseases.) Fortunately, many new treatment modalities (discussed below) have been devised that not only decrease the patient's chance of reinfecting the new liver with HBV, but can also significantly prolong their survival time.

　　　Administration of the hepatitis B immune globulin (HBIG) (see chapter 24) has proven to be effective in preventing, or at least delaying, reinfection of the new liver in many people. When HBIG is given both before and after transplantation, the risk of recurrence of hepatitis B may be reduced to between 10 and 40 percent. And the five-year survival rate after transplantation for people with hepatitis B who receive HBIG is now equivalent to that of people undergoing transplantation for other liver diseases. However, since recurrence of hepatitis B may still occur even with HBIG therapy, other treatment options are being tested.

Alfa interferon (discussed in chapters 11, 12, and 13) given in small doses—1.5 million units, three times per week—may be beneficial for some people with decompensated cirrhosis due to hepatitis B in that it may lessen or possibly eradicate HBV DNA prior to transplantation. This may decrease the likelihood of post-transplant reinfection with HBV. However, alfa interferon may prompt rejection of the new liver, and therefore after transplant it should be used with extreme caution.

Lamivudine (an oral antiviral medication discussed in chapter 12) has also been proven to be beneficial in preventing reinfection when given before and after transplantation. In fact, lamivudine has eradicated detectable HBV DNA levels in people who suffered a recurrence of HBV after a transplant, despite having received preventive therapy with HBIG. Whether people will need to continue lamivudine therapy lifelong is being evaluated. The biggest challenge to lamivudine therapy appears to be the development of mutations of HBV DNA that are resistant to further therapy. Possibly, lamivudine in combination with HBIG or the use of adefovir (another oral antiviral medication discussed in chapter 12) in combination with HBIG may be the optimal regimen for the prevention of hepatitis B after liver transplantation.

Ganciclovir (an intravenously administered nucleoside analogue) and famciclovir (an oral nucleoside analogue) appear to decrease HBV DNA levels after transplantation in some people. (These drugs were discussed in chapter 12.) While these treatments may cause an improvement in liver inflammation due to recurrent hepatitis B, HBV DNA levels may return after these agents are discontinued. Further study on these drugs is necessary in order to determine optimum dose and duration of use.

Combination therapy using HBIG and lamivudine appears to be very promising and may be the therapy of choice if further study confirms existing results. Other combinations, such as HBIG and adefovir, as well as the simultaneous use of two nucleoside analogues, are currently being investigated.

In conclusion, all people with hepatitis B, especially those with high HBV DNA levels, need to be treated with some form of viral suppressive therapy prior to undergoing liver transplantation.

Hepatitis D

People who are coinfected with the hepatitis B virus (HBV) and the hepatitis delta virus (HDV) have a lower incidence of reinfection of the new liver compared with people infected with HBV alone. (Coinfection with HBV and HDV was discussed in chapter 9.) If reinfection does occur, it is usually mild. When coinfected people receive HBIG prior to undergoing liver transplantation, the incidence of reinfection is only approximately 13 percent.

Hepatitis C

Liver failure due to chronic hepatitis C is the most common reason for liver transplantation in the United States. Recurrence of the hepatitis C virus (HCV) in the newly transplanted liver occurs in practically all cases, and within one year of transplantation approximately 80 percent of people will have evidence of inflammation due to HCV on liver biopsy specimens. (This does not apply to hepatitis C patients who were cured—those who achieved long-term eradication of HCV.) Reinfection with HCV leads to fulminant liver failure in 10 percent of cases, and to cirrhosis, liver failure, or death in five to ten years. Accordingly, retransplantation (a second transplant) is often necessary. Despite this fact, five-year survival rates among people who receive a transplant due to hepatitis C are comparable to survival rates for people who receive transplants for other liver diseases. However, recurrence of HCV may have an impact on long-term survival after transplant.

Levels of HCV RNA are generally higher after transplantation than before transplantation, to the tune of approximately ten to two hundred times the pre-transplant level. This is presumably due to the fact that immunosuppressive therapy (such as the corticosteroid prednisone) administered after a liver transplant increases viral replication and thereby enhances the risk of recurrent hepatitis C. Therefore, if the amount of immunosuppression is either decreased or discontinued soon after transplantation, the HCV RNA load should decrease. In fact, some transplant centers routinely discontinue corticosteroid therapy within six months after transplantation. Furthermore, the antirejection immunosuppressive agent tacrolimus, as opposed to the antirejection immunosuppressive agent cyclosporine, requires significantly lower doses of prednisone to achieve adequate immunosuppression. Therefore, it is recommended that people who undergo transplantation due to chronic hepatitis C be placed on tacrolimus for immunosuppression.

Overall, approximately 15 to 20 percent of people with hepatitis C develop a rapidly progressive course of disease within five years after transplantation. Cirrhosis has occurred in less than two years from transplantation in some people, and it develops in five to seven years in as many as 30 percent of people. People coinfected with both HCV and HIV do particularly poorly after a liver transplant, and recurrence of hepatitis C in the new liver typically causes liver failure within three years. Other people found to do poorly after transplantation include those having high pretransplant HCV RNA loads and those having genotype 1b and genotype 4. Different immunosuppressive regimens after transplantation may account for a rapid progression of disease among some people. Also, the use of older liver donor organs may be associated with a poorer outcome.

Some people develop failure of the new liver within several months of transplantation, thereby making retransplantation necessary. Unfortunately, retransplantation for people with hepatitis C has been associated with a poor outcome. Less than 40 percent of these people survive for one year. Therefore, the focus in patients transplanted for HCV is on prevention, or at least suppression, of viral replication after transplantation. It appears that treatment with interferon after transplantation is quite effective. Many transplant centers routinely start patients on interferon and ribavirin therapy soon after transplantation—some centers as soon as three months following transplantation. When given early—approximately three to six months after transplantation (when HCV RNA levels are typically still low)—interferon therapy has been shown to reduce the incidence of HCV RNA, liver inflammation, and damage due to recurrent hepatitis C. Further studies are being conducted to confirm the efficacy of pegylated interferon and ribavirin and to determine if all people, or strictly those at high risk for a poor outcome, should start this after transplant.

Some new antirejection medications, such as Daclizumab, may be associated with a less severe HCV infection after transplantation. The same applies to the drug azathioprine. Treatment with interferon and ribavirin immediately prior to transplantation has been associated with a lower incidence of HCV recurrence after transplantation. Studies on people with HCV who were cured (i.e., those who experienced long-term eradication of HCV) have not been done. However, I believe that it is doubtful that these patients experienced HCV recurrence after transplantation.

Autoimmune Hepatitis (AIH)

Despite the availability of successful medical therapy, approximately 20 percent of people with autoimmune hepatitis (discussed in chapter 14) become candidates for a liver transplant. This may be due to the development of complications of cirrhosis or to failure to respond to medical therapy (for example, corticosteroids and azathioprine) after attempting treatment for approximately four years. The success rate of transplantation in people with AIH is excellent, with approximately 92 percent of people living at least five years after liver transplantation. Autoantibodies generally disappear within two years from the time of transplantation. The disease recurs after transplantation approximately 17 percent of the time. Recurrence can usually be managed successfully by adjustment of immunosuppressive drug dosages. Although dosages of immunosuppressive drugs may be decreased after transplantation, total discontinuation is not recommended.

Primary Biliary Cirrhosis (PBC)

People with primary biliary cirrhosis (discussed in chapter 15) have a very slow yet relentlessly progressive disease course that spans approximately twenty years. Medical therapy (ursodeoxycholic acid, for example) has been shown to slow the progression of the disease, thus delaying the need for a liver transplant in some people with PBC. Nonetheless, these people continue to advance to cirrhosis and its complications or to have symptoms associated with PBC, such as osteoporosis, severe fatigue, or uncontrollable pruritus, any of which may necessitate liver transplantation. In fact, between 5 and 18 percent of people who undergo liver transplantation for PBC do so because fatigue or pruritus has significantly diminished their quality of life. Liver transplantation ultimately leads to improvement in bone strength. However, this benefit is not seen until at least a year after the transplant, due to the use of high doses of corticosteroids and the initial period of inactivity after transplantation, each of which weakens bones.

PBC accounts for about 10 percent of liver transplants in the United States. People with PBC do very well after liver transplantation. Approximately 88 percent of them survive at least five years. Typically, these people enjoy a good quality of life and can return to their normal lifestyles.

Unlike the disappearance of the antinuclear antibody after transplant in people with AIH, the antimitochondrial antibody remains positive in people who receive transplants due to PBC. It appears that PBC can recur in the new liver. However, since the disease is so slowly progressive, it will take many years for any significant symptoms to occur, if they occur at all.

Nonalcoholic Steatohepatitis (NASH)

NASH accounts for approximately 2 to 3 percent of transplantations in the United States. However, this percentage is perhaps a gross underestimation, as most cases of cirrhosis referred for liver transplantation that have no definable cause are most likely due to NASH. Patients with NASH are often poor candidates for liver transplantation due to their obesity and diabetes. NASH recurs in the new liver approximately one-third of the time and may cause a rapid progression to cirrhosis in approximately 13 percent of people. This is most likely due to the fact that after transplantation it is common to gain weight as a result of post-transplant medications, such as prednisone, as well as from a feeling of well-being. Furthermore, prednisone in itself can cause a fatty liver. And diabetes, another cause of NASH, may occur post-transplant. All transplant recipients, especially those transplanted due to NASH or those prone to NASH, must be diligent about maintaining a normal weight, exercising, and eating a low-fat diet. Medical treatment for NAFLD occurring post-liver transplant have not been evaluated.

Alcoholic Liver Disease (ALD)

The subject of liver transplantation for people with alcoholic liver disease (discussed in chapter 17) has been an ongoing area of controversy. Some have argued that since livers are such a scarce resource, a person who recklessly caused her liver failure by deliberately abusing alcohol should not be permitted to be listed for a transplant. Others have argued that alcoholism is a disease and, as such, it is not a person's "fault" that she has liver failure due to excessive alcohol use and should therefore be given the same chance at a new liver as anyone else with liver disease.

A viewpoint somewhere in the middle currently prevails on the issue of transplantation for people with ALD. Once the patient is aware of the consequences that have occurred due to alcohol abuse, it is then considered to be her responsibility to successfully complete a rehabilitation process and to adhere to lifelong abstinence. The rehabilitation process may include Alcoholics Anonymous (AA), an inpatient rehabilitation program, and psychiatric treatment. After sobriety has been achieved for a sustained duration, the person may then be considered a candidate for a liver transplant. While UNOS does not utilize a defined abstinence interval, the length of time of documented abstinence has been arbitrarily chosen to be six months by many transplantation centers. The person with ALD must also demonstrate that she has a stable social support system in the form of loved ones or friends, and that she does not have other substance abuse problems or psychiatric disorders. A patient is removed from the list if she does not comply with medication instructions, office visits, medical advice, dietary restrictions, or, of course, if she returns to alcohol use.

Numerous people with ALD have undergone successful liver transplants. In fact, transplantation due to ALD accounts for approximately 20 percent of transplants performed in the United States. Survival rates after transplant are excellent and are similar to that of people transplanted due to other types of liver disease.

After transplantation, people typically live active and productive lives, provided that there is no *recidivism* (relapsing back to drinking alcohol). Within three years of transplantation, return to alcohol abuse occurs in approximately 15 to 20 percent of people. The patient is advised to continue Alcoholics Anonymous (AA) meetings post-transplant until a psychiatrist has determined that the risk of recidivism is unlikely.

Hemochromatosis

When the diagnosis of hemochromatosis (discussed in chapter 18) is made early and treatment is begun promptly (and prior to the development of cirrhosis), people with hemochromatosis usually have a normal life expectancy. However, when hemochromatosis is not discovered until after cirrhosis has already developed or if a person does not adhere to a strict phlebotomy schedule, long-term complications of liver disease may occur, thereby necessitating liver transplantation. Although hemochromatosis is a common disease, it is an uncommon indication for liver transplantation.

Liver transplantation for people with hemochromatosis has not been as successful as transplantation due to other liver diseases. People with hemochromatosis appear to have an increased incidence of developing infections and heart failure after transplantation. This accounts for the poor survival rate post-transplant. In fact, the chance of surviving one year after transplant is only approximately 60 percent. For such people the chance of surviving five years after transplant is approximately 55 percent. Survival after transplant is significantly improved if iron depletion is performed prior to transplant. In these cases, there is a one-year survival rate of 75 to 83 percent.

People with both hemochromatosis and cirrhosis are two hundred times more likely to develop liver cancer compared with the general population. In fact, approximately 27 percent of people who receive transplants due to hemochromatosis have been found to have liver cancer, and approximately 19 percent of liver cancers in these people are not even diagnosed until the time of transplant. Surprisingly, the discovery of an incidental liver cancer found during transplantation in people with hemochromatosis does not appear to significantly decrease the chances of living for one year beyond transplant.

It is unknown whether hemochromatosis recurs in the new liver. Since iron stores increase slowly in people with hemochromatosis, a study monitoring a large number of people for ten to twenty years after transplantation is needed to accurately answer this question.

Liver Tumors

People discovered to have a malignant liver tumor (discussed in chapter 19) should consider surgical resection (the removal of the tumor) as the first treatment option. Unfortunately, only approximately 30 percent of people with liver cancer have surgically resectable tumors at the time they are diagnosed. When the tumor's size or location prevents resection, or if cirrhosis is present, liver transplantation should be considered. Since the entire liver is being replaced, liver transplantation has the potential to remove not only the tumor, but also the underlying cirrhosis. Unfortunately, most people in the United States with liver cancer who undergo transplantation have cirrhosis due to hepatitis C or B, and these viruses invariably recur in the newly transplanted liver. Thus, the underlying disease usually recurs, thereby setting the stage for another tumor to grow.

The same prognostic factors that are associated for survival that apply to transplantation apply to surgical resection. The best outcomes normally occur in young, otherwise healthy people who have one small tumor (less than 5 centimeters in size) or two to three tiny tumors (all less than 3 centimeters in size) limited to the liver alone—meaning that the cancer has not spread to lymph nodes, surrounding vessels, or other organs. In fact, for liver transplantation performed on otherwise healthy people with small, isolated tumors, the survival rate is approximately 75 percent at four years. Similarly, 90 percent of people who undergo liver transplantation and are incidentally discovered to have a small tumor survive for at least five years.

The long waiting time for a liver transplant often prevents people with liver cancer from becoming candidates for transplantation due to the rapid spread of the tumor during this waiting period. Thus, a living-donor liver transplant (if available to the patient) is an excellent alternative option, as it minimizes the waiting time.

For people who do not possess the above-mentioned ideal characteristics, recurrence of liver cancer is high and long-term survival after transplantation is low. Much research is being conducted with the aim of decreasing recurrence and improving survival times for these people. One promising therapy involves the use of chemotherapy drugs at various intervals before, during, and/or after transplantation. Studies utilizing therapies such as cryosurgery or ethanol injections in combination are also being conducted.

LIVER DONORS

Despite the growing success and acceptance by doctors and patients alike of liver transplantation, the average number of donor organs available at any given time has continued to remain the same. This has caused the demand for livers to far outweigh the supply. In this respect, liver transplantation has become a victim of its own success. And each year the gap widens further. The number of people placed on the transplant list continues to grow at a faster rate than the number of available donor organs. Each year in the United States approximately 12,500 to 27,000 potential organ donors die without having donated their livers. That's a lot of livers—enough to cover all the people on a waiting list. So why is there a shortage of livers? Well, for various reasons only 15 to 20 percent of suitable organ donors become actual organ donors. This section discusses some issues associated with organ donation and some ways that have been devised to increase the number of livers available for transplantation.

General Criteria for Organ Donation

One of the most important steps toward ensuring a successful outcome of a liver transplant is choosing an appropriate donor liver. Thus, it is crucial to eliminate those donors whose livers have a poor chance of functioning properly.

The major source of livers for donation is brain-dead people with a functioning heart and circulatory system. A designated family member must sign a witnessed consent form allowing donation. If the potential donor has AIDS, is infected with HIV, has cancer (except of the skin or brain), or has evidence of active hepatitis B, the liver may not be used as a donor under any circumstances. Ideally, the donor's liver function tests (LFTs) should be normal, and the donor's liver should contain no more than 30 percent fat. It has been shown that donated fatty livers (see chapter 16) function quite poorly and are often rejected soon after transplantation. The body size and blood type of the donor and the recipient should be compatible. The donor's age should preferably be under fifty.

Recently, in an effort to increase the number of suitable donor livers available for transplantation, some of the above criteria have become less stringent. Livers from donors over the age of fifty, and sometimes from those as old as seventy, are now being used and generally with favorable results. Livers from donors who have hepatitis C are being utilized in cases where the patient undergoing the transplant also has hepatitis C.

Increased awareness of organ donation among laypeople and healthcare professionals is needed to help expand the donor pool. In the United States, in order for a person to donate an organ, she must obtain and sign an organ donor card. The donor must carry this card at all times. Finally, it is important for the potential donor to inform family members of her wish to donate organs. This will eliminate any confusion or uncertainty on this issue at the time of the donor's death.

Living Donors

Living liver donation involves the removal of one lobe of the liver from a donor (typically the right lobe in adult-to-adult transplantation) and its transplantation into the recipient with liver disease. This technique offers an additional means of expanding the existing liver donor pool. Furthermore, waiting time on the transplant list is eliminated and transplantation may be performed at a time when the patient is not exceedingly ill. And not only does living donor transplantation diminish the waiting time for the living donor recipient but also reduces the waiting time for those on the transplant list. The donor may be either related (living-related liver donor) or not related (living-unrelated liver donor) to the recipient. In either case, the donor must have a blood type that is compatible to the recipient. The first successful living-related liver transplant in the United States occurred in 1989 from a parent to a child. More than two thousand living-donor transplants have been performed in the United States since that time. The success rate of this type of liver transplantation appears to be comparable to that of conventional liver transplantation. Complications to the living donor, which can conceivably include death, are exceptionally infrequent. Any potential risks will be discussed with the donor in advance of the operation. The donor must weigh any such risks against the potential benefit to the donor. Within approximately one year's time, the donor's liver will regenerate the segment that was donated.

The living-donor recipient must meet the same qualifications as the recipient of a conventional liver transplant. In addition, an extensive evaluation of the donor is undertaken. The donor must be between twenty and fifty years old, must have a blood type that is compatible with the recipient, and must pass extensive psychological testing. A complete blood evaluation, electrocardiogram, chest radiograph, sonogram of the abdomen, CT scan to assess the volume of the liver, and special type of MRI to evaluate the bile ducts must all be performed. A consent form must be reviewed carefully by the donor, who must also be clearly informed that withdrawal from the process is always an option. A liver biopsy may need to be performed on those donors with risk factors for a fatty liver. This is because fatty livers carry an increased risk of complications including rejection for the recipient. (See chapter 16 for more information about fatty livers.) The donor's hospital stay lasts approximately five to seven days, and most donors are back to work and their usual activities in two to three months.

Split-Liver Transplantation

Sometimes, one viable donor liver is split in two, with each half being transplanted into a separate person. This procedure, known as split-liver transplantation, obviously has the capacity to double the number of livers available for donation. Usually, an adult receives the larger right side of the liver, and a child or small adult receives the smaller left side of the liver. However, new techniques are enabling a more even split, so that one donor liver can be utilized for two adult patients. The first split-liver operation was performed in 1988. Since that time, major advances in surgical and technical expertise have occurred, allowing this procedure to be employed with increasing frequency and success. So far, this procedure appears to be very promising. Patients appear to have a survival rate after transplant that approximates the survival rate after conventional whole-liver transplantation. Some experts are lobbying to have liver splitting mandated as the first option in the transplantation of cadaver livers.

Auxiliary Transplants

An auxiliary liver transplant involves placing a small portion of a functioning liver from a donor into the body of a person with liver failure without removing the recipient's liver. This technique has been used on people with irreversible liver failure, as well as people with fulminant, potentially reversible, liver failure. While there have been some isolated reports of success with this procedure, further study is needed to confirm its efficacy.

Hepatocyte Transplantation and Gene Therapy

Hepatocyte transplantation involves the infusion of a small number of liver cells (hepatocytes) from a donor liver into a person who has either a genetic defect of the liver (such as Crigler-Najjar syndrome) or fulminant liver failure. The use of hepatocyte transplantation might even eliminate the need for transplantation in some people with fulminant liver failure by promoting spontaneous recovery. While there have been only limited attempts to implement this procedure in humans, the results in animal-based studies appear promising.

Another exciting procedure that is still in the experimental stage is one that involves taking samples of one's liver cells, altering the genetics, and then reconstituting it back into the person's genetically defective liver. Known as gene therapy, this procedure is also being evaluated for use in preventing the rejection of a transplanted liver, thereby eliminating the need for post-transplant immunosuppressant medications. This promising technique is undergoing extensive testing.

Liver Dialysis—The Bioartificial Liver (BAL)

Whereas people with chronic kidney failure can be maintained on dialysis for long periods of time until a donor kidney is located, a comparable form of long-term dialysis for people with liver failure has not been devised. However, there is a method of temporarily treating people with fulminant irreversible liver failure who are awaiting an imminent liver transplant (within a few days) or who have fulminant, potentially reversible, liver failure. The apparatus used for liver dialysis is known as a *liver-assist device*. Such a device is designed to remove toxins from the blood of people who have liver failure. Preliminary results show that this type of device may be effective in improving the liver function and mental status of some patients with reversible fulminant liver failure, thereby allowing their injured liver sufficient time to completely recover. Furthermore, this device may serve as a time-sparing method—by keeping people who are awaiting imminent liver transplantation alive for several extra days.

A recent advance in this type of device may enable it to provide entire liver function instead of merely removing toxins. This is achieved by adding functioning liver cells to the liver device. There are a few such devices currently in use. Although some promising results have been reported, additional studies are required before this type of device can be recommended.

Use of Hepatitis-Infected Livers

As a result of the donor shortage, some transplant units have started using the livers of hepatitis C antibody positive as well as hepatitis B core antibody positive donors. This section discusses the issues pertaining to this policy.

Hepatitis C Antibody (HCV Ab) Positive Donors

Up to one-third of patients listed for transplant are awaiting transplant due to hepatitis C. Many potential organ donors are infected with hepatitis C, even though this is typically a contraindication for organ donation. However, in situations in which an uninfected donor is not available, an HCV-infected donor liver is sometimes used. When this takes place, the predominant hepatitis C strain—whether it be the donor's or the recipient's—totally overtakes the other strain. So, even though these people have a "double" hepatitis C infection, the body reacts as if infected with only one strain of HCV. In fact, in cases in which the donor HCV strain predominates, a milder course of liver disease usually results. There have been no studies on patients who eradicated HCV (as a result of interferon therapy) prior to transplantation. Therefore, it is important that these patients not receive a hepatitis C–infected liver.

Hepatitis B core Antibody (HBcAb) Positive Donors

Donors who are positive for hepatitis B core antibody (HBcAb) are ineligible to have their livers used for transplantation. Due to the severe immunosuppression, a small percentage of recipients would become infected with hepatitis B after receiving such a liver as a result of a reactivation of the HBV from the donor. This creates a dilemma in that the exclusion of HBcAb positive donors represents a loss of numerous potential donor livers. In fact, in areas where hepatitis B is endemic, approximately 10 to 15 percent of the population is positive for HBcAb. Thus, some transplant centers have begun to permit HBcAb positive individuals to be liver donors. Thus far, transplants of this nature have been largely successful, and recipient survival rates have been similar to those receiving livers from HBcAb negative donors. Approximately 5 percent of those who receive a liver from an HBcAb positive donor go on to acquire hepatitis B themselves. But these recipients typically have a benign course of the disease. Treatment after transplantation with lamivudine, either with or without hepatitis B immune globulin (HBIG), typically has yielded excellent results in controlling (or even preventing) hepatitis B infection in these patients. Finally, it is advisable for all patients undergoing liver transplantation to be vaccinated against hepatitis B. In fact, it is recommended that anyone with a chronic liver disease receive the hepatitis B vaccine. (See chapter 24 for more information on the hepatitis B vaccine.)

POST-TRANSPLANT MEDICATIONS AND THEIR SIDE EFFECTS

The major hurdle that a person faces after a liver transplant is whether her body will accept the new liver as if it were its own. Rejection of the liver occurs if the patient's body does not recognize the new liver as belonging to itself. Therefore, similar to the situation that occurs in people with autoimmune hepatitis (discussed in chapter 14), the body's immune system may attack the new liver in an attempt to reject it from the body. When this happens, the new liver may become damaged, or, even worse, it may become totally nonfunctional (rejected by the body).

Since 1983, however, a powerful group of effective medications have become available to help reduce the likelihood of rejection. These medications are known as immunosuppressants. Beyond the first year after transplantation, rejection of the new liver is very uncommon. And within the first year of transplantation, the incidence of rejection has been on the decline. While rejection rates were once approximately 15 to 20 percent, they are now as low as 2 percent in many transplant centers. (People with primary biliary cirrhosis and autoimmune hepatitis have a higher incidence of rejection.)

There are now a number of medications available to blunt a person's immune system so that the new liver will not be rejected by the body. These medications are known as *antirejection immunosuppressive agents*. The regimen of post-transplant immunosuppression usually includes a corticosteroid (such as prednisone) combined with either cyclosporine or tacrolimus. Sometimes a third immunosuppressive drug is used, such as mycophenelate mofetil. These medications are not without side effects. Furthermore, cyclosporine and tacrolimus may interact with other drugs, which can lead to toxic levels or to less-than-therapeutic levels of these immunosuppressants. Fortunately, due to the number of immunosuppressive agents now available, each patient can have a regimen individually tailored to her case. This can be of great help in minimizing side effects, maximizing potency, and improving the patient's quality of life. It should be noted that in approximately 5 percent of patients, immunosuppression medications are totally withdrawn at some point. Thus, approximately 95 percent of patients need lifelong immunosuppressive therapy. The following is a discussion of the medications that a person may need to take after a transplant in order to prevent rejection. Included in the discussion are the potential side effects of each medication.

Cyclosporine (Neoral)

The immunosuppressive properties of cyclosporine were discovered in 1972, and, as of 1983, cyclosporine (originally known as Sandimmune) was routinely used as an antirejection drug. In 1996 Sandimmune was replaced by Neoral, an improved oral form of cyclosporine that provides better gastrointestinal tract absorption and, as such, allows for easier management of dosing.

There are many side effects associated with cyclosporine. Kidney failure may occur but is readily reversible upon lowering the dosage. Due to changes in sugar (glucose) and fat (*lipid*) metabolism caused by cyclosporine, the patient may be at increased risk of hypertension and heart disease. Cyclosporine may also affect the central nervous system—seizures, numbness, confusion, and hallucinations have been experienced by some people while on therapy. Increased hair growth, especially in brunettes, is common. Enlargement of the gums may occur, often necessitating surgical correction. There also appears to be an increased risk of cancer associated with cyclosporine use.

Tacrolimus (FK-506 or Prograf)

The immunosuppressive properties of tacrolimus were discovered in 1984, and ten years later it was approved by the FDA, specifically for use in antirejection therapy. Side effects associated with tacrolimus are similar to those of cyclosporine. Tacrolimus has been associated with greater kidney and neurological damage as compared with cyclosporine, according to some (but not all) studies. People may experience insomnia, headaches, and decreased alertness while taking tacrolimus. A high glucose level or even the development of diabetes may occur to those taking tacrolimus, thereby requiring an adjustment of dosage. Hypertension and high cholesterol levels can occur while on treatment, but this occurs less frequently than with cyclosporine. Less weight gain after transplantation has been noted in patients who were placed on tacrolimus as compared with those on cyclosporine. It has been noted that people on tacrolimus may experience an increased incidence of infections. Other associated symptoms that can occur while on tacrolimus include stomach upset, hair loss, and itching.

. . .

Which immunosuppressant medications are used is determined on a case-by-case basis and depends, as well, upon the preference of the transplantation center. Tacrolimus has some advantages over cyclosporine (as noted above) and is the primary immunosuppression drug for most large liver transplant programs in the United States. In fact, some studies have shown that a higher percentage of people live longer after transplant if placed on tacrolimus (approximately 80 percent of people treated with tacrolimus are alive three years after transplant versus approximately 73 percent of people treated with cyclosporine).

Corticosteroids (Prednisone)

Prednisone is a corticosteroid (steroid) that possesses both anti-inflammatory and immunosuppressive actions (prednisone was discussed in detail in chapter 14). This medication is routinely used post-transplant in all patients as part of the antirejection regimen. Steroids were originally part of lifelong immunosuppressive therapy, once standard after liver transplantation. However, there is now a growing trend toward discontinuation of steroids after transplantation. This is advantageous, as there are numerous side effects of long-term prednisone use, and the discontinuation of steroids will minimize, or totally eliminate, the potential for developing these side effects.

Results have been excellent for people taken off steroids approximately three months after liver transplantation. It does not appear that the discontinuation of steroids adversely affects either patient survival or the likelihood of rejection of the new liver. Furthermore, the incidence of medication-induced side effects is significantly less for people taken off prednisone three months after transplantation than for those who stay on longer.

The underlying liver disease leading to transplantation must also be taken into consideration when making a decision concerning withdrawal of steroids. For instance, since steroids stimulate the replication of both the hepatitis B and C viruses, early steroid withdrawal is quite advantageous for people with either hepatitis B or hepatitis C. However, people with autoimmune hepatitis (AIH) may not benefit from early withdrawal of steroids due to the potential for recurrence of AIH in the new liver. In general, determining the best time to withdraw the administration of steroids is determined on a case-by-case basis.

Mycophenolate Mofetil

Mycophenolate mofetil (CellCept, manufactured by Roche Laboratories) is a new antirejection drug that works like azathioprine (discussed in chapter 14), once a popular post-transplantation drug. It is now being used in place of azathioprine as an immunosuppressant. Mycophenolate mofetil has been shown to be effective for people experiencing rejection of a new liver despite their being treated with prednisone and other immunosuppressive agents. It is also used as an alternative immunosuppressant for people experiencing intolerable side effects from cyclosporine and/or tacrolimus.

Side effects of mycophenolate mofetil include digestive disturbances and bone marrow suppression (decreased white and red cell levels).

Sirolimus

Sirolimus (Rapamune), an antibiotic similar to tacrolimus, was initially used to fight fungal infections. At some point it was then found to have immunosuppressive properties. Sirolimus, when combined with either tacrolimus or cyclosporine, allows reduced levels of prednisone to be used post-transplantation. In this way, it acts as a steroid-sparing medication. Sirolimus decreases the incidence of rejection of the new liver in the first few months after transplantation. It may be a useful treatment for liver recipients suffering from chronic rejection. Side effects include low white blood cell counts, low platelet counts, high cholesterol levels, fluid retention, and joint aches. Further studies are being performed on this new antisuppressive medication.

COMPLICATIONS AFTER TRANSPLANT

During the first year after liver transplantation, approximately 85 to 90 percent of people have an excellent course with little or no serious complications. Any deaths that occur happen primarily during the first three months after transplantation. These deaths are mainly due to rejection of the new liver, infection, and technical complications. Approximately 55 percent of people are alive ten years after transplantation. The most common causes of death after the first three months include cancers, recurrent liver disease, chronic rejection, and cardiovascular disease.

Cancers

Cancers may occur in people after liver transplant due to a depressed immune system, infections, genetic predisposition, age, and possibly the use of multiple immunosuppressive medications. People who are transplanted due to alcoholic cirrhosis are most likely to develop cancer after liver transplantation. It has been noted that approximately 3 to 15 percent of all transplant recipients develop cancer within five years and as much as 55 percent develop cancer within fifteen years of liver transplantation. Non-Hodgkin's lymphoma and skin cancer are the cancers most commonly developed by transplant recipients. Other cancers that have been noted to occur include those of the head and neck, bladder, colon, lung, and breast. Leukemia, as well, can occur. Risk factors include smoking cigarettes, drinking alcohol, and inflammatory bowel disease (such as ulcerative colitis and Crohn's disease). After transplantation it is especially important to avoid excess sun exposure (including tanning beds), as well as to avoid cigarette smoking and alcohol consumption.

Recurrent Liver Disease

Liver disease may recur after transplantation and with a variable course. Patients transplanted due to HCV typically experience the most severe recurrence of disease (especially if recurring HCV is left untreated).

Chronic Rejection

Chronic rejection may also occur, and this may lead to death even more than eight years after transplantation. It appears that African Americans experience chronic rejection more frequently and therefore appear to have a poorer long-term survival rate than Caucasians.

Cardiovascular Disease

As a liver transplant recipient's survival time increases, cardiovascular complications may become likely. This increased risk is attributable to the side effects of chronic use of prednisone, tacrolimus, and cyclosporine. Additional risk factors for cardiovascular disease include obesity, diabetes, hypertension, and high cholesterol. Thus, post-transplant it is especially important to maintain a normal weight, exercise regularly, eat a healthy diet, and avoid smoking cigarettes. Following these recommendations will also help reduce the likelihood of bone disease such as osteoporosis, a common disorder post-transplant. The treatment of osteoporosis is covered in chapter 20.

LIVING WITH A NEW LIVER

Most people have a normal lifestyle and a good quality of life after a liver transplant. For women who have undergone a transplant, menstruation typically returns within one year of transplantation. Therefore, women usually are capable of becoming pregnant as of one year from the date of transplantation (see chapter 24 for more information concerning this matter). The social functioning, sexual activity, and mental health of people who have undergone a transplant seem to be equal to that of the general public. Most people are able to return to work, with little or no decrease in workload. While transplant recipients occasionally experience some degree of physical limitation, overall there appears to be a significantly improved quality of life after transplantation.

CONCLUSION

The advances made in the field of liver transplantation have been truly miraculous. Better surgical skills, increased use of living donor transplantation, better choice of transplant candidates, improved immunosuppressive medication regimens, and improved treatments for recurrent viral hepatitis after transplantation are just some of the reasons liver transplantation has become so successful and why it has become the accepted standard treatment for people with liver failure. People usually return to a normal lifestyle after the transplant and typically enjoy a good quality of life. Future advances in the field of liver transplantation may allow the discontinuation of all medications after a transplant. This would be truly remarkable.

The next chapter discusses ways that people can take active roles in improving their health and possibly prevent some complications of liver disease through diet, nutrition, and exercise.

Twenty-three

DIET, NUTRITION, AND EXERCISE

After being diagnosed with liver disease, some of the first questions that a person typically asks concern nutrition and exercise. Commonly asked questions include: What foods are good for the liver? Are there foods that can harm the liver? Are vitamin supplements helpful? How much protein should I get in my diet? Is it a good idea to exercise? Should certain exercises be avoided? Unfortunately, many doctors lack the expertise to supply knowledgeable answers to these and similar questions. One reason for this is that most medical schools do not spend enough time on the topics of diet, nutrition, and exercise.

As you learned in chapter 1, everything that enters the body must pass through the liver to be processed. The liver functions as a filter to protect the body from harmful substances and is responsible for the production and use of most nutrients. Therefore everything that is ingested has an effect on the liver—some positive, some negative. That's why it is advisable for people to eat foods with an eye toward promoting liver health. This is especially true when the liver is damaged. Understanding the basics of nutrition is necessary in order to make intelligent food choices that will benefit the liver. Due to FDA regulations, food labels contain nutritional information. A person with liver disease should always read these labels carefully. Also, most people with liver disease need to restrict some foods from their diets. This should not be viewed as a punishment but rather as a step in the direction of a healthier liver. Exercise is an important practice in the fight against liver disease. Regular exercise will increase energy levels, decrease stress on the liver, and, in many cases, even delay the onset of certain complications associated with liver disease.

The more people know about nutrition and exercise, the more likely they will be to institute and adhere to lifestyles that maximize health and minimize disease. That's why this chapter discusses these important issues. It provides pertinent details concerning protein, carbohydrates, fats, vitamins, and minerals and discusses how nutritional requirements differ depending upon the particular liver disease. Of course, a person—in accordance with her own specific dietary needs and limitations—may vary the recommendations contained in this chapter. This chapter also provides other nutritional information, such as tips on how to dine out while on a restricted diet and how to get through the holiday season and social events while on a restricted diet. It discusses some popular nutritional supplements, such as glucosamine chondroitin and SAMe. Finally, the importance of exercise, both aerobic and weight-bearing, for people with liver disease is discussed.

IS THERE AN OPTIMAL DIET FOR THOSE WITH LIVER DISEASE?

Unfortunately, a person cannot expect to walk into the doctor's office and request "a diet for liver disease." Such an across-the-board diet simply does not exist. Many factors account for the unfeasibility of a standardized liver diet, including variations among the different types of liver disease (for example, alcoholic liver disease versus primary biliary cirrhosis) and the stage of the liver disease (for example, stable liver disease without much damage versus unstable decompensated cirrhosis). One's other medical disorders even if unrelated to their liver disease, such as diabetes or heart disease, must also be factored into any diet. Each person has her own individual nutritional requirements, and these requirements may change over time.

Most people with liver disease find that eating multiple small meals throughout the day is the best approach, as it maximizes energy levels and the ability to digest and absorb food. However, if one insists on eating three meals per day, try to follow the saying, "Eat breakfast like a king, lunch like a prince, and dinner like a pauper."

It is important to keep in mind the difference in calorie content among different food groups. While protein and carbohydrate each supplies 4 calories per gram, fat supplies 9 calories per gram. It is also important to know that 1 gram of alcohol is equivalent to 7 calories. So alcohol actually supplies more energy in the form of calories to the body than protein and carbohydrates and just slightly less than that supplied by fat. However, while alcohol may provide a person with some degree of energy, it has absolutely no nutritional value. Therefore, alcohol has been said to provide "empty calories."

GENERAL NUTRITIONAL GUIDELINES FOR LIVER DISEASE

Notwithstanding the above information, an optimal diet for a person with stable liver disease (modifications to be made as per individualized needs) might contain all of the factors listed below. (You'll note that this diet resembles a generalized healthy diet for all people—even those without liver disease. And, in fact, that's exactly what it is!)

- 60 to 70 percent carbohydrates—primarily complex carbohydrates, such as pasta and whole-grain breads

- 20 to 30 percent protein—only lean animal protein and/or vegetable protein

- 10 to 20 percent polyunsaturated fat

- 8 to 12 eight-ounce glasses of water per day

- 1,000 to 1,500 milligrams of sodium per day

- Avoidance of excessive amounts of vitamins and minerals, especially vitamin A, vitamin B_3, and iron

- No alcohol

- Avoidance of processed food

- Liberal consumption of fresh, organic fruits and vegetables

- Avoidance of excessive caffeine consumption—no more than one to three cups of caffeine-containing beverages per day

- Vitamin D and calcium supplement

- Vitamin C

- An antioxidant such as vitamin E or CoQ_{10}

- Glucosamine chondroitin

Since people typically eat a wide variety of foods, the liver must constantly be engaged in an intricate balancing act to ensure that the right nutrients get to the right parts of the body in the right amounts. In a healthy person, this balancing act occurs automatically. But when the liver has been weakened or damaged, it has trouble juggling the various nutrients. This is where the diet of a person with a liver problem comes into play. If she eats the right balance of foods, her already burdened liver won't have to work as hard. Nutrition is one aspect of disease where a person has some degree of control and can actively participate in speeding recovery and minimizing the likelihood of additional injury. The following sections discuss different nutrients in detail.

Protein

Proteins are the major building blocks that the body uses to make body components, such as muscles, hair, nails, skin, and blood. Proteins also make up important parts of the immune system called antibodies, which help fight off disease. Proteins are themselves made up of smaller building blocks called amino acids. An adequate protein intake is important to build and maintain muscle mass and to assist in healing and repair. The liver bears primary responsibility for making sure that old proteins get broken down and recycled and that new proteins are always available. Proteins can also be used as an energy source, although they are not as efficient as carbohydrates and fat. They are used as an energy source only under extreme circumstances, such as during starvation or at the end stages of liver disease, when the body begins breaking down its own muscles in a desperate attempt to stay alive. Known as *muscle wasting,* this is manifested on the body as decreased, and sometimes almost total lack of, muscle. People with muscle wasting are often referred to as looking like "skin and bones."

Since protein is such a vital component of the body, many people mistakenly believe that the more protein they consume, the better. Not only is this belief misguided, but for someone with liver damage such an approach to nutrition can actually be downright dangerous. The trouble is that a damaged liver cannot process as much protein as a healthy liver. And when a damaged liver gets unduly overloaded with protein, encephalopathy may occur. Finally, diets high in protein have been demonstrated to enhance the activity of the cytochrome P-450 enzyme system, which is responsible for drug metabolism. This enhanced activity increases the likelihood that a drug may be converted into a toxic by-product capable of causing liver injury. This is discussed in more detail in chapter 24.

Dietary Recommendations for Protein

When a person thinks of protein, a juicy hamburger or a roast chicken may come to mind. However, remember that protein has vegetable sources as well as animal sources (see table 23.1 for the protein content of some common foods). Protein intake must be adjusted in accordance with a person's body weight and the degree of liver damage present. Approximately 0.8 grams of protein per kilogram (2.2 pounds) of body weight is recommended in the diet each day for someone with stable liver disease. As such, total protein intake would range between about 40 and 100 grams per day—equaling the approximate 20 to 30 percent of daily calories derived from protein that a person should ideally consume.

When choosing animal protein, it is important to choose lean (low-fat) cuts of meat such as fish, white-meat chicken, and white-meat turkey. Keep in mind that even the leanest cuts of red meat are high in fat content. In fact, approximately 50 to 75 percent of calories from most red meats actually come from fat! Even a carefully trimmed cut of fine lean red meat probably derives about 50 percent of its calories from fat. This becomes especially significant for people with liver disease due to being overweight, as a diet high in fat may contribute to such a person's liver-related abnormalities (see "Fat" on page 386 for more information).

People with unstable liver disease (decompensated cirrhosis) need to lower the percentage of animal protein they consume and need to eat mostly vegetable sources of protein. A diet high in animal protein (which contains a lot of ammonia) may precipitate an episode of encephalopathy among these people. Researchers aren't exactly sure what causes encephalopathy, but they suspect that an excess of ammonia in the body may be one of the triggers. Some popular weight-loss diets involve the consumption of a very high amount of red meat (animal protein). People with cirrhosis are advised to avoid any such diets.

Table 23.1. Protein Content of Common Foods

Food	Portion Size	Protein Content
Bread (whole wheat)	1 slice	2.5 g
Broccoli (boiled, drained)	4 ounces	3.4 g
Cheese (Cheddar)	1 ounce	7.1 g
Chicken (dark meat, roasted without skin)	4 ounces	31.0 g
Chicken (white meat, roasted, without skin)	4 ounces	35.1 g
Egg (hard-boiled)	1 large	6.0 g
Flounder (baked, broiled, or microwaved)	4 ounces	27.4 g
Ham (roast)	4 ounces	28.4 g
Hamburger (cooked medium)	4 ounces	27.3 g
Lamb (cooked)	4 ounces	27.8 g
Milk (whole)	1 cup	8.0 g
Peas (frozen, boiled)	4 ounces	4.0 g
Potato (baked, with skin)	4 ounces	2.6 g
Rice (white, cooked)	4 ounces	3.1 g
Shrimp (steamed)	4 ounces	23.7 g
Spaghetti (cooked)	4 ounces	5.4 g
Steak (sirloin, broiled)	4 ounces	34.4 g
Tuna (chunk light in vegetable oil, drained)	6 ounces	49.8 g

Vegetarian diets, on the other hand, have a low ammonia content and have been shown to be much less likely than animal protein diets to induce encephalopathy. Also, vegetable fiber plays a role in helping to eliminate harmful waste substances, such as ammonia, from the body. Therefore, people prone to encephalopathy are advised to maintain a high intake of vegetable protein and a low intake of animal protein or, even better, to become vegetarians. This type of diet will help control mental symptoms in people suffering from some degree of chronic encephalopathy. Also, high-fiber, vegetable protein diets may reduce sugar levels in some people and may, therefore, be especially useful to diabetic people with cirrhosis and possibly in people with nonalcoholic fatty liver disease (NAFLD). However, even vegetable proteins are not perfect and also may be subject to dietary restriction. For instance, if a person suddenly develops encephalopathy, it may be necessary to limit any type of protein consumption to 20 grams or less per day, until this episode resolves.

The Importance of Avoiding Protein and Amino Acid Supplements

It's very easy for people with liver disease to consume too much protein. It's just as important to realize that the ingestion of protein supplements, such as those commonly found in health-food stores and supermarkets, can similarly be dangerous to people with a liver condition. Protein supplements force the liver and kidneys to work overtime in order to get rid of the excess protein ingested. Furthermore, excess protein can increase the risk of dehydration, as extra fluid is required to eliminate the by-products of protein metabolism from the body. Lastly, protein supplements, which are not regulated by the FDA (see chapter 21), often contain a variety of vitamins, minerals, and other food supplements that may cause dangerous excesses of these items in the body. Protein supplements are only required for people who are malnourished and unable to obtain adequate protein intake through their regular diets.

Amino acid supplementation is also potentially dangerous for people with liver disease. Although amino acids are indeed natural, it doesn't mean that they're always safe, especially for people with liver disease. Most of the amino acid supplements that are available over the counter come in quantities that are far greater than the amount the body needs. Consumption of excessive amounts of amino acids may cause serious side effects. Probably the best-known example of this involves L-tryptophan, an aromatic amino acid (AAA) used as a supplement to aid sleeping. Promoted for many years as safe and natural, L-tryptophan was eventually banned for sale by the FDA in 1990 because many people who consumed this amino acid developed a serious muscle disorder. Death even occurred in some people as a result of L-tryptophan ingestion. Some other amino acid supplements are high in AAA (for example, phenylalanine, tyrosine, and tryptophan), which have been demonstrated to be detrimental to some people with liver disease. Another amino acid, methionine, may induce encephalopathy in people with liver disease. Vegetables contain very little methionine yet have a high content of the branched-chain amino acids (BCAAs, such as leucine, isoleucine, and valine). Some experts believe BCAAs are beneficial to people with encephalopathy. However, under no circumstances should any form of amino acid supplement be added to the diet of a person with liver disease.

Carbohydrates

The major function of carbohydrates is to provide a ready supply of energy to the body. Carbohydrates supply this energy in the form of glucose (blood sugar). There are two separate categories of carbohydrates. The first category is known as simple carbohydrates (sugars that can be easily broken down by digestion). Simple carbohydrates may consist of only one sugar unit, known as a monosaccharide, and they include glucose, fructose (fruit sugar), and galactose (a component of milk products). Or they may consist of two sugar units, known as a disaccharide, and they include maltose (used in the fermentation of beer), sucrose (table sugar), and lactose (milk sugar).

Complex carbohydrates consist of polysaccharides (hundreds of simple sugars linked together) and are commonly known as starches and fibers. Complex carbohydrates cannot be immediately used by the body as energy. They must first be broken down into glucose, either by cooking or the digestive process. Exam-

Table 23.2. Carbohydrate Content of Common Foods

Food	Portion	Carbohydrate Content
Apple	1 medium	21.1 g
Banana	1 medium	26.7 g
Bread (pumpernickel)	1 slice	14.7 g
Bread (wheat)	1 slice	10.6 g
Bread (white)	1 slice	13.0 g
Milk	1 cup	11.7 g
Peanut butter	2 tablespoons	5.7 g
Potato (baked with skin)	1 medium	51.0 g
Potato (mashed)	½ cup	18.4 g

ples of complex carbohydrates include grains, nuts, seeds, breads, pasta, rice, cereals, and potatoes.

Dietary Recommendations for Carbohydrates

People with liver disease should strive for a diet consisting of approximately 60 to 70 percent carbohydrates, with complex carbohydrates predominating. For such people, a well-balanced diet will include at least 400 grams of carbohydrates (see table 23.2 for the carbohydrate content of some common foods). If there are too few carbohydrates in a person's diet, this will likely result in excessive protein and fat intake. If too much protein is consumed and not enough carbohydrates, the liver will be forced to use protein as an energy source. This is an unwise and inefficient use of protein, as protein will be diverted from its primary job of building cells and tissues. Furthermore, this will put undo stress on the liver, as it is more taxing for the liver to convert protein into energy than it is to convert carbohydrates into energy. If too much fat and not enough carbohydrates are consumed, many health disorders, including obesity, may result. This may eventually lead to fatty liver or nonalcoholic fatty liver disease (NAFLD) (see "Fat" on page 386). It is also important to keep in mind that a meal of complex carbohydrates, such as pasta, should not be drowned in sauces loaded with cream, butter, or oil. Doing so introduces too much fat into an otherwise healthy dish. Keep in mind that excessive complex carbohydrates, on the other hand, may lead to bloating and malabsorption of certain vitamins and minerals. This underscores the importance of adhering to the recommended balance of nutrients listed on pages 380–381.

Simple carbohydrates, such as raisins, hard candy, or honey, may stick to teeth. In people suffering from dry mouth, this is particularly likely, thereby increasing the likelihood of cavities for these people. Therefore, it is especially important that people suffering from dry mouth (sometimes present as a symptom in people with primary biliary cirrhosis or in people with chronic hepatitis B or C on interferon treatment) brush their teeth immediately after eating or snacking.

This may require that these people bring a toothbrush, toothpaste, and floss to restaurants, work, and school. Also, these people may want to use a prescription dental cream specifically made for people prone to dental cavities.

People with alcoholic liver disease (ALD) often suffer from abnormal carbohydrate metabolism. Approximately one-third of them have diabetes. A diet rich in high-fiber, complex-carbohydrate foods may improve their condition somewhat.

Carbohydrates and the Liver

The liver plays a crucial role in carbohydrate metabolism. Before sugars are able to supply energy to the body, they are routed to the liver, which is in charge of deciding their fate. The liver makes every effort to correct any nutritional imbalances attributable to poor eating habits. Thus, it may immediately send sugar (in the form of glucose) into the bloodstream to provide an instant energy boost to a person who needs it. Or the liver may send glucose to the brain or muscles, depending upon what activities are being performed at the time (for example, taking a test versus exercising). Or it may decide to store glucose (in the form of the starch glycogen) for later use when the body requires more energy. If too much carbohydrate is consumed, the liver transforms it into fat (in the form of triglycerides). In this case, excess fat accumulates in the body—usually in places where it is least wanted. Excess fat may be deposited directly into the liver, resulting in fatty liver or NAFLD (see "Fat" below).

Converting foods other than carbohydrates into energy is stressful even to a normal liver. By eating an unbalanced diet that is low in complex carbohydrates, a person with liver disease will add to the stress that the disease has already caused her liver. In fact, this is one reason why so many people with liver disease feel fatigued. Simply put, their diets are working against them. A well-balanced diet can help combat the fatigue associated with liver disease. (See "Exercise for Those with Liver Disease" on page 411 for other tips on combating fatigue.) Eating multiple small meals throughout the day instead of three large meals is recommended. Each meal should focus on complex carbohydrates, such as a plain baked potato or high-grain breads. By using such an eating strategy, a healthy energy source will be constantly supplied to the body. A diet rich in complex carbohydrates as opposed to one focused on simple sugars will provide a person with more sustained energy. For example, eating a candy bar provides a quick burst of energy because the body easily converts all those simple sugars into glucose. But the pick-me-up doesn't last long and is often followed by a swift energy drop as the liver tries to readjust energy levels. A plate of pasta, on the other hand, is a good source of complex carbohydrates. It takes more time to digest and thus provides a slower, more sustained release of energy.

Fat

Fats are the body's most efficient means for storing excess energy. They are a very concentrated source of calories. Gram for gram, fats contain more than dou-

Table 23.3. Percentage of Fat Found in Some Common Foods

Food	Percentage of Fat	Food	Percentage of Fat
Avocado	86	Hot dog	83
Bacon	92	Margarine	100
Butter	100	Mayonnaise	98
Chicken (with skin)	56	Milk (whole)	49
Chicken (without skin)	35	Peanut butter	75
Egg	69	Pecans	89
Hamburger	61		

ble the amount of calories of other nutrients. Thus, a diet high in fat is likely to result in more weight gain than a diet high in protein or carbohydrates.

It is important for people with liver disease to minimize their fat intake by avoiding foods that are high in fat (see table 23.3 for the percentage of fat found in some common foods). Excess fat on the body can result in NAFLD (see chapter 16). Although it is uncommon, it is possible for someone with NAFLD to develop cirrhosis and liver failure. Fatty livers are so unhealthy that they are not even considered viable for use in transplantation. A fatty liver may cause liver disease or may contribute to the worsening of other liver diseases. People with alcoholic liver disease who are obese appear to be particularly prone to developing cirrhosis. And people with hepatitis C and a fatty liver are likely to develop liver scarring at an accelerated rate. Fortunately, most cases of fatty liver due to being overweight can be reversed with a low-fat diet, exercise, and weight loss. Some people with liver disease don't have to worry about obesity. Some are even underweight. But even these people should not feel free to eat excessive amounts of fats, since fat deposits can accumulate in the liver no matter how much, or how little, a person weighs.

People with primary biliary cirrhosis (PBC) often have difficulty absorbing fats. This is because the destruction of the bile ducts within the liver causes a failure to secrete the bile salts that are necessary to absorb fats. This can result in steatorrhea, a condition of fat malabsorption. Therefore, people with PBC should adhere to a diet low in fat (see chapter 15 for more information on this disorder).

Dietary Recommendations for Fat

As a general rule, no more than 30 percent of a person's caloric intake should come from fat. That's the absolute maximum. Ideally, a person should aim for something in the neighborhood of 10 to 20 percent. People who are overweight should aim for 10 percent. While it is important to eat as little fat as possible, eating a small amount of the more healthy fats does have some benefit. Fat supplies the body with a source of reserve energy. In emergency situations, stored body fat is transformed into energy. It is this stored fat that keeps people warm on cold winter days. Also, certain fatty acids are necessary for the normal functioning of some bodily processes. These fats, which are known as essential fatty acids, perform (as the name suggests) a variety of duties that are essential to the proper functioning of the body. However, it should be pointed out that as little as a tablespoon of polyunsaturated fat a day can provide all of the essential fatty acids that the body needs. In addition, people need some fat in order to properly absorb the four fat-soluble vitamins—A, D, E, and K. Without some fat, these vitamins may become deficient in the body, even if they are taken in supplemental form. This type of vitamin deficiency sometimes occurs in people with cholestatic diseases, such as primary biliary cirrhosis. Lastly, fat helps make food tastier. This is important for people who suffer from a suppressed appetite due to chronic liver disease.

Most people are familiar with the fact that saturated fats are less healthy than unsaturated fats. What accounts for this? Well, most saturated fats tend to be hard or solid at room temperature. Therefore, they have the ability to clog arteries and boost cholesterol levels. Polyunsaturated fats, which are liquid at room temperature, don't do this. So it's best to stay on a diet that is low in saturated fats. (Keep in mind that fish fat is more liquid than chicken fat, which is more liquid than beef fat.)

Cholesterol and the Liver

Cholesterol is related to, but not synonymous with, fat. Cholesterol, which is found only in animal products, is not all bad. In fact, in some respects, it is essential to maintaining life. Cholesterol is needed to build sex hormones and bile salts. In the skin, it is made into vitamin D with the help of sunlight. However, people do not need to consume any cholesterol in order to facilitate these processes. The liver is capable of making most of the cholesterol required by the body—only about 15 percent of blood cholesterol comes from the diet. Yet many factors other than diet may account for high blood cholesterol levels. These include cigarette smoking, lack of exercise, and a genetic susceptibility to this condition. Triglyceride levels are a measurement of how much fat is circulating in the bloodstream.

High-density lipoprotein (HDL) is often referred to as the "good cholesterol" and low-density lipoprotein (LDL) is often referred to as the "bad cholesterol." HDL cholesterol seems to be responsible for sending all cholesterol to the liver to be broken down and then either recycled or excreted from the body. Overweight people tend to have low levels of HDL and high levels of LDL. Excess fat located around the abdomen (more so than fat deposited elsewhere in the body) seems to be related to elevated blood cholesterol levels. While not established with certainty, it is believed that the fatty acids released by abdominal fat tend to flow directly into the portal vein and from there directly into the liver. The liver then receives a signal to increase cholesterol output.

People with primary biliary cirrhosis (PBC) generally have high cholesterol levels (sometimes in the range of 500 to 1,000 mg/dl) that are not attributable to dietary indiscretions. However, they are not at increased risk for heart disease or heart attacks due to these elevated levels.

VITAMINS AND MINERALS

The liver is the body's main warehouse for storing nutrients. It absorbs and stores excess vitamins and minerals from the blood. If a person's diet does not supply an adequate amount of these nutrients on a given day, the liver releases just the right amount of them into the bloodstream. However, the liver has a limited capacity for processing vitamins and minerals. Any excess amounts that the liver is unable to process are generally eliminated from the body. Yet, at some point, the liver can become damaged due to the strain of processing an overabundance of certain vitamins and minerals.

If a person eats a healthy, well-balanced diet, all the vitamins and minerals required for daily needs and activities should be amply supplied. Despite this, many people feel that they should take vitamin and/or mineral supplements just to be on the safe side. While this may be fine for an overall healthy person, it may be downright dangerous for someone with liver disease. Thus, excessive doses of vitamin and mineral supplements may do much more harm than good to an already damaged liver.

However, there are exceptions to this rule: First, not everyone eats a healthy, well-balanced diet. Also, some people follow strict vegetarian diets. Under these circumstances, vitamin and mineral supplementation may be necessary. People with certain liver diseases, especially cholestatic diseases such as primary biliary cirrhosis, absorb some vitamins poorly. These people may also require supplementation. People with alcoholic liver disease have a need for vitamin supplementation due to the nutrient-depleting effects of alcohol on the body. On the other hand, some liver diseases actually result in an overload of a certain vitamin or mineral. An example of this is hemochromatosis (discussed in chapter 18), which is a liver disease of iron overload. Alternatively, some liver diseases are associated with iron deficiency from internal bleeding, for example, which can occur in people with bleeding esophageal varices due to decompensated cirrhosis. Therefore, the requirements of vitamins and minerals in the diet of a person with liver disease must be evaluated on an individualized basis. Lastly, it is important to keep in mind that vitamins and minerals are considered food supplements, and thus they are not regulated by the FDA, as per the DSHEA Act (see chapter 21).

Vitamins

Vitamins are organic substances that come from animals and plants. They are essential to human development, growth, and functioning. Vitamins are known as *micronutrients* because they are required by the body only in small amounts (compared with protein or water for example) to maintain health. Normally, the required amount is supplied by eating a well-rounded diet.

Just like foods and medications, vitamins must pass through the liver to be metabolized. If taken to excess, any vitamin has the potential to cause serious health problems. This is true even for people with normally functioning livers.

However, for people with liver disease, the potential for damage is much greater. Depending upon the severity of liver damage, certain people may even need to eliminate from their diets foods that have been fortified with certain vitamins. These may include commonly consumed foods, such as some breakfast cereals.

On the other hand, some people with liver disease are prone to vitamin deficiencies and must take vitamin supplements. If your doctor has recommended a specific vitamin supplement, make sure that it is taken with meals in order to be absorbed into the body properly. Furthermore, vitamin supplements should be kept in a cool, dry place, as its potency may be diminished by sunlight and dampness.

Vitamins can be categorized based on their solubility characteristics—fat soluble and water soluble. This difference has important implications for people with liver disease and will be covered in the following sections on the different types of vitamins.

Fat-Soluble Vitamins

Fat-soluble vitamins include vitamins A, D, E, and K. They are absorbed by the body only with the help of fats or bile. These vitamins are stored in fat cells. In people with cholestatic liver disease (liver disease in which there is an impairment or failure of bile flow within the bile ducts), they may be poorly absorbed by the body. In such cases, vitamin supplementation is necessary. The best type of vitamin to take in this case is the water-soluble form of a fat-soluble vitamin. Often, baby vitamins are totally water soluble. Since infants have immature digestive tracts, supplements designed specifically for them tend to be easiest to digest. Each of the fat-soluble vitamins is discussed in more detail below.

Vitamin A. Vitamin A is needed to maintain normal vision, especially night vision, and is essential to the immune system. It also plays a vital role in building and maintaining healthy skin, bones, and teeth. Vitamin A belongs to a group of compounds known as *retinoids* (also referred to as retinol, retinoic acid, or retinyl esters). About 80 to 90 percent of the total body stores of retinoids are found in the liver. The liver makes the ultimate decision as to where vitamin A is needed most in the body.

For people without liver disease, 1,000 mcg per day (3,333 IU per day) for men and 800 mcg (2,667 IU per day) for women should be the maximum amount of vitamin A consumed. This can easily be obtained from a well-balanced diet. Still, approximately one-quarter of American adults take supplements that contain vitamin A. This vitamin is found in abundance in the following foods: liver, egg yolks, fortified milk and other dairy products, margarine, liver oil, and fish oil. A person with advanced liver disease should never take vitamin A supplements and should not consume excessive quantities of the above-mentioned foods.

Plant forms of vitamin A are known as *carotenoids* (also called carotene). Carotene is also referred to as provitamin A, because the body must convert this substance to vitamin A before it can be utilized by the body as active vitamin A. The most common carotenoid found in food is beta-carotene. Foods high in beta-carotene include cantaloupes, carrots, sweet potatoes, and green leafy vegetables such as spinach.

Excessive consumption of vitamin A (doses of approximately 25,000 to 50,000 IU per day) is extremely dangerous to the liver as it may cause a liver disease known as *hypervitaminosis A*. In fact, this condition can lead to cirrhosis. Hypervitaminosis A may result from excessive vitamin A supplementation or from unusual dietary habits, such as excessive consumption of liver, egg yolks, or dairy products. People with liver disease should avoid eating liver since it contains a superabundance of vitamin A, more than any other organ meat. Interestingly, hundreds of years ago, doctors believed that some eye disorders could be cured by applying a piece of liver directly to a patient's eye, due to its high vitamin A content. Medications such as Accutane (isoretinoin) and Retin-A (tretinoin), both of which are used in the treatment of acne, are derived from vitamin A and therefore should not be used by people with advanced liver disease. Oral contraceptives may increase the absorption of vitamin A, thereby leading to dangerously high levels.

Vitamin A's potential to cause liver toxicity may be enhanced by alcohol consumption or by excessive intake of other fat-soluble vitamins (such as vitamin E) or by a vitamin C deficiency. Time wise, vitamin A toxicity may manifest only a few hours after a person has taken a massive dose. However, hypervitaminosis A can also develop slowly in a person who takes moderate doses of vitamin A over a long period of time. Symptoms of vitamin A overload may include nausea, vomiting, visual disorientation, headaches, and bone and joint pain. The liver can become enlarged and scarred, eventually leading to cirrhosis. Portal hypertension accompanied by jaundice and ascites can occur (see chapter 6). Vitamin A toxicity is often, but not always, reversible with a cessation of vitamin A consumption.

The bottom line is that people with liver disease are advised to minimize their intake of this vitamin. An exception to this rule applies only to people in advanced stages of cholestasis who are suffering from night blindness. An example would include a person with stage 4 primary biliary cirrhosis (PBC) who is also taking cholestyramine, a medication used to control itching that further impairs absorption of vitamin A. It has been noted that approximately 20 percent of people with PBC are deficient in vitamin A. Most of these people show no obvious symptoms of a vitamin A deficiency. Therefore, people with PBC should have their vitamin A levels checked. Even if found to be deficient, only those people experiencing difficulty with night vision should receive vitamin A supplements. When supplementing with vitamin A it is important to add zinc supplementation to maximize absorption of vitamin A. The water-soluble form of vitamin A—Aquasol—one capsule daily (50,000 IU) is best absorbed (see chapter 15 for more information on PBC).

Unlike retinoids, carotenoids are not toxic to the liver and cannot cause hypervitaminosis A. However, beta-carotene can turn a person's skin an orange-yellow color, giving her the mistaken appearance of being both jaundiced and in danger of liver failure. Also, excessive beta carotene may put a person with liver disease at additional risk for bone loss and osteoporosis (see chapter 20).

Vitamin A is found in animal livers and green and orange fruits and vegetables such as asparagus, broccoli, carrots, and cantaloupe. Animal sources of vitamin A tend to contain much greater quantities of this vitamin (six times as much) than vegetable sources. Therefore, it is advised that people with liver disease avoid cod liver oil and animal liver. Vegetables may be consumed freely. However, the practice of daily juicing of large quantities of fruits and/or vegetables should be avoided in people with severe liver disease.

Vitamin D. Vitamin D, a fat-soluble vitamin, is often referred to as the "sunshine vitamin." This is because sunlight is required to transform cholesterol into vitamin D. In order to ensure an adequate supply of vitamin D, most people need only expose themselves to sunlight for approximately fifteen minutes several times a week. Vitamin D is essential for the absorption and metabolism of calcium. This vitamin enables calcium to be available to bones. Vitamin D is especially important for people with chronic liver disease who are prone to osteoporosis or osteomalacia. These conditions were discussed in chapters 2 and 20. People prone to these disorders include those with primary biliary cirrhosis, those with cirrhosis due to any liver disease especially when complicated by cholestasis, and those taking an immunosuppressive medication such as prednisone. These people are advised to take a vitamin D supplement or to eat foods high in vitamin D. This is especially important if a person's sun exposure is limited due to weather conditions or geographic location. It is probably a good idea for all people with chronic liver disease to supplement their diets with calcium and vitamin D.

Foods containing an abundant amount of vitamin D include milk (which is fortified with vitamin D), cold-water fish, fish oil, cod liver oil, and egg yolks. The U.S. government's recommended daily intake of vitamin D is 5 mcg (200 IU). People with liver disease found to be deficient in vitamin D should take a supplement of between 400 and 800 IU per day. Keep in mind that excessive supplementation with vitamin D can lead to dangerous deposits of calcium in the kidneys, heart, and blood vessels. The need for vitamin D supplementation should be determined on a patient-by-patient basis by monitoring blood levels of 25-hydroxy vitamin D and the level of calcium in the blood and urine. The water-soluble form of the vitamin—vitamin D_2 (ergocalciferol)—should be used when possible.

Vitamin E. Vitamin E, also known as tocopherol, acts as an antioxidant in the body. It protects red blood cells and bodily tissues against damage. Some studies have shown that supplementation with vitamin E may protect the liver from free-radical–mediated injury arising from excessive alcohol intake. Therefore, people who regularly drink alcohol and, in particular, people with alcoholic liver disease, may benefit from supplementation with vitamin E. Since vitamin E requires bile for absorption, people with blockages of bile may suffer a deficiency. Deficiency of vitamin E is most frequently seen in people whose bilirubin has risen above 3 mg/dl and whose alkaline phosphatase (AP) is above 1,000 IU/l. Thus, people with cholestasis (such as those with primary biliary cirrhosis) or people with decompensated cirrhosis (due to any liver disease) may benefit from supplementation with vitamin E. A vitamin E deficiency may lead to a compromised immunity, a feeling of imbalance, and a lack of coordination. In fact, vitamin E deficiency can cause neurological dysfunction after liver transplantation. In cases of severe, prolonged vitamin E deficiency, blindness may occur.

The U.S. government's recommended daily allowance of vitamin E is most commonly 100 IU per day (although it can range from 30 to 400 IU per day). This amount of vitamin E can usually be obtained through a balanced diet. Foods containing abundant amounts of vitamin E include vegetable oils, whole grains, dark leafy vegetables, nuts, and legumes. These foods fall under the category of polyunsaturated fatty acids. Most vitamin E supplements contain only alpha-tocopherol, which is the most potent form of vitamin E. To get full benefit from a vitamin E supplement, it should contain both alpha- and gamma-tocopherol and be taken with zinc. If possible, try to obtain the water-soluble ester of vitamin E (d-alpha-tocopheryl-polyethylene glycol succinate [TPGS]). Vitamin E is best absorbed when it is in this form, which is especially important if cholestasis is present.

Some researchers believe that vitamin E therapy may be a beneficial adjunct to the treatment of viral hepatitis. In some studies done on patients with chronic hepatitis C, response rates were improved by the addition of vitamin E to interferon and ribavirin. Furthermore, it has been suggested that vitamin E may slow progression of liver disease; delay the onset of, and reduce the degree of, ribavirin-induced anemia in some patients; help relieve leg cramps; diminish memory loss; and increase male sexual performance—benefits that are of particular relevance to those on interferon and ribavirin treatment. While further study is needed to confirm the effectiveness of vitamin E as an adjunctive liver disease therapy, it is probably a good idea to consume a vitamin E supplement in a dose of between 400 and 800 IU each day. Bear in mind that the above-mentioned potential benefits of vitamin E have not been confirmed in people with hepatitis C and therefore should be considered speculative.

Vitamin E supplementation may cause excessive bleeding and bruising if taken while one is on an anticoagulant medication (blood thinner) such as Coumadin or Plavix or if taken in combination with herbs such as garlic or ginkgo. People with decompensated cirrhosis should refrain from vitamin E supplementation, especially if they have experienced variceal bleeding or if they have a vitamin K deficiency manifested by a prolonged prothrombin time. Finally, vitamin E supplementation should be discontinued about one month prior to any surgical or invasive procedure (such as a liver biopsy).

Vitamin K. Vitamin K is used by the liver to manufacture the protein prothrombin. Prothrombin, as discussed in chapter 3, is essential for proper blood clotting.

Without vitamin K, people would hemorrhage as the result of a cut. Vitamin K also helps keep bones strong. Vitamin K plays an important role in converting glucose into glycogen. Glycogen is then stored in the liver, creating a reserve of energy. Half of the vitamin K in the body is made by "friendly" bacteria that naturally live in the intestines. The remainder comes from dietary sources. Abusing certain laxatives, such as mineral oil, or taking antibiotics for prolonged periods of time may result in a depletion of vitamin K.

When a vitamin K deficiency is due to poor absorption, the deficiency may be corrected by taking water-soluble vitamin K orally, known as Synkayvite (5 to 10 mg per day), until the factor that was causing the malabsorption has been eliminated. People with cholestatic liver disease tend to have a vitamin K deficiency that is impossible to correct with oral supplementation. In situations where bleeding is a potential risk (such as for those people requiring surgery), intravenous infusions of fresh frozen plasma (FFP) must be given to these patients to temporarily correct this problem. In people with obstruction of the bile ducts outside the liver, the deficiency can often be corrected with an injection of vitamin K.

Foods containing an abundance of vitamin K include spinach and other leafy green vegetables, carrots, potatoes, cereals, and liver. There is no recommended daily allowance of vitamin K.

Water-Soluble Vitamins

Water-soluble vitamins include vitamin C and vitamin B complex. Vitamin B complex consists of eight different B vitamins. Neither fat nor bile is needed to absorb water-soluble vitamins from the digestive tract, and therefore a deficiency of these vitamins does not normally occur in people with cholestatic liver diseases. Water-soluble vitamins are stored in the body or are used to meet its daily requirements. Reserves of these vitamins can last many months. Therefore, people with liver disease rarely develop a deficiency of a water-soluble vitamin. One exception to this rule: people with alcoholic liver disease. This group often requires water-soluble vitamin supplementation due to the nutrient-depleting effects of alcohol on the body. Toxicity due to water-soluble vitamins is uncommon, as excessive doses of these vitamins can easily exit the body through perspiration or in the urine.

Vitamin C. Vitamin C, also known as ascorbic acid, is an antioxidant. This vitamin aids in the healing of cuts and bruises and also strengthens bones, cartilage, teeth, and skin. In addition, vitamin C enhances the absorption of iron. Therefore, people suffering from an iron overload disease such as hemochromatosis, and people with chronic hepatitis C who have elevated iron levels, must be careful not to consume excessive amounts of this vitamin. However, since vitamin C aids in the production of interferon, an immune system protein made by the body, supplementation with this vitamin may be beneficial in the treatment of people with hepatitis B and C. Furthermore, some experts feel that vitamin C may delay the onset of and reduce the degree of ribavirin-induced anemia in some patients with hepatitis C treated with interferon and ribavirin. The addition of pros as well as cons underscores the importance of discussing supplementation with a knowledgeable hepatologist.

Most fresh fruits and vegetables contain abundant amounts of vitamin C. It should be noted that cooking destroys vitamin C within food. The recommended amount of vitamin C is approximately 60 to 72 mg per day. This amount is easily obtained through a healthy diet. People with liver disease who do not consume a healthy diet, such as those with alcoholic liver disease whose primary intake of calories in the diet is from alcohol, need to take vitamin C supplements. Also, people with liver disease who use oral contraceptives, use certain antidepressants, or smoke cigarettes may have reduced levels of vitamin C in the body and require supplementation. For all other people with liver disease, supplementing with vitamin C is generally not necessary unless recommended for specific situations as determined by their doctor.

Supplemental vitamin C should be taken in the esterfied form (Ester C) for maximum absorption and effectiveness. Chewable vitamin C may cause damage to the teeth and should be avoided. This is especially important for people with liver diseases associated with dry mouth (such as PBC) and for people taking interferon for hepatitis, who are also prone to dental cavities.

Vitamin B Complex. The B complex vitamins consist of eight different vitamins: thiamine (vitamin B_1), riboflavin (vitamin B_2), niacin (vitamin B_3), pantothenic acid (vitamin B_5), pyridoxine (vitamin B_6), cyanocobalamin (vitamin B_{12}), folate, and biotin. All of these, with the exception of excessive doses of niacin (vitamin B_3), are safe for people with liver disease. The following is a discussion of each B vitamin.

- Thiamine (vitamin B_1) is essential for metabolizing carbohydrates into energy to be used by the brain and the nervous system. It also aids appetite and digestion. Symptoms of a thiamine deficiency include a loss of appetite, confusion, and disequilibrium (a feeling of imbalance). This vitamin is frequently deficient in people with alcoholic liver disease. Excessive caffeine use may decrease thiamine levels in the body. When neurological signs of a thiamine deficiency occur in people with alcoholic liver disease, hospitalization and immediate intravenous thiamine replacement are often required.

  Thiamine can be found in whole-grain or enriched cereals, breads, brown rice, pork, liver, and soybeans. About 5 mg is the maximum amount of thiamine that can be absorbed per day from supplementation. Some "stress tablets" that purport to boost energy levels contain more than 5 mg of thiamine. The excess is simply eliminated from the body unused.

- Riboflavin (vitamin B_2) is important for energy production. It helps promote the growth and repair of tissues and organs, specifically the skin, mucous membranes, eyes, and nerves. It is also essential to proper digestion. It has been found to be effective in preventing the onset of migraines. Deficiency can lead to cracks and sores in the corner of the mouth and visual problems. The use of oral contraceptives and strenuous exercise occasionally lead to a riboflavin deficiency. Riboflavin can be found in both whole-grain and enriched-grain products, as well as in liver, milk, and leafy green vegetables. If too much riboflavin is ingested, urine will turn a bright yellow color, but this is not medically significant.

- Niacin (vitamin B_3), which is also known as nicotinic acid or nicotinamide, helps transform carbohydrates and fats into energy. It is needed for healthy skin. Large doses of niacin are sometimes prescribed for people with high cholesterol. This can be very dangerous for people with liver disease, as dosages exceeding 500 mg per day can cause liver damage if taken over a prolonged period of time. Thus, people with liver disease are advised to refrain from excessive consumption of this vitamin. Niacin can also cause a reddened flush on the face, arms, and chest which, although somewhat alarming, is harmless. Good sources of niacin include milk, eggs, meat, vegetables, and peanuts.

- Pantothenic acid (vitamin B_5) is needed to convert proteins, carbohydrates, and fats into energy. Pantothenic acid also promotes immune function. It is known as the "anti-stress vitamin." Supplementation has been found to be helpful for people with rheumatoid arthritis. Deficiency is uncommon, since pantothenic acid is synthesized by microorganisms that live in the small intestine. However, deficiency does occur occasionally in people who drink alcohol excessively. Megadoses of this vitamin can produce severe diarrhea. Deficiency can cause fatigue and depression. Food sources of this vitamin include fresh vegetables, brewer's yeast, eggs, nuts, and meat.

- Pyridoxine (vitamin B_6) is needed for efficient metabolism of proteins, carbohydrates, and fats. It aids in the production of hormones and red blood cells. Vitamin B_6 is found in so many foods (for example, liver, salmon, nuts, brown rice, most vegetables, and meat) that a deficiency is rare, except among people with alcoholic liver disease. Occasionally, the use of oral contraceptives can increase the requirement of this vitamin. Excessive doses of pyridoxine can lead to nerve damage.

- Cyanocobalamin (vitamin B_{12}) is needed to make blood cells. Therefore, a deficiency of this vitamin often leads to anemia and associated fatigue. This explains why people with liver disease who suffer from excessive fatigue often ask about vitamin B_{12} injections. However, the expectation that such an injection will provide an "extra boost" of energy is misguided. Since this vitamin is commonly found in animal food products such as meat, fish, milk, and eggs, a vitamin B_{12} deficiency is a very uncommon cause of fatigue in people with liver disease.

 A few exceptions to the above statement exist. One exception applies to those people with alcoholic liver disease (ALD) for whom the bulk of nutrients are obtained from alcohol. A vitamin B_{12} deficiency may develop among these people. Furthermore, since alcohol interferes with absorption of vitamin B_{12}, a vitamin B_{12} deficiency may develop if a person consumes an excessive amount of alcohol even if she maintains a well-balanced diet (see chapter 17 for more information on ALD). A deficiency of this vitamin may also occur in people with chronic liver disease who must maintain a strict vegetarian diet for long periods, such as is the case for those suffering with chronic encephalopathy. Finally, the older a person is, the more likely a vitamin B_{12} deficiency is to develop. This is because stomach acid is needed to absorb this vitamin from food, and as a person ages, the amount of acid in the stomach diminishes. Therefore, people with liver disease who are over the age of sixty should be checked for a vitamin B_{12} deficiency. Also, people with liver disease who are chronically on medications that block stomach acid—such as H_2 blockers (for example, Pepcid, Axid, Tagamet, and Zantac) and proton-pump inhibitors (for example, Prilosec, Prevacid, Aciphex, Nexium, and Protonix)—should be checked as well. Symptoms of a vitamin B_{12} deficiency include mood swings, irritability, rapid heart rate, fatigue, short-term memory loss, and severe psychosis.

- Folate is needed for proper brain functioning and is crucial to the formation of red blood cells. As with vitamin B_{12}, a folate deficiency can also produce anemia. In fact, vitamin B_{12} must be present in order to activate folate, which accounts for the fact that a deficiency of one tends to simultaneously cause a deficiency of the other. Folate deficiency is very common in people with alcoholic liver disease. Women taking oral contraceptives and people taking the chemotherapy agent methotrexate may require folate supplementation. Symptoms of folate deficiency include a sore red tongue, fatigue, and memory loss. Megadoses of folate can interfere with the absorption of certain medications and zinc, and can mask signs of a vitamin B_{12} deficiency. Sources of folate include leafy green vegetables, oranges, barley, brown rice, cheese, and whole grains.

- Biotin is needed for healthy hair, nails, and skin. It is produced by microorganisms living in the small intestines.Therefore, deficiency is uncommon unless excessive quantities of raw egg whites are eaten, as they may prevent the body's ability to absorb biotin. Biotin at a dose of 100 mg per day may help to prevent or diminish the hair loss that is sometimes associated with interferon therapy. Keep in mind that this benefit is merely anecdotal and has not been proven, although it's probably worth a try. Preliminary studies have shown that biotin may decrease insulin resistance. Thus, biotin supplementation may be beneficial for people with nonalcoholic fatty liver disease (NAFLD). However, this needs to be confirmed by further studies. Good sources of biotin include brewer's yeast, poultry, and milk.

Minerals

Minerals are inorganic substances, which means that they are not manufactured by either plants or animals. They originate in soil and water and become incorporated, in varying degrees, into all plant and animal life. Minerals are essential for almost all of the body's functions. They play a crucial role in energy production, heartbeat regulation, and control of muscle tone. A well-rounded diet will typically provide ample amounts of all the minerals needed to carry out daily activities. Macrominerals include those minerals that the body needs in large quantities. Macrominerals that are of special relevance to people with liver disease include calcium and sodium. Microminerals are those minerals that the body needs in trace amounts. Microminerals that are of particular relevance to people with liver disease include iron, zinc, and selenium. The following is a discussion of these minerals.

Calcium (Ca)

Calcium is essential for healthy teeth and bones, normal muscle contraction, and blood clotting. Almost all of the calcium in the body resides in the bones. Without an adequate amount of calcium, the bones become soft and brittle. Osteoporosis is characterized by reduced bone mass and the resulting increased risk for bone fractures. Osteoporosis is common to many liver diseases, especially cholestatic liver diseases such as primary biliary cirrhosis (see chapters 2 and 20). It is important for all people with chronic liver disease to consume foods rich in calcium and/or to supplement their diets with this mineral. However, it is important to remember that calcium supplementation alone will not prevent osteoporosis. Other factors, such as cigarette smoking, lack of exercise, excessive alcohol consumption, and abnormal hormone levels, play roles in the development of bone loss. Alcohol has been shown to be directly toxic to bone cells and may impair calcium absorption. Thus, it is especially important for people with alcoholic liver disease to take calcium supplementation. In fact, as stated above, it is a good idea for all people with chronic liver disease to take both calcium and vitamin D supplements.

Good sources of calcium include dairy products, dark green leafy vegetables (except spinach), tofu, and canned sardines with bones. Also many foods, such as orange juice, have been fortified with calcium. Excessive calcium consumption may interfere with the absorption of iron and zinc. In addition, excessive calcium intake may cause a variety of medical problems, including kidney stones, constipation, and fatigue. As with all supplements, regardless of how much is consumed, the body will only use the amount needed. Any surplus will be eliminated from the body unused or will accumulate and perhaps cause medical problems. If calcium supplementation is taken, it should be limited to no more than 1,000 to 2,500 mg per day in two divided doses and should be taken with a vitamin D supplement (which is usually included in the calcium tablet). Since stomach acid is needed to properly absorb calcium, antacids such as Tums, which reduce stomach acid, are poor sources of this mineral. Thus, H_2 blockers (such as Zantac, Pepcid, Axid, and Tagamet) and proton-pump inhibitors (Protonix, Nexium, Prevacid, Prilosec, and Aciphex) can cause decreased absorption of calcium. Simultaneous intake of biphosphonates (such as Fosamax) and calcium, both of which are used in the treatment of osteoporosis, may decrease the absorption of the biphosphonate, and thus should be taken at different times of the day.

Sodium (Na)

Sodium is a mineral that the body requires to maintain precise water balance. Sodium occurs in nature only in combination with chloride, another mineral. Sodium chloride is commonly known as *salt*. The body requires about 50 to 400 mg of sodium per day. Yet the average American consumes about twenty-five to thirty-five times that amount! While this overconsumption of salt is not necessarily dangerous for most healthy people, it can create problems for a person with advanced liver disease.

Decompensated cirrhosis may lead to ascites (an abnormal accumulation of fluid in the abdomen). If not treated in a timely manner, this ascitic fluid may become infected (a condition known as spontaneous bacterial peritonitis, or SBP). People with ascites must be placed on a severely salt-restricted diet. For every gram of sodium consumed, the accumulation of 200 ml of fluid results. The lower the consumption of sodium in the diet, the better controlled this excessive fluid accumulation is. For people with ascites, sodium intake should be restricted to less than 1,000 mg per day and preferably under 500 mg. This goal is difficult, yet attainable.

In order to successfully adhere to a salt-restricted diet, it is necessary to become a knowledgeable food shopper and to diligently read all food labels. People are often surprised to discover which foods are high in sodium (see table 23.4 for the sodium content of some common foods). General guidelines regarding sodium consumption are as follows: The amount of sodium in fresh foods is significantly less than that in the same foods after they have been processed, cured, canned, or frozen; therefore, choose fresh foods whenever possible. Table salt and salt used for cooking should be totally eliminated from the diet. One teaspoon of table salt contains 2,325 mg of sodium! All canned foods and food from fast-food restaurants should be avoided. Some over-the-counter medications have high sodium contents. For example, one tablet of Rolaids contains 53 mg of sodium, two tablets of Alka-Seltzer contain 567 mg of sodium, and one serving of Bromo-Seltzer contains 717 mg of sodium. These medications should be substituted with products that have a lower sodium content. If the label on a medication or other product does not clearly state the sodium content, a pharmacist should be able to supply this information or offer a way to obtain it. Meats, especially red meats, have a high sodium content. Consequently, adherence to a vegetarian diet may become necessary for people who develop severe ascites. Spices, such as basil, dill pepper, and vinegar, to name a few, may be used in place of salt as a food seasoning. Salt substitutes containing potassium chloride

Table 23.4. Sodium Content of Common Foods

Food	Portion	Sodium Content
Alka-Seltzer	2 tablets	567 mg
Anchovies (canned)	5	734 mg
Baking soda	1 teaspoon	821 mg
Big Mac	1	1,510 mg
Butter	1 tablespoon	116 mg
Chicken noodle soup (some types)	1 cup	1,106 mg
Corn (canned)	½ cup	285 mg
Cornflakes	1 ounce	351 mg
English muffin	1	378 mg
Frankfurter	1	504 mg
Ketchup	1 tablespoon	156 mg
Margarine	1 tablespoon	132 mg
Milk	1 cup	121 mg
Sauerkraut	½ cup	780 mg
Soy sauce	1 tablespoon	1,029 mg

should be avoided. These substitutes tend to raise potassium levels in the body. This can be especially dangerous to people taking spironolactone (Aldactone), a potassium-sparing diuretic (water pill) used in the management of ascites.

It is fortunate that many foods on the market have been specifically manufactured as low sodium products. Furthermore, as of 1986, the FDA has required that the sodium content of all processed foods be listed on the package label. This regulation has been a boon to the consumer. People with liver disease without ascites are advised to refrain from excessive salt intake, although they need not limit their consumption as severely as those who have ascites.

Iron (Fe)

There are two types of dietary iron. Heme (animal) iron found in animal foods, such as red meat, is well absorbed from the diet. Nonheme (plant) iron found in plant foods, such as spinach, is poorly absorbed into the body. Popeye was wrong: Spinach is not a good source of iron. In fact, only about 15 percent of ingested animal iron and only 3 percent of ingested plant iron are actually absorbed by the body. The average American consumes about 10 to 20 mg of iron per day. In order to increase the absorption of plant iron in the body, a vitamin C supplement should be consumed at the same time. On the other hand, tea, which contains tannins (a plant substance), inhibits the amount of iron absorbed from the diet. And iron decreases the effectiveness of vitamin E when taken together.

The quantity of iron in the body usually amounts to about 3 to 4 grams (50 mg/kg in men and 40 mg/kg in women). People have a limited ability to eliminate excess iron from the body. In fact, only about 1 to 2 mg of iron is capable of being excreted each day. Therefore, if too much iron is ingested (whether in the form of food or supplements), excess iron in the body results. This excess iron is stored primarily in the liver. As such, the liver is the part of the body that is most susceptible to the toxicity of iron.

Iron is an essential component of hemoglobin, a protein responsible for delivering oxygen to the body's cells and organs. (One red blood cell carries approximately 270 hemoglobin molecules, each of which contains 4 iron molecules.) Iron is also a component of myoglobin, a protein responsible for delivering oxygen to the muscles. Finally, iron helps make adenosine triphosphate (ATP), an important component of energy. Thus, it is common to associate iron with energy and strength. Interestingly, the link between fatigue and iron deficiency was brought to the attention of the American public by a 1960s commercial for the supplement Geritol, which popularized the term iron-poor blood. People with liver disease often assume that when they feel weak and tired, they need to take iron supplements. But taking iron supplements under such circumstances is not always a wise move and may, in fact, be dangerous. The symptoms of iron deficiency and iron overload can be quite similar—fatigue, headaches, and shortness of breath. Also, the fatigue associated with liver disease is more likely to be due to something other than the amount of iron in the body. Therefore, prior to taking an iron supplement, it is crucial that a person with liver disease get her blood tested to obtain her iron profile. If it is determined that an iron supplement is needed, one should be aware that it may turn the stools black. This may be confused with melena—black stools due to upper gastrointestinal bleeding from esophageal varices, for example. Always check with your doctor if this occurs (see chapter 18 for more information on iron studies).

Excessive iron in the body of a liver patient can be extremely dangerous. In extreme excess, iron is toxic to the liver and can lead to cirrhosis, liver failure, and liver cancer. Furthermore, there is growing evidence that even mildly increased (or sometimes even normal) amounts of iron may cause or enhance the amount of injury to the liver when one has a liver disease. This applies especially to people with alcoholic liver disease and chronic hepatitis C. In fact, iron overload is sometimes seen in people with alcoholic liver disease as well as people with chronic hepatitis C and has been found to worsen the outcome of these diseases and to decrease the responsiveness to treatment. Liver scarring and liver cell damage are directly related to the iron content of the liver. Since a person's body is unable to eliminate an overabundance of iron, neither iron supplements nor vitamins containing iron should be included in the diet of a person with liver disease, unless it has been determined that she has an iron deficiency.

Hemochromatosis is an inherited disease of iron overload (see chapter 18). People with this disease and those with high iron levels due to other liver disorders should avoid cooking with cast-iron cookware and should avoid eating with

Table 23.5. Iron Content of Some Common Foods

Food	Portion	Iron Content
Beef	3 ounces	6.1 mg
Cereal (iron-fortified)	1 ounce	4.5 mg
Chicken	3.5 ounces	1.1 mg
Liver	3.5 ounces	14.2 mg
Shrimp	3 ounces	2.5 mg
Spinach	1 cup	0.8 mg

cast-iron utensils. These people should consume only moderate amounts of foods that are high in iron content (see table 23.5 for the iron content of some common foods). Furthermore, some herbs commonly taken to treat liver disease (for example, milk thistle, dandelion, and licorice) may contain iron. Therefore, people with hemochromatosis or other diseases associated with iron overload should avoid these herbs.

Zinc (Zn)

Zinc is essential to the normal functioning of the immune system, is important for the senses of taste and smell, and may protect the liver from chemical damage. Some researchers believe that zinc may even protect the body from viruses, including the common cold.

Zinc is necessary for enabling the effects of vitamin A activity. Therefore, it is often the case that people who are deficient in zinc are also deficient in vitamin A. A zinc deficiency may occur in people with cirrhosis, especially when cirrhosis is due to excessive alcohol use. This may stem from insufficient dietary intake of zinc or from a reduced intestinal absorption of zinc. Such a deficiency may also be due to an increased excretion of zinc in the urine. A zinc deficiency may contribute to a decreased appetite, fatigue, brittle nails, hair loss, and poor wound healing. These symptoms are experienced by some people with alcoholic liver disease. Supplementation with zinc is recommended if a deficiency is discovered. Some studies show that zinc may help improve mental status in people with encephalopathy.

The addition of zinc to interferon treatment in patients with hepatitis C may increase the response rate for viral eradication. Although this benefit has not been proven, it is advisable to supplement the diet with a 30-mg tablet of zinc taken once or twice a day while on interferon therapy. While daily dosages up to 100 mg of zinc may boost the immune system and improve one's chance of response to interferon, an excess of this amount may be dangerous and may even depress the immune system. In addition, excessive zinc consumption may lead to nausea, vomiting, and diarrhea.

Good sources of zinc include beef, liver, brewer's yeast, seafood, egg yolks, fish, and lima beans.

Selenium (Se)

Selenium is an antioxidant that may improve the immune system and protect against certain cancers. Selenium and vitamin E act together to help maintain a healthy heart and liver and to assist in the production of antibodies. Selenium may help protect the livers of people with alcoholic liver disease. It has been found to increase both red and white blood cells in people with AIDS. Even though no studies have been conducted on the subject, it can be speculated that selenium may similarly decrease the incidence of low red and white cell counts that are potential side effects of interferon and ribavirin therapy for chronic hepatitis C (see chapter 13).

Selenium deficiency has been associated with fatigue, heart disease, liver disease, and sterility. Low selenium levels have been found in some people with hepatitis B and C, and it has been postulated that this deficiency may speed progression to cirrhosis and liver cancer. Sources of selenium include brazil nuts, brewer's yeast, broccoli, brown rice, and chicken. If selenium supplements are needed, the recommended dose is 100 mcg per day. Do not exceed 200 mcg per day, as high selenium levels have also been associated with liver disease, in addition to brittle nails, hair loss, and bad breath.

OTHER DIETARY SUPPLEMENTS

The discussion of all dietary supplements is beyond the scope of this book. This section will cover four dietary supplements that are commonly used and frequently inquired about by people with liver disease: S-Adenosyl-L-Methionine (SAMe), glucosamine chondroitin, and Coenzyme Q_{10}. Alpha-lipoic acid (ALA) was covered in chapter 21.

S-Adenosyl-L-Methionine (SAMe)

SAMe is a derivative of the amino acid L-methionine. It is made in the body when methionine combines with energy (adenosine triphosphate [ATP]). In Europe, SAMe is considered a drug to treat liver disease, fibromyalgia, and depression. SAMe may improve liver enzyme elevations and may reverse or even prevent liver toxicity that is caused by various drugs as well as alcohol and some chemicals. It may increase natural levels of glutathione, an antioxidant enzyme produced by the liver that protects it from free-radical damage. And it has also been postulated that SAMe may prevent liver tumors. Further study needs to be conducted with SAMe before it can be routinely recommended for people with liver disease. Dosages should not exceed 800 mg twice per day and should be taken on an empty stomach.

Glucosamine Chondroitin Sulfate

Glucosamine is a substance classified as an amino sugar. It is made from the simple carbohydrate glucose in combination with the amino acid glutamine. Amino sugars are not used as a source of energy like other sugars; rather they are incorporated into the body to help form nails, tendons, eyes, bones, and ligaments. Chondroitin sulfate is part of a group of substances known as glycosaminoglycans (formerly called mucopolysaccharides). It is found in cartilage, bone, cornea, and skin. In clinical trials it has been shown that glucosamine can build and possibly repair joint cartilage. Thus, it may alleviate some joint pains associated with liver disease or the treatment of liver disease.

Glucosamine may also have anti-inflammatory properties. Glucosamine in combination with chondroitin sulfate has been shown to be helpful in treating the symptoms of and halting the progression of osteoarthritis. Some people have found relief of muscle and joint aches, a side effect often associated with interferon therapy. Some studies have postulated that glucosamine chondroitin may be useful proactively, meaning that it may help prevent osteoarthritis from occurring in the first place. Glucosamine should probably not be taken by people with NAFLD, as this substance has been shown to increase insulin resistance. The usual dose of glucosamine chondroitin is 1,500 mg of glucosamine and 1,200 mg of chondroitin once per day. Readers should note that glucosamine and chondroitin sulfate are typically combined within the same tablet.

Coenzyme Q_{10} (CoQ_{10sw})

Coenzyme Q_{10} is a vitaminlike antioxidant found in all parts of the body. This substance aids in the production of energy and stimulates the immune system. It has been used to reduce the side effects of cancer chemotherapy. Thus, it may be helpful in reducing interferon-related side effects, although no studies have been performed to assess its efficacy in this area. CoQ_{10} has been used to treat allergic disorders such as asthma, mental disease such as Alzheimer's, and heart disease. The amount of CoQ_{10} in one's body decreases with age. Therefore, it is recommended that people over the age of fifty supplement their diets with this substance. Deficiency of this substance may lead to tooth decay and diabetes. CoQ_{10} has been found to be effective at dosages ranging from 50 to 200 mg daily. Foods that are good sources of CoQ_{10} include mackerel, salmon, sardines, beef, peanuts, and spinach.

OTHER DIETARY CONCERNS

Some foods and supplements have been associated with hepatitis and liver disorders. Therefore, it is recommended that people with liver disease avoid the foods and supplements discussed in this section. Other nutritional concerns that people often have include how the consumption of water and caffeine affects the liver. These concerns will be addressed in this section. Gas-related problems, some thoughts on gluten intolerance, and finally some nutritional tips will conclude this section on nutrition.

Foods and Supplements to Avoid

Raw shellfish (oysters and clams) have been the source of many outbreaks of hepatitis A. People with chronic liver disease are at increased risk of complications and poor outcomes if they become infected with hepatitis A. Therefore, all people with chronic liver disease who intend to eat shellfish should get the hepatitis A vaccination (see chapter 24 for more information on vaccinations). There have been some reports of people with hemochromatosis dying from eating raw shellfish that was contaminated with the bacteria *Vibrio vulnificus*. High iron levels have been linked to fatal infection with this bacteria; therefore, it is probably wise for people with hemochromatosis, other liver diseases with high iron levels such as hepatitis C, and cirrhosis due to any liver disease to avoid raw or poorly cooked shellfish. Well-cooked shellfish on the other hand is not dangerous.

Many wild mushrooms found in North America and Europe contain deadly toxins known as phallotoxins (phalloidin and alpha amanitin). These mushrooms are renowned for causing liver failure, or even death, when consumed. As a precaution, all patients with liver disease are advised to avoid eating wild mushrooms, especially if self-picked. See chapter 21 for more information concerning these mushrooms.

Shark cartilage is a nutritional supplement that has been purported to be of benefit to some people with cancer. There is a possible, although unproven, association between shark cartilage and drug-induced hepatitis. People with chronic liver disease are best advised to avoid this supplement until it has been evaluated further.

Aflatoxin, a hepatotoxin (common in Asia and southern Africa but uncommon in the United States), is produced by a fungus (*Aspergillus*). This fungus is a potential contaminant of foods that have been stored for prolonged periods of time in damp, warm conditions. The most commonly infected foods are peanuts and corn. In some countries, aflatoxins have been linked to hepatitis, cirrhosis, and liver cancer. This is discussed in more detail in chapter 19.

Saccharin, a sweetener, has been associated with acute hepatitis. Even though this association has not been conclusively proven, people with liver disease are best advised to avoid saccharin.

Adequate Water Consumption

The body consists of about 70 percent water. It requires water in order to carry out its essential functions. It is important for people to drink at least six to eight 8-ounce glasses of water per day. It is especially important for people with chronic hepatitis B or C who are on interferon therapy to stay well hydrated. These people should probably increase their water intake beyond the recommended amount to at least one gallon of water per day. People with liver disease often find that drinking abundant amounts of water helps give them an improved sense of well-being. And people on interferon often find that liberal water consumption helps them with some of the side effects of the medication. On the other hand, people with ascites are prone to excessive water retention. These people are advised to restrict their water intake to approximately three to four 8-ounce glasses of water per day, depending upon the degree of fluid accumulation present. When drinking bottled mineral water, it is important to take note of the water's sodium content. In some instances, the sodium content may present a problem for people on sodium-restricted diets. Also one may consider purchasing a filtration system for the kitchen faucet for more purified water.

Caffeine's Effect on Those with Liver Disease

Caffeine is present in coffee, tea, chocolate, cola, and some over-the-counter medications. Caffeine is metabolized through the liver. However, caffeine itself is not directly harmful to the liver. In fact, one study even suggested that coffee, but not other caffeine-containing drinks, may delay progression of liver disease to cirrhosis. (This result has not been substantiated by other studies.) In moderation (one to two cups of a caffeine-containing beverage per day), caffeine may suppress the fatigue associated with liver disease to some extent. However, higher amounts of caffeine may cause irritability, restlessness, and insomnia. Some people may experience a rapid heartbeat and/or palpitations from caffeine consumption. Excessive intake of caffeine may put people with chronic liver disease at increased risk for osteoporosis and bone fractures. And, in people with cirrhosis, the metabolism of caffeine is slowed, resulting in higher concentrations of caffeine in the blood. Thus, people with cirrhosis should limit their caffeine intake to one cup of coffee or tea per day. In fact, it is best for all people with liver disease to consume caffeine in moderation. This is especially important for people taking interferon, as this medication may, by itself, cause symptoms similar to those caused by caffeine.

Gas-Related Problems

Some people with liver disease complain of increased gas production (*flatulence*), abdominal bloating, and abdominal distention. These symptoms may stem from malabsorption and/or maldigestion of certain nutrients by the body. These symptoms are especially likely to occur in people with alcoholic liver disease and cholestatic liver diseases, such as primary biliary cirrhosis. Such symptoms may also be caused by the medications used in the treatment of liver disease. Cholestyramine (Questran) is one example of a medication that is likely to cause increased gas production. Alternatively, flatulence may not be related to a liver disorder at all but instead may stem from increased consumption of foods that have a tendency to cause gas (see the list below) or from the development of a food intolerance, such as lactose intolerance.

    To remedy these symptoms, people can try decreasing their consumption of gas-containing foods and foods that they are having difficulty digesting. Often, elimination diets are helpful. An elimination diet involves eliminating one food at a time from the diet to determine whether that food is solely responsible for the gas production. It is usually best to begin by eliminating milk and milk products, as they are the foods most commonly not tolerated. One approach that will cut down on the gas-producing potential of fruits is to peel off the skins. Another is to cook fruits and vegetables until they are soft and soggy. Unfortunately, these methods of preparation also significantly reduce the nutritional value of these foods. Finally, taking an antigas remedy (typically containing simethicone) can sometimes help.

Foods that can cause gas include:

- Dairy products, such as milk (including skim and low-fat), yogurt, milk chocolate, cheese, and cheese pizza

- Raw vegetables, especially onions, carrots, cabbage, lettuce, broccoli, and cauliflower

- Beans

- Bagels

- Pretzels

- Soups

- Fruits with skins

- Dried fruits, such as raisins and prunes

- Fatty foods

- Artificial sweeteners, such as sorbitol

- Carbonated beverages, such as soda

- Chewing gum

Gluten's Effect on the Liver

Gluten, a protein found in wheat, oats, barley, and rye, is often unable to be absorbed in people with primary biliary cirrhosis. An inability to absorb gluten, known as a *gluten intolerance,* occurs in the autoimmune disease known as *celiac sprue.* Celiac sprue typically causes diarrhea and weight loss. Celiac sprue is approximately ten times more likely to occur in people with PBC than among the general population. Treatment consists of eliminating all gluten products from the diet. Both PBC and celiac sprue are discussed in chapter 15. People with celiac sprue often have elevations in liver enzymes even if they do not have PBC.

How to Enjoy a "Liver-Friendly" Holiday

For most of us, the holidays bring an increase in the amount of time spent visiting with friends and relatives and shopping at the mall. Yet, along with the merriment that surrounds this season comes the likelihood of above-normal stress. This is especially true for a person with liver disease. Important concerns include how a person with liver disease (who may already be suffering from fatigue, irritability, insomnia, and headaches) can best enjoy the holiday season and how he or she can maintain a healthy diet and avoid the temptations of alcohol throughout the holiday season. The following are some helpful tips for people with liver disease as to how they may enjoy the holidays without compromising the health of their livers.

- Opt for nonalcoholic beer, wine, or champagne or sparkling water, seltzer, or ginger ale

- Steer clear of eggnog and cakes, desserts, or coffee that may include alcohol as a hidden ingredient

- Munch on crudités as an appetizer, but avoid the dip

- Eat white-meat turkey or chicken basted in its own juices as opposed to precooked or preseasoned meats

- Use fresh cranberries instead of those from a can

- Eat fresh, plain, steamed vegetables instead of those cooked in butter or margarine

- Use whole-grain breads instead of white bread

- Only eat nuts of the unsalted or dry-roasted variety

- Eat small portions throughout the day

- Steer clear of holiday candies made with simple sugars

In some cases the cause of these liver enzyme elevations is probably due to NAFLD. However, once a gluten-free diet has been instituted, liver enzyme elevations typically normalize. In fact, one study demonstrated that dietary treatment with gluten restriction may have contributed to the prevention of progression to cirrhosis and liver failure.

WEIGHT PROBLEMS AND LIVER DISEASE

Many people have problems related to weight. Well, people with liver disease are no different, but with one exception: Weight problems are often related to their liver diseases. Therefore, it is important for anyone with liver disease who is experiencing an unexpected weight gain or loss to consult a doctor about this change. The following sections provide information about weight loss and gain in people with liver disease. See chapter 16 for information on obesity, BMI, and the liver.

The Causes of Weight Gain and Loss

If a person with liver disease experiences weight gain, it is important to determine the underlying cause. This is because the cause of the weight gain may have significant implications. While fat is the most common cause of weight gain, weight gain can also be due to ascites. Ascites is a sign of worsening liver disease. Weight gain may also be due to protein gain in the form of enlarged muscle mass. This should be construed as a healthy development. Muscle weighs more than fat, and therefore if bodybuilding has been incorporated into a person's lifestyle, this type of weight gain is the reward. It is advisable to be evaluated by a specialist if unexpected weight gain occurs. The specialist will determine what treatment, if any, is necessary under the circumstances.

As with weight gain, weight loss can be due to a variety of factors. If one is on a fat- and/or calorie-restricted diet, then any weight loss is probably attributable to the diet. However, weight loss, especially if unexpected, can be due to protein or muscle loss. This can be a sign of worsening liver disease or liver cancer. It is important to consult with a doctor before starting a weight-reduction diet and to remain under a doctor's supervision while the diet is ongoing. It is especially important to inform the doctor if an unexpected weight loss occurs.

The Reason Why People with Liver Disease Have a Hard Time Losing Weight

Many people with liver disease have a difficult time losing weight. This may be attributable to any of the following factors. First, some medications used in the treatment of liver disease can actually cause weight gain. The most common example of this is the medication prednisone. Prednisone is used to treat autoimmune hepatitis (discussed in chapter 14) and is part of the panoply of antirejection medications used after a liver transplant. Prednisone is notorious for causing weight gain, both by increasing the percentage of body fat and through its tendency to promote fluid retention.

Second, people with liver disease often have hypothyroidism (a slow thyroid condition). This leads to a sluggish metabolism typically resulting in weight gain. Thyroid abnormalities are often seen in people with AIH and in people on interferon treatment for chronic hepatitis B or C. Thyroid abnormalities are easily correctable with medications.

Third, many people with liver disease are chronically fatigued. Consequently, they may rarely exercise and tend to lead relatively sedentary lifestyles. This creates a cycle that perpetuates further weight gain.

Finally, it is common for a person to experience considerable weight gain after receiving a liver transplant. This occurs because medications used in the prevention of liver graft rejection, such as cyclosporine and prednisone, can cause an increase in body fat and fluid retention. This problem can be remedied in many instances by slowly decreasing the dosage of prednisone until it is discontinued and changing from cyclosporine to tacrolimus. Liver transplant recipients are prone to adopt a diet high in fatty foods. This most likely occurs because their diets may have been severely restricted prior to the transplantation or their appetites may have been suppressed due to their illness and associated depression. After transplantation, a new sense of well-being, accompanied by an improved outlook on life, often leads to an increased appetite.

A Warning About Crash Diets and Diet Pills

The recommended way to lose weight is to adopt a healthy, balanced diet and to exercise regularly. It is easy to be tempted to take a shortcut to this goal via the use of crash diets or diet pills. This is definitely not recommended. These mass-market solutions may produce serious adverse or perhaps even fatal consequences in a person with liver disease. Many fad diets emphasize one particular category of nutrient, say protein, or even just one specific type of food, like grapefruit, to the exclusion of everything else. A healthy person's liver might be able to tolerate this approach, but a damaged liver often cannot. The nutritional imbalance that an ill-advised fad diet can create can easily throw a weakened liver into failure and land a person in the hospital. The same applies to some diet pills. Remember, everything that is ingested eventually has to be processed by the liver. Diet pills may add to the stress of an already burdened liver, thereby increasing the likelihood that a person's condition will worsen rather than improve. Despite spending approximately $33 billion annually on commercial weight-loss products, there has been an increase in the prevalence of obesity in the United States over the last two decades. This underscores the point that these products do not work and should not be tried.

The Reason Why People with Liver Disease Have a Hard Time Gaining Weight

Some people with liver disease have a hard time gaining weight. This more commonly occurs in people with cirrhosis. As noted above, during this time, protein is used as an energy source as the body begins breaking down its own muscle in a desperate attempt to stay alive. This results in a loss of fat, and eventually of muscle. This occurrence is called protein-energy malnutrition (PEM), a condition that mimics a state of starvation. PEM is believed to occur in approximately 20 percent of people with compensated cirrhosis and in 80 percent of people with decompensated cirrhosis (those with encephalopathy, variceal bleeding, or ascites). See chapter 6 for more about cirrhosis.

People with cirrhosis often have decreased appetites, nausea, and a feeling of fullness even after eating small meals. When calorie counts are performed on these people, they are often found to be consuming a suboptimal amount, even though these people often believe that they are eating enough. People who have trouble gaining weight should make sure that they are eating multiple small meals in addition to a bedtime snack. If a person's appetite is poor, she can try eating baby food. That's right—baby food. Baby food is a nutritious source of calories and is easy to digest. Decreased appetite may be due to an unpalatable diet. Thus, a sodium and/or animal protein–restricted diet should be adhered to only if one is suffering from ascites and encephalopathy, respectively.

A zinc deficiency can cause a diminished appetite. One's zinc levels should be determined and if a deficiency is found, zinc supplementation will be necessary. Approximately 37 percent of people with cirrhosis develop diabetes, which is often a cause of an inability to gain weight. Once glucose levels are corrected with medication, patients find it easier to put on pounds.

People with cholestatic liver disease such as primary biliary cirrhosis (chapter 15), or anyone with cholestasis (impairment of bile flow), which can occur in any end stage liver disease, may be unable to absorb fats efficiently. This condition is known as fat malabsorption. This is caused by a failure to secrete bile salts necessary to absorb fats. The fats that these people are unable to absorb are eliminated from their bodies in their stools, which tend to be multiple, light in color, loose in consistency, and frothy in texture. This type of stool is known as steatorrhea. People with fat malabsorption are unable to absorb the fat-soluble vitamins— A, D, E, and K. Such people should be checked for deficiency of these vitamins as well as for a magnesium deficiency. Supplementation is recommended, as needed, so as to avoid further complications. Medium-chain triglycerides (such as NutriHep Enteral Nutrition, Nestle, Deerfield, Il) should be added as a dietary supplement.

EXERCISE FOR THOSE WITH LIVER DISEASE

Regular exercise is an important component in the fight against liver disease. This isn't something that can be found in any medical textbook or that is taught in medical school classrooms. This may explain why most liver doctors don't realize how important exercise can be to maintaining their patients' health. But I've seen the benefits over and over again in my practice. People who are in good shape and who exercise on a regular basis not only feel better, but often respond more positively to medical treatment. People do not have to do a lot of exercise in order to reap its benefits. Nor does it make sense to overdo it. The main thing is simply to get going. Regular exercise will increase energy levels, decrease stress on the liver, and, in many cases, even delay the onset of certain complications associated with liver disease. For people with liver disease, it is crucial to consult with a doctor before beginning any type of exercise program.

Some of the Benefits of Exercise

The benefits of exercising are numerous. First, exercise gives people a general sense of well-being and an improved self-image. It is a known fact that if a person feels well mentally, her immune system will be stronger and give her that extra edge needed in the fight against disease.

Second, as previously discussed, exercising gives a person a boost of energy. Fatigue is probably the most common as well as one of the most bothersome symptoms that plagues people with liver disease. Many people with liver disease frequently feel like they don't have enough energy to make it across the room, let alone around the block. However, the best way to fight this seemingly relentless exhaustion is to exercise. Yes, the notion of exercising when you are fatigued may seem counterintuitive—like a vicious cycle—but most people find that it actually works. In part, fatigue may have to do with the fact that both the heart and liver are working overtime to keep a good supply of filtered blood circulating throughout the body. Adding a regular exercise routine enables both organs to work more efficiently. Over time, this will boost energy levels. While most people find it tough going at first, they eventually realize that the benefits make it well worth it.

Third, exercise improves cardiovascular function. As the body gets stronger and more aerobically fit, the cardiovascular system will be able to work more efficiently. Less effort will be required of the heart to pump blood to the liver and other body organs. Less effort on the heart equals stronger cardiovascular function and an increased overall energy level for a person with liver disease. It is extremely important to attempt to do some exercise while on interferon treatment, as this will decrease the fatigue, irritability, and depression often associated with this medication.

Fourth, exercise results in a reduction of total body fat. While nearly everyone knows that being overweight places a great deal of stress on the heart, most people don't realize that it also makes it harder for the liver to do its job. When total body fat is reduced, fat content in the liver is simultaneously reduced. This often results in a significant reduction of elevated liver enzymes, no matter what the underlying liver disorder is. Eating right and getting plenty of exercise is undoubtedly the slowest way to lose weight known to humanity, but it's also the safest and surest. This is especially true for people with liver disease. Even intermittent exercise has been shown to be beneficial in obese women. Combining a healthy diet with regular exercise is also the best way to keep from regaining the weight.

The Benefits of Exercise for Osteoporosis

Exercise is essential in order to decrease the incidence of potentially detrimental bone disorders. Osteoporosis is a bone disorder frequently associated with liver disease. It results in decreased bone density, thereby leading to fragile, easily fractured bones. While osteoporosis is a disease that most frequently affects post-menopausal women, it can also affect premenopausal women and men with liver disease. Postmenopausal women are particularly susceptible to osteoporosis because, as estrogen production stops, bone loss accelerates. Furthermore, women naturally have a lower percentage of muscle and bone mass than men. This further increases their risk of developing osteoporosis. Other risks for osteoporosis in people with liver disease include excessive alcohol use, primary biliary cirrhosis, advanced cirrhosis from any liver disease typically resulting in muscle wasting, and the use of prednisone. Fortunately, people can reduce the likelihood of developing osteoporosis by making exercise and a healthy diet part of their lifestyles.

Just as muscles grow in response to muscle contractions, bone strength and density increase when the muscles attached are contracting. Studies have shown that muscle and bone growth promoted by frequent weight-bearing exercise is vital to the prevention of osteoporosis. Supplementing the diet with at least 1,000 to 1,500 mg per day of calcium in combination with vitamin D is also important. If a person already has osteoporosis, it needn't keep her from exercising, but she will have to use more caution so as to keep from breaking any bones. High-impact aerobic exercises, which involve jumping and twisting, can increase the risk of injury and should be avoided. Low-impact exercises, such as swimming and walking, are the safest choices for aerobic exercise. Weight-bearing exercises with light weights can generally be safely performed. Close attention should always be paid to proper form. Running on a hard surface, such as concrete pavement, should be avoided. Soft surfaces, such as specially designed running tracks, a treadmill, or a sandy beach, are preferable.

The Types of Exercise for Liver Disease

People with liver disease should take up both aerobic and weight-bearing exercises, as they each play a different role in fighting liver disease. It is fortunate that there are an abundance of books, videotapes, and television programs that teach, step-by-step, both types of exercises. It is important to use these self-help materials prior to starting any exercise regimen. Other helpful ideas include scheduling a few appointments with a personal trainer to design a fitness routine that personally meets the needs of a person with liver disease. Many fitness trainers will even work in their clients' or the trainer's homes. And recently, one-on-one fitness training facilities have become widespread. They offer both privacy and personalized attention. This is important, as many people are too self-conscious or too shy to exercise in a crowded gym and/or lose self-motivation after the first few sessions at a gym. A welcome development has been the appearance very recently of gyms geared specifically to individuals who are not in good shape. In these facilities, embarrassment is mitigated and the convergence of similarly situated clientele creates an environment akin to a combination support group/health club. Finally, the likelihood of success is increased if a person adopts an exercise program that she already enjoys and that can easily be adhered to with consistency at least three times a week.

Timing is also important. It is fine to exercise at any time of the day that is personally convenient. However, by the end of the day, most people are usually too mentally and physically tired to do anything, least of all run on a treadmill! That is why most people with liver disease find that they need to do their exercises first thing in the morning. While some people may find it difficult to get up in the morning in the first place, once they get started with an exercise regimen, it will become easier and easier. And people usually find that exercising in the morning helps give them an extra boost of energy to make it through the day. Finally, don't overdo it. It's more important to maintain a regular routine than to set any records.

Aerobic Exercises

Aerobic exercise trains the heart, lungs, and entire cardiovascular system to process and deliver oxygen more quickly and efficiently to every part of the body. It's the kind of exercise that gets the heart pumping. As one becomes more aerobically fit, the heart won't have to work as hard to pump blood to the rest of the body, including the liver. The pulse will begin to slow down, making it easier for the liver to send back to the rest of the body the blood it has just filtered. The benefits of being an aerobically fit person include an overall improved energy level, which translates into decreased fatigue. Fortunately, a person does not have to purchase high-fashion workout clothes or go to a fancy gym to get aerobic exercise. Walking briskly, bicycling (either stationary or regular), swimming, or using a treadmill all provide solid aerobic benefits. Many people start off with something easy, such as walking around the block. A helpful hint is to start by walking up and down the street close to home. In that way, if a bout of fatigue suddenly occurs, it won't take long to get home.

Weight-Bearing Exercises

Weight-bearing exercises build up both bones and muscles. For many reasons, it is important for all people with liver disease to incorporate weight-bearing exercises into their daily exercise routines. First, because they are prone to osteoporosis, people with liver disease need good strong bones. Weight training is the best way to fight against this, as stronger muscles equal stronger bones. Second, in advanced stages of liver disease, the body is forced to recruit muscle as a source of energy, and people are at risk of developing severe muscle wasting and greatly diminished strength. However, if a person has a reserve of muscle built up on her body, it will take a much longer time for this complication of liver disease to develop. Third, people who have too much fat on their bodies are at risk of worsening their underlying liver condition by developing nonalcoholic fatty liver disease (NAFLD). Weight training reduces the amount of fat on the body and increases muscle mass. Therefore, the chance of developing NAFLD will be reduced. Finally, since muscle weighs more than fat, weight training is the perfect means of gaining lean healthy weight for those people who are underweight.

One exception to weight training should be mentioned. People with cirrhosis complicated by esophageal varices should avoid weight training. This is because wall tension in the esophagus may drastically increase with weight training, which puts this group at increased risk for esophageal variceal rupture and hemorrhage.

Once again, there are lots of self-help books and videotapes that describe how to create a personalized weight-bearing exercise routine. It's a good idea to hire a personal fitness trainer who can design a personalized routine specific to an individual's needs. It is important that the trainer be aware of the client's liver disorder and realize that consequently the client will not always be able to exercise to her fullest capacity. A person with liver disease should never push herself excessively, nor should she allow herself to be pushed by a trainer. If she feels too tired or if a body part feels strained, she should stop exercising until she feels better. Fitness training has become a field that requires certification, so make sure that the trainer is certified.

It is important to remember to work out every part of the body evenly. Did you know that there are eleven distinct body parts to work out?! In that way, the chances of injury are decreased. A few stretching exercises should always be performed first to warm up the muscles before doing weight-bearing exercises. The amount of weight being lifted should allow for eight to twelve repetitions. Each repetition (rep) is defined as one full and individual execution of a particular lifting exercise. A set is a distinct grouping of repetitions, followed by a brief rest interval. Three sets of a given type of exercise should be performed. Aim to work out each body part at least once a week. Twice a week is ideal.

Putting Together an Exercise Program

Nobody expects a person beginning an exercise regimen to run a marathon or enter a bodybuilding contest. Setting impossibly high standards only guarantees failure. But if a person starts with easy goals and works her way up, she is much more likely to make exercise part of her daily routine. A good beginning regimen might include ten to twenty minutes of aerobic exercise, followed by a few weight-bearing exercises three times a week. Everyone should work at her own pace until she is working out daily or at least three to five times per week. But even if a person can exercise only for a few minutes at a time, there is no need to despair. Doing a little exercise is better than doing none at all. It will get easier as time goes on.

When a person is in an acute phase of hepatitis or is experiencing a severe exacerbation or relapse of disease, any form of intense exertion should be avoided. There's no need for enforced bed rest, however. A person should listen to her body. If she is exhausted, then it's time to rest. If she's up to physical activity, then by all means she should be active. But she must be aware of her personal limitations and know when it's time to call it quits. The liver has only so much energy to distribute to the rest of the body, so it's never wise to overdo it. Again, it is essential to consult with your doctor prior to commencing any exercise program.

CONCLUSION

While a healthy diet and suitable exercise regimen should not be a substitute for conventional medical treatment, it should be considered an essential addition to therapy. In fact, following the appropriate regimen could actually improve the long-term outcome of some people with liver disease and can help prevent or delay the onset of some complications associated with liver disease. Furthermore, proper nutrition and exercise can also minimize the need for the use of excessive medications in many cases. Since everyone has individual needs and requirements related to diet and exercise, it is important to seek out a liver specialist, nutritionist, and/or fitness trainer who has the expertise to guide you in the right direction. This chapter provided a general guideline upon which to form a basis for a personalized nutrition and exercise program.

The next and last chapter of this book provides the answers to lifestyle-related questions commonly asked by people living with liver disease, their friends, and their loved ones.

Twenty-four

PREGNANCY, SEX, MEDICATIONS, AND PREVENTION

In most cases, a person who has been diagnosed with liver disease can continue to live a normal, active life. However, there is some information that people with liver disease should know in order to keep themselves healthy, to protect themselves from additional liver damage, and to help keep their loved ones and close contacts free of liver disease. This chapter discusses four topics that commonly concern people living with liver disease—pregnancy, sex, medications, and prevention.

First, people with liver disease and their spouses invariably want to know to what extent the liver disease will impact pregnancy and the health of their offspring, and if pregnancy will have an effect on the course of the disease. Typically, they are surprised to learn that most women with liver disease have had successful, uncomplicated pregnancies and healthy children without further damage to their livers. The first section of this chapter discusses these issues and also covers what the consequences may be if a woman develops liver disease during pregnancy.

The second topic discussed in this chapter concerns sex-related issues. Although most people with liver disease experience normal sexual functioning and interest, some people do suffer from sexual dysfunction, ranging from a decreased interest in sex to an inability to achieve an erection. In addition, the forms of contraception that are safest for people with liver disease and which types of hepatitis and liver disease can be sexually transmitted are covered under this topic as well.

The third topic discussed in this chapter relates to the impact that certain medications unrelated to the treatment of liver disease may have on the liver. Which medications are safe and which medications are potentially dangerous for people with liver disease will be discussed. Some people are more susceptible than others to drug-induced (medication-induced) liver problems. While many of these factors are alterable (such as reducing the amount of alcohol consumed), other factors (such as age) cannot be changed. Also covered under this topic are the effects of acetaminophen (Tylenol) and aspirin and other nonsteroidal anti-inflammatories (NSAIDs) on the liver. Also, since many people do not realize that recreational drugs can be harmful to the liver and that they can sometimes cause hepatitis or decrease the effectiveness of medications used to treat liver disease, this subtopic is also addressed.

The last section of this chapter discusses a topic of special importance—the prevention of liver disease. Two separate issues will be covered: how to prevent the spread of liver disease to others and how to prevent the occurrence of additional liver diseases in a person who already has liver disease. This section focuses on the importance of obtaining the hepatitis A and B vaccinations and also discusses some general preventive strategies that are recommended for those living with liver disease and for the people in their lives.

PREGNANCY AND THE LIVER

The issues surrounding pregnancy and the liver are many. This section will address several of these issues, including how pregnancy may affect the liver and the general health of a woman with preexistent chronic liver disease. Another issue covered is what impact chronic liver disease may have on the fetus. This section will also discuss some liver diseases that may occur in pregnant women with no prior history of liver disease.

Pregnancy in Women with Preexistent Chronic Liver Disease

Most women with liver disease can become pregnant, have uncomplicated pregnancies, and go on to give birth to healthy babies. However, in some circumstances, liver disease may adversely affect pregnancy and childbirth. The following pages discuss pregnancy in women with preexistent chronic liver diseases, including decompensated cirrhosis, chronic hepatitis B and C, autoimmune hepatitis, and others.

Decompensated Cirrhosis and Pregnancy

Cirrhosis (see chapter 6) is often associated with amenorrhea (lack of menses) and infertility. Consequently, women with cirrhosis—especially decompensated cirrhosis—may have difficulty conceiving. As a result of their advanced liver disease, women with decompensated cirrhosis who do conceive have an increased risk of serious complications during pregnancy. Approximately 15 to 20 percent of these women suffer spontaneous abortion (miscarriage). Also, there is an increased risk for premature childbirth or stillbirth. Furthermore, women with decompensated cirrhosis are at an increased risk for the development of liver failure during pregnancy, although it is unknown how often this occurs.

Bleeding from esophageal varices is probably the biggest pregnancy-related health risk for women with decompensated cirrhosis. Variceal bleeding is most common during the second trimester, occurring in approximately 20 to 45 percent of women with portal hypertension. Ten percent of the time, women with decompensated cirrhosis experience variceal bleeding during labor and immediately after childbirth. Death of the mother from uncontrollable variceal hemorrhage occurs approximately 10 to 18 percent of the time during the course of pregnancy. Depending on the trimester, the baby may nevertheless have a chance for survival. Women with decompensated cirrhosis who are thinking about becoming pregnant should undergo an upper endoscopy, which can assess the presence and degree of esophageal varices. If a woman has esophageal varices, she should be placed on a beta-blocker such as propanolol (Inderal). It should be kept in mind that beta-blockers may pose risks to a fetus, including a slow heart rate and potential growth retardation. Such risks must be weighed against the potential benefit to be gained by preventing bleeding from esophageal varices. Women who have previously bled from esophageal varices are advised to refrain from becoming pregnant. For these women, if pregnancy is still desired despite the high risks, it is recommended that a transjugular intrahepatic portosystemic shunt (TIPS) or other shunt procedure be considered before pregnancy occurs—as this may decrease the risk of bleeding from esophageal varices. It has been noted that for pregnant women with chronic liver disease, those with alcoholic cirrhosis appear to have the worst prognosis. Those with primary biliary cirrhosis appear to have the best prognosis.

Despite the increased risk of complications, many women with decompensated cirrhosis successfully proceed through pregnancy and childbirth without any complications. It is important for these women to be monitored regularly by a liver specialist and to choose an obstetrician who has experience with high-risk pregnancies. Fetuses should be very closely monitored during pregnancy. If there are signs of fetal distress or if bilirubin levels become very high in the mother, early delivery should be considered. Infants born alive generally do very well.

Chronic Hepatitis B and Pregnancy

Women with chronic hepatitis B (see chapter 9) generally do quite well during pregnancy, providing that they have not progressed to decompensated cirrhosis. Although it has been reported, a flare-up of hepatitis B during pregnancy is very uncommon. Transmission of the hepatitis B virus (HBV) to the fetus during pregnancy is rare. The placenta is usually an efficient barrier to transmission of HBV to the fetus. However, approximately 15 percent of the time, transmission transplacentally (through the placenta) occurs, apparently in cases where the placenta has leaked blood into the fetus (for example, during a pregnancy in jeopardy of a miscarriage). However, prenatal transmission (transmission from mother to infant during childbirth) is very common, occurring in more than 90 percent of the cases if the mother is HBeAg and/or HBV DNA positive. In fact, transmission to the fetus at childbirth accounts for approximately 40 percent of the world's chronic carriers in endemic areas (such as Asia and Africa). The incidence of transmission is similar regardless of whether delivery is by Cesarean section or vaginally. Newborn infants are usually asymptomatic (without symptoms). Some will eventually develop symptoms, whereas others will not (see chapter 9).

Universal vaccination of all newborns whose mothers are HBsAg positive, with both the hepatitis B immune globulin (HBIG) shot and the hepatitis B vaccine within twenty-four hours of birth is now mandatory (see page 434 for a discussion of vaccinations). In fact, universal screening of pregnant women for HBsAg is now standard practice. This prevents transmission of HBV from the infected mother to the infant approximately 80 to 90 percent of the time. New mothers are advised to avoid breast-feeding if they are infectious, even though this mode of transmission is not considered very likely. Of course, if the mother has bleeding nipples, the risk of transmission increases.

Treatment of pregnant women who have actively infectious chronic hepatitis B should be delayed until after childbirth because the medications used to treat this disease are teratogenic.

Chronic Hepatitis C and Pregnancy

Women with chronic hepatitis C (see chapter 10) usually have uneventful pregnancies, provided that the liver disease is stable and the pregnant woman has not progressed to decompensated cirrhosis. As a general rule, a stable liver equals a safe pregnancy. Transmission of the hepatitis C virus (HCV) to the newborn is very uncommon, occurring between 3 and 7 percent of the time. The likelihood of transmission is increased if HIV is present. It has been demonstrated that in cases where a woman is HIV-positive, aggressively treating the HIV prior to pregnancy greatly reduces the risk of transmitting HCV to the infant. The risk of transmitting HCV may also be increased by the presence of a high HCV viral load (for example, greater than 2 million viral RNA copies/ml) in the third trimester or at the time of childbirth. However, some studies have shown that transmission of HCV to the newborn does not occur regardless of the mother's HCV viral load. Invasive procedures such as amniocentesis and the use of fetal-blood monitoring via scalp vein catheter should be avoided, as they entail a risk of spreading HCV to the fetus. A complicated delivery with prolonged rupture of the membranes (greater than six hours) has also been associated with an increased risk of transmission to the infant. Some experts believe that delivery by Cesarean section (C-section) may reduce the risk of transmission of HCV to the newborn. However, there is currently not enough evidence of this to warrant routinely recommending C-section over vaginal delivery.

It is not necessary to test infants for the presence of the HCV Ab during their first eighteen months of life. Due to passive transfer of this antibody from the mother during childbirth, HCV antibodies will usually be present in the newborn during this time. However, this in no way indicates that the infant has hepatitis C. In fact, in most cases, HCV Ab disappears in infants after six months. Transmission is determined by a positive HCV Ab in the infant at greater than eighteen months of age and/or a detectable HCV RNA level tested after the infant is two months of age and confirmed at least twice additionally at intervals of three to four months apart. Although HCV can be detected in breast milk (colostrum), breast-feeding has not been associated with the transmission of HCV and is considered safe, unless nipples are traumatized, cracked, or bleeding. Infants appear to have a high rate of spontaneous remission of HCV. In one study, up to 75 percent of children cleared HCV spontaneously by two years of age. Thus, it appears that children are more likely to spontaneously clear HCV than adults; however, more data are needed before this conclusion can be definitively drawn.

Treatment of pregnant women with hepatitis C should be delayed until after they have given birth. This is because ribavirin, a medication used in the treatment of hepatitis C, has been shown to be teratogenic (capable of causing birth defects). Interferon, another medication for hepatitis C, may also be teratogenic.

Autoimmune Hepatitis and Pregnancy

In many cases, severe autoimmune hepatitis (discussed in chapter 14) causes women to stop menstruating, and, as a result, these women cannot become pregnant. However, when treated with corticosteroids and azathioprine, menstrual cycles usually return to normal and pregnancy can be achieved. Women with AIH generally have successful pregnancies and deliveries.

Flare-ups of AIH may occur during pregnancy, although such occurrences are usually rare due to the immunosuppressive effects of pregnancy. In fact, some women have even experienced a remission of AIH during pregnancy. To further minimize the chance of an AIH flare-up, a pregnant woman should remain on therapy during pregnancy. At low dosages, both prednisone and azathioprine have been demonstrated to be safe for use during pregnancy. However, as a precaution, it is probably wise to discontinue using azathioprine as soon as pregnancy is discovered, as some studies have found this medication to be teratogenic. Furthermore, if contemplating pregnancy, one should probably discontinue azathioprine approximately six months before conceiving. Ursodeoxycholic acid and cholestyramine, two other medications often used in the treatment of AIH, are considered safe during pregnancy. For women with AIH, there are a few instances in which pregnancy should be delayed at least one year because a poor outcome is likely. These situations include an AIH flare-up, any liver-related complication such as variceal bleeding, or the recent withdrawal of prednisone.

Although rare, stillbirths and premature labor have been reported among women with AIH. Conservative management during pregnancy, which should include fluid and sodium restriction and the elimination of all unnecessary medications, enhances the likelihood of a successful outcome for both the mother and her unborn baby.

Alcoholic Liver Disease and Pregnancy

Women with alcoholic liver disease (see chapter 17) are often infertile. Women with ALD who do become pregnant and continue to drink alcohol during pregnancy put their infants at high risk for a number of abnormalities. These abnormalities are collectively referred to as *fetal alcohol syndrome.* Infants suffering from fetal alcohol syndrome may be born with enlarged, scarred livers and elevated transaminase levels. It thus appears that alcohol intake during pregnancy may cause chronic liver disease in the newborn. Other abnormalities often found in these newborns include mental retardation, delayed maturity and growth, and defects in the skull, face, and brain. It is extremely important for all women, especially those with ALD, to avoid alcohol during pregnancy.

Primary Biliary Cirrhosis and Pregnancy

Women with primary biliary cirrhosis (see chapter 15) generally have uneventful pregnancies and deliveries. However, some studies have noted a greater-than-average incidence of stillbirths, spontaneous abortions (miscarriage), and worsening liver function among these women. These events more commonly occurred in women with advanced liver disease. Pruritus can worsen during pregnancy and may be successfully and safely treated with cholestyramine. On the other hand, pruritus sometimes improves during pregnancy. Ursodeoxycholic acid, which is used to treat PBC, is generally considered to be safe during pregnancy.

Liver Tumors and Pregnancy

Most liver tumors (see chapter 19) found in women who are of child-bearing age are benign (noncancerous). These tumors include hepatic adenomas, focal nodular hyperplasia, and hemangiomas. They may enlarge and rupture when exposed to high levels of estrogen, which can occur during pregnancy. Fortunately, such complications during pregnancy are very rare. If rupture does occur, immediate surgery is required, which may put the fetus at risk. Thus, if these tumors are large (greater than 5 centimeters) and symptomatic, surgical resection should be considered prior to becoming pregnant.

Liver Transplantation and Pregnancy

After liver transplantation, approximately 90 percent of premenopausal women regain menstruation within one year, and menstruation may return as early as six weeks from the date of transplant. Thus, despite having undergone a liver transplant (see chapter 22), women may become pregnant and can successfully complete their pregnancies. However, it is advisable that they wait at least one year and preferably at least two from the time of transplantation before becoming pregnant. Immunosuppressive medications should be continued during pregnancy as there is little risk that they will adversely affect the fetus. Blood levels of immunosuppressive drugs, especially cyclosporine, should be monitored carefully due to potential changes in drug metabolism during pregnancy. In general, there is an increased incidence of premature delivery and low infant birth weight among women who have undergone liver transplantation. Women who become pregnant after liver transplantation must be carefully observed by a liver specialist, as well as by an obstetrician who specializes in high-risk pregnancies. Approximately 70 percent of pregnancies result in live and healthy births. Liver transplantation rarely needs to be performed during pregnancy. This usually results in miscarriage.

Liver Diseases That May Develop During Pregnancy

During pregnancy, liver disease can develop in a women who did not have anything wrong with her liver before becoming pregnant. When viral hepatitis occurs during pregnancy, it is no different from viral hepatitis as it occurs in nonpregnant women—with the exception of pregnant women infected with the hepatitis E virus (HEV). Viral hepatitis is the most common cause of jaundice occurring during pregnancy. Other causes of jaundice can include drug-induced liver disease and gallstones. Gallstones commonly occur during pregnancy, and women with certain liver diseases (such as PBC) have an increased risk of developing gallstones. Furthermore, due to the gallbladder's close proximity to the liver (see figure 1.1 on page 9), the presence of gallstones often mimics liver disease by causing elevations in LFTs.

SEX AND LIVER DISEASE

Two sex-related issues that commonly concern people with liver disease are sexual function/dysfunction and methods of contraception. This section discusses these issues in detail. The medical treatment of sexual dysfunction in men and which types of hepatitis can be transmitted sexually are also addressed.

Sexual Function and Dysfunction

Most people with chronic liver disease have normal sexual function and normal interest in sex. However, some people do complain of decreased libido, decreased ability to achieve and maintain an erection (a condition known as *erectile dysfunction*), and decreased satisfaction with sex.

Decreased sexual interest and erectile dysfunction occur in approximately 2 percent of healthy, middle-aged males without liver disease. This is about the same incidence noted in males in the early stages of liver disease. Men with advanced liver disease, however, are more likely to experience testicular dysfunction, loss of body hair, gynecomastia, redistribution of body fat, a female configuration of pubic hair, decreased muscle mass, decreased sexual desire, and erectile dysfunction. These characteristics are due to the changes in hormone levels that can occur in such men with advanced liver disease. The male hormone, *testosterone,* is typically low, and the female hormone, *estrogen,* is typically high in such men. These findings are particularly applicable to men with alcoholic liver disease, as alcohol abuse (even in the absence of liver disease) may cause decreased testosterone levels and thereby lead to sexual dysfunction.

Women with liver disease appear to have normal sexual function, with the exception of women whose liver disease is due to excessive alcohol consumption. Women who have undergone a liver transplant generally experience improved sexual interest, body image, and sexual intimacy.

Any chronic illness may be associated with sexual dysfunction. This is particularly true for liver disease, since it is so often associated with fatigue and depression, each of which can contribute to a decreased interest in sex. In addition, medications used in the treatment of liver disease, particularly interferon, may cause sexual dysfunction and decreased libido—especially in men. Sexual dysfunction is also a common side effect of many of the antidepressant medications often used to treat the depression and anxiety that arise from treatment with interferon and ribavirin. When medication is discontinued, the medication-induced sexual dysfunction abates. Certain herbs often taken by people with liver disease, such as licorice, can cause decreased testosterone levels in men, thereby contributing to sexual problems. Other medical conditions unrelated to liver disease may also cause or worsen sexual dysfunction. Therefore, people should openly discuss any sexual problems with their doctors so that it can be determined whether some other medical condition, such as a prostate disorder or a psychiatric disorder, exists.

Women on interferon and ribavirin therapy for chronic hepatitis C often experience vaginal dryness. This may cause pain upon intercourse, vaginal irritation, and vaginal burning and itching. This results in decreased sexual interest. Vaginal discomfort may become particularly severe if a condition known as atrophic vaginitis—a condition of decreased estrogen in the body common in postmenopausal women—is present. Women should be aware of this potential side effect and should use a vaginal moisturizing cream. A topical estrogen and progesterone cream may be needed to improve or alleviate these symptoms. However, oral estrogen supplements should generally be avoided, as they carry a risk of causing or worsening jaundice and cholestasis. "Natural" soy estrogen, which has been linked to causing hepatitis, should be avoided. Please refer to chapter 11 for more information on women and decreased libido.

Treatment for Sexual Dysfunction in Men

Viagra (silenafil citrate) was the first oral medication for the treatment of erectile dysfunction to be approved by the FDA. The effects of Viagra on people with liver disease or on people who have undergone liver transplants have not been specifically studied. Moreover, Viagra's interaction with medications used to treat liver disease or with medications used after transplantation has not been evaluated. Therefore, the adverse effects of Viagra, if any, in people with liver disease (whether pre- or post-transplant) are not conclusively known. It has been noted, however, that about 2 percent of men experience abnormal liver function tests as a result of taking Viagra.

For people without liver disease, the recommended dose of Viagra is 50 mg taken one hour prior to sexual activity. Since this drug is metabolized through the liver, people with liver disease are advised to decrease this dose to 25 mg. Careful monitoring by a doctor, preferably a liver specialist, of a patient's liver function is essential for anyone with liver disease who uses this drug. People using

Viagra post-liver transplant are advised additionally to have the levels of their antirejection medications checked with increased frequency. However, it may be best to refrain from using Viagra until studies documenting the effects of this drug on people with liver disease and on those who have received liver transplants have been published.

Studies have failed to conclusively determine whether testosterone replacement treatment improves sexual function in men with chronic liver disease. Furthermore, testosterone may even be dangerous for those with liver disease. Therefore, this type of treatment cannot be recommended until further research has confirmed its effectiveness.

Vitamin E may increase male sexual performance. This potential benefit of vitamin E has not been confirmed in people with hepatitis C. However, since vitamin E may increase response rates in people with hepatitis C treated with interferon and ribavirin, it is probably a good idea to consume a vitamin E tablet if suffering from decreased libido (see chapter 23 for more information on vitamin E).

Contraception

People often assume that most forms of hepatitis are easily transmitted through sexual contact. Such an assumption is incorrect. In fact, only one hepatitis has a high rate of sexual transmission—namely, hepatitis B. Men with infectious hepatitis B should use a condom until such time as their partners have completed the hepatitis B vaccination series (see page 437) and have demonstrated *immunity*—as evidenced by the presence of HBsAb in their blood. Likewise, any woman with infectious hepatitis B should have their partners use condoms until such time as their partners have completed the hepatitis B vaccination series and have demonstrated immunity.

The incidence of sexual transmission of hepatitis C is very low, and most such cases likely stem from a mingling of blood during sexual contact. It appears that it is easier to transmit hepatitis C from men to women than vice versa. Since there is no vaccination available for hepatitis C, men with chronic hepatitis C who are not in long-term monogamous relationships should wear condoms. This is especially important for those men who have multiple sex partners, who engage in anal sex (where the incidence of bleeding is higher than with vaginal sex), who have breaks or sores on their genitals (such as herpes sores, which may bleed), or who have frequent prostate infections. Similarly, women with chronic hepatitis C who are not in long-term monogamous relationships should have their partners wear condoms, especially if any of the above-mentioned circumstances apply. Extra precautions should be taken in situations where a woman with chronic hepatitis C is menstruating. However, it should be emphasized that for people in stable, monogamous relationships, the incidence of sexual transmission of the hepatitis C virus (HCV) to the partner is extremely low. In fact, only about 3 to 6 percent of sex partners of HCV-infected people are also positive for

HCV. And since this statistic is based on indirect evidence, it is unclear whether the sex partners of the HCV-infected people quoted in these studies became infected through sexual acts or by some other route.

People with liver diseases other than hepatitis B or hepatitis C (as well as the sex partners of these people) need not take any special sexual precautions. Auto-immune hepatitis, primary biliary cirrhosis, nonalcoholic fatty liver disease (NAFLD), alcoholic liver disease, and hemochromatosis are not liver diseases that can be transmitted sexually. As these diseases probably, to some degree, have a genetic basis, people with one of these diseases may pass on the susceptibility for the disease to their offspring.

Although birth control pills are an effective form of contraception, they will not prevent the spread of a sexually transmitted disease nor do they lessen the likelihood of such a disease being transmitted. Women with a benign liver tumor (hemangioma, focal nodular hyperplasia, or hepatic adenoma) are advised to avoid birth control pills containing estrogen, as estrogen may cause enlargement or rupture of these tumors. Furthermore, estrogen has been shown to cause and also worsen jaundice and cholestasis. Therefore, it is advisable for all women with liver disease to avoid taking estrogen-containing birth control pills. As an alternative, women may wish to consider the long-acting contraceptive medroxyproges-terone (Depo-Provera), which is preferable because it does not contain estrogen. Instead, it contains the hormone progesterone. However, women should be aware that progesterone-containing birth control pills may cause sodium retention, thereby making these contraceptives unsuitable for women with ascites. In-trauterine devices (IUDs) are associated with an increased tendency to bleed when used by a woman with cirrhosis who has a decreased platelet count. Such women are advised to avoid the use of IUDs.

MEDICATIONS AND THE LIVER

There are over one thousand drugs and chemicals that are capable of causing injury to the liver, some of which appear in table 24.1. The terms *drug-induced liver disease, drug hepatotoxicity,* and *drug-induced hepatitis* are used to describe those instances in which a medication or chemical substance has caused injury to the liver. Drug-induced liver injury may account for as many as 10 percent of hepatitis cases in adults overall, 40 percent of hepatitis cases in adults over fifty years old, and 25 percent of cases of fulminant liver failure.

As noted in chapter 11, there is a rigorous process, known as clinical trials, that a drug must go through before it is determined to be safe for the public. These clinical trials are conducted on a carefully selected group of people who have met a long list of criteria in order to be able to participate in the testing of the medication. However, after the FDA has approved a particular drug, a larger and more varied group of people will be taking the drug. This more diverse group of people may have additional medical problems that were not encountered during the testing of the medication. This is why occasionally a drug originally thought to be safe may be discovered to cause severe liver injury. In fact, drug-induced liver injury is the most common reason for the withdrawal from the market of an already FDA-approved drug. Two examples of drugs withdrawn from the market due to severe liver injury include Duract (bromfenac), a nonsteroidal anti-inflammatory medication, and Rezulin (troglitasone), a diabetic medication.

Since all medications are processed through the liver at least to some degree, people with liver disease must become aware of which medications can cause liver damage, which medications can worsen pre-existing liver disease, and which medications are safe to take. It is the liver's job to detoxify any substances that are potentially harmful to the body. An already damaged and weakened liver must work much harder than a healthy liver in order to accomplish this task. When a person with liver disease ingests a potentially hepatotoxic drug, this puts an additional strain on the liver and can result in further liver injury or possibly even liver failure. Even people with a healthy liver can develop liver disease as a consequence of ingesting a toxic medication or drug.

In general, people with liver disease should avoid medications known to be hepatotoxic. People who must be treated with a medication that is potentially hepatotoxic should have their LFTs closely monitored by their doctors. If a person's LFTs become greater than three times baseline values, the medication causing these elevations should be discontinued. Also, it is essential that people with liver disease inform their liver specialists of every medication or drug that they are taking—including herbs, over-the-counter drugs, and/or recreational drugs. There is no reason for the patient to expect the doctor to be judgmental. Her goal is the same as the patient's. Therefore, complete information should be provided to the doctor concerning prescription medications, over-the-counter medications, and herbal and alternative therapies. Remember, a doctor's objective is to help her patient get better and to help protect her patient from unintentional additional liver damage.

People with cirrhosis must be particularly aware of which drugs are hepatotoxic, as they are typically more sensitive to drugs side effects due to the inability of the liver to clear the drug from the body (excretion rate). Even drugs that are not known to be hepatotoxic may have a prolonged excretion rate. This means that the drug and its metabolites will stay in the body longer. Therefore, usual dosages of these drugs should not be taken—the dosage should be decreased. Examples of such drugs that require a decrease in the dosage when used for a prolonged period of time in people with cirrhosis include Benadryl (diphenhydramine), morphine, Demerol (meperidine), and methadone.

How Drugs Cause Liver Disease

A particular drug may cause liver damage for many reasons. First, there are some drugs that are intrinsically toxic to the liver. These drugs can cause liver injury when the drug is taken in a dosage that exceeds the recommended dosage. This form of drug hepatotoxicity is what is known as "dose dependent." The greater the amount by which the dosage taken exceeds the recommended dose, the more likely it is that the drug will cause liver injury. Drugs in this category are usually broken down by the cytochrome P-450 enzyme system discussed in chapter 1. Under normal circumstances, the cytochrome P-450 enzyme system usually converts toxic substances into nontoxic ones. However, in situations of drug hepatotoxicity, the reverse happens. A nonhepatotoxic drug is broken down into hepatotoxic by-products. These by-products cause liver damage as they begin to accumulate. An example of a drug in this category is the headache and minor pain reliever acetaminophen (Tylenol), which is discussed on page 430. The drugs in this category may also cause liver injury if taken in excess in combination with another hepatotoxic substance, such as alcohol.

Second, there are some drugs that can trigger an *idiosyncratic reaction* (an abnormal, unexpected hypersensitivity) to a normal dose of the drug similar to an allergic reaction, even though a normal dose may have been taken. Such a reaction is not related to the quantity of the drug ingested, and, furthermore, the ensuing liver injury is unpredictable. This type of drug hepatotoxicity is often accompanied by fatigue, fever, and rash. It usually develops after a person has already been taking the drug for a few weeks. An example of a drug in this category is the anticonvulsant phenytoin (Dilantin).

Finally, a person's susceptibility to a potentially hepatotoxic drug is enhanced by many factors. Some of these factors are within the person's control, such as cigarette smoking and excessive alcohol intake. But other factors cannot be altered. These include advancing age and being of the female gender. Many of the relevant factors, both alterable as well as permanent, are listed below (see table 24.1 for more information concerning most of the medications mentioned in this list).

- *Age.* Adults are more prone to liver injury from certain hepatotoxic drugs such as isoniazide (INH), a drug used to treat tuberculosis.

- *Gender.* Females are more susceptible than males to most forms of drug-induced liver disease—especially drugs that can cause chronic hepatitis, such as methyldopa (Aldomet), a drug used to treat hypertension (high blood pressure).

- *Genetics.* Some people have a genetically based impaired ability to break down potentially hepatotoxic drugs into safe by-products, such as phenytoin (Dilantin)—a drug used to treat seizures.

- *Dose.* The higher the dose, the greater the risk of liver toxicity. This applies to drugs such as acetaminophen (Tylenol), which are by nature potentially toxic to the liver.

- *Duration.* For some drugs, such as methotrexate (a type of chemotherapy), the longer it is used, the greater the likelihood of liver damage or even cirrhosis.

- *Kidney damage.* People with poorly functioning kidneys are more prone to the hepatotoxicity of some drugs, such as tetracycline, an antibiotic.

- *Alcohol.* Alcohol consumption enhances the hepatotoxicity of certain drugs, such as acetaminophen.

- *Cigarettes.* Cigarette smoking enhances the hepatotoxicity of certain drugs, such as acetaminophen.

- *Drug interactions.* Taking two hepatotoxic drugs in combination can greatly increase the likelihood of liver damage compared with taking one hepatotoxic drug alone.

- *Hepatitis C.* The presence of hepatitis C may increase the hepatotoxic potential of certain drugs such as the NSAID ibuprofen (Motrin) and certain medications used in the treatment of HIV.

- *HIV.* The presence of HIV increases the likelihood of hepatotoxicity from certain drugs, such as sulfamethoxazole-trimethoprim (Septra).

- *Rheumatoid arthritis (RA) and systemic lupus erythematosus (SLE).* People with these autoimmune disorders are more prone to the hepatotoxic effects of aspirin than people without these disorders.

- *Obesity.* Obesity increases the susceptibility of halothane-induced liver injury (halothane is a type of anesthesia).

- *Nutritional status.* Either fasting or a high-protein diet can increase a person's susceptibility to acetaminophen-induced liver injury.

Characteristics of Drug-Induced Liver Disease

Many drugs have the ability to cause any form of liver disease, including acute and chronic hepatitis as well as a fatty liver and nonalcoholic fatty liver disease (NAFLD). And many drugs can cause cirrhosis, liver failure, or even liver tumors. People with drug-induced liver disease may be asymptomatic with only mildly elevated LFTs, or they may be severely ill with liver failure and consequently in need of a liver transplant. Or they may be somewhere in between. Drug-induced liver disease can result in exactly the same symptoms and signs as those that characterize the same disease when not induced by drugs. It is essential for both the patient and the doctor to consider the potential hepatotoxicity of all drugs that the patient is taking and to promptly discontinue the use of such medications whenever an adverse effect on the liver is suspected. Continuing to use a drug after liver-related symptoms and signs have appeared greatly increases the chances of serious liver damage.

Drug-induced liver injury may be diagnosed through blood work. Some medications may cause hepatocellular liver injury. This is manifested by elevations in the transaminases AST and ALT. Other medications may cause cholestatic liver injury. This is manifested by elevations in AP and GGTP. And some medications may cause both types of liver injury. In addition, there are medications that may cause elevated bilirubin levels. Patients with elevated bilirubin levels exhibit signs of jaundice, including yellowing of the skin and eyes and a darkening of the urine.

Drug-induced liver disease can be expected to occur in most but not all cases within the time frame of between five and ninety days from initial exposure to the hepatotoxic drug. Thus, people taking potentially hepatotoxic drugs should be monitored with blood tests during this time period. If a greater than threefold increase from baseline LFT levels occurs, the medication should be discontinued. LFTs should improve within two to four weeks from when the medication was discontinued.

Since more than one thousand drugs are potentially hepatotoxic, a comprehensive list detailing every hepatotoxic drug is beyond the scope of this book. However, table 24.1 lists some commonly used medications that may cause liver injury in some people. It is important to remember that not everyone will sustain liver injury as a result of using one of these drugs. And it is important to keep in mind that, as discussed on page 427, there are numerous variables that increase a person's susceptibility to the hepatotoxicity of these medications. Still, any person with liver disease who is using one or more of these medications needs to be carefully monitored. Careful monitoring is particularly crucial when such a person is using two or more hepatotoxic drugs in combination with alcohol. People with liver disease are best advised to use an alternative to one of these potentially hepatotoxic medications whenever possible.

Painkillers and Liver Disease

Acetaminophen (Tylenol) is a medication used to control pain (known as an *analgesic*) and fever (known as *antipyretic*). It does this without producing the stomach discomfort often experienced with aspirin and other NSAIDs. This characteristic has made acetaminophen a very popular alternative to NSAIDs. In small doses (less than 4 grams per day, or eight pills taken over a twenty-four-hour period of time) acetaminophen is quite safe for the liver—unless combined with alcoholic beverages (see below). (Note: Each acetaminophen tablet or pill typically contains 500 mg of acetaminophen.) In fact, acetaminophen is the recommended medication for relieving minor aches, pains, and headaches in people with liver disease.

However, when taken in excessive quantities or when combined with alcohol, acetaminophen may cause death due to liver failure. In fact, an overdose of acetaminophen is the most common cause of fulminant hepatic failure as well as the most common cause of drug-induced liver disease in the United States. After acetaminophen became readily available in 1960 as an over-the-counter medication, it became one of the most popular means of attempting suicide. For liver injury to occur, acetaminophen must generally be consumed in quantities exceeding 15 grams within a short period of time, such as in a single dose. Although uncommon, ingestion of 7 to 10 grams at one time may cause liver damage.

Table 24.1. Some Medications with Potential Hepatotoxicity

Medication	Use	Possible Liver Disorder
Anabolic steroids	For muscle growth	Liver tumor
Chlorpromozine (Thorazine)	Antipsychotic	Pseudo-PBC
Cimetidine (Tagamet)	Treats ulcers	Acute hepatitis and cholestasis
Ciprofloxin	Antibiotic	Cholestatic hepatitis
Clindamycin (Cleocin)	Antibiotic	Acute hepatitis
Cocaine	Psychotropic	Acute hepatitis
Corticosteroids (prednisone)	Anti-inflammatory	Fatty liver
Coumadin	Blood thinner	Acute hepatitis and cholestasis
Cyclosporine A	For immunosuppression	Cholestasis
Diazepam (Valium)	Psychotropic	Acute hepatitis and cholestasis
Erythromycin estolate	Antibiotic	Cholestasis
Estrogens and androgens (testosterone)	Varied uses	Liver tumor
Halothane	Anesthesia	Acute/chronic hepatitis
Ibuprofen (Motrin)	Analgesic	Acute hepatitis
INH (isoniazid)	Treats tuberculosis	Hepatitis
Methotrexate	Treats rheumatoid arthritis	Cirrhosis
Methyldopa (Aldomet)	Treats hypertension	AIH
Metronidazole (Flagyl)	Antibiotic	Acute hepatitis
Naproxen (Anaprox)	Analgesic	Acute hepatitis and cholestasis
Omeprazole	Treats ulcers	Hepatitis
Oral contraceptives	Birth control	Liver tumor
Phenytoin (Dilantin)	Anticonvulsant	Acute hepatitis
Rosiglitazone (Avandia)	Treats diabetes	Liver failure
Salicylates (aspirin)	Analgesic	Acute/chronic hepatitis
Tamoxifen	Treats breast cancer	Acute hepatitis
Tetracycline	Antibiotic	Fatty liver

The consumption of alcohol in conjunction with acetaminophen significantly increases the likelihood that a person will incur severe liver damage. Therefore, people who consume alcohol on a regular basis should probably limit acetaminophen intake to a maximum of 1 to 2 grams per day (that is, two to four pills within a twenty-four-hour period). Still, the best advice for people with liver disease is to totally abstain from alcohol.

People should take special note that acetaminophen is also an active ingredient in more than two hundred other medications, including Nyquil and Anacin 3. Therefore, it is essential to read the labels of all over-the-counter medications carefully. Other commonly used medications, such as omeprazole (Prilosec), phenytoin (Dilantin), and isoniazid (INH), may increase the risk of liver injury caused by acetaminophen. It is always in the liver patient's best interest to consult with a liver specialist prior to taking any medication.

Acetylsalicylic acid (aspirin) and other NSAIDs are drugs that are widely used for their anti-inflammatory and analgesic effects. They also have the potential to cause drug-induced liver disease. In fact, many NSAIDs have been withdrawn from the market due to their hepatotoxicity. All NSAIDs have the potential to cause liver injury. However, some NSAIDs are more hepatotoxic than others. NSAIDs presently on the market that have been frequently associated with liver injury are aspirin (ASA), diclofenac (Voltaren), and sulindac (Clinoril). Ibuprofen (Motrin) has been reported to cause severe liver injury in people with hepatitis C. A new generation of NSAIDs, known as the cyclooxygenase-2 (COX-2) inhibitors, has recently been approved by the FDA. This group of NSAIDs has the advantage of having fewer gastrointestinal side effects—less abdominal discomfort and less risk of gastrointestinal bleeding—than conventional NSAIDs. There are three different COX-2 inhibitors currently available to the public— Vioxx, Celebrex, and Bextra. COX-2 inhibitors have been associated with some liver dysfunction, although not as commonly as other NSAIDs.

It is recommended that people with liver disease avoid using all NSAIDs. If NSAIDs are medically required for the treatment of another medical disorder, a reduced dose should be used for a limited period of time and only by people with stable liver disease. Older women with liver disease seem to be particularly susceptible to the hepatotoxicity of NSAIDs and are advised to avoid NSAIDs altogether. Since NSAIDs may cause salt and water retention, people with fluid retention problems (such as ascites or leg swelling) may suffer worsening of these conditions. People with decompensated cirrhosis are at increased risk for kidney damage stemming from the use of NSAIDs. Since this may lead to hepatorenal syndrome (see chapter 6), people with advanced liver disease are advised to totally avoid all NSAIDs. Furthermore, people with ascites (fluid accumulation) may not respond to treatment with water pills (diuretics) while on NSAIDs, as they counteract their actions (see chapter 20). People with liver disease who have had internal bleeding from an ulcer or esophageal varices, for example, may be at risk for recurrent bleeding induced by NSAIDs and should totally avoid this class of medications. People who are also taking corticosteroids (such as prednisone) or anticoagulants (such as Coumadin) may have an increased risk of complications from NSAIDs. Finally, people with liver disease who smoke cigarettes or drink alcohol should avoid NSAIDs as they are also at increased risk for complications.

Recreational Drugs and Liver Disease

It is important for people with liver disease to refrain from using any recreational drugs. In fact, it has been shown that cocaine and ecstasy (an amphetamine) each has the potential of causing hepatitis. Furthermore, cannabis (marijuana) may decrease the effectiveness of interferon therapy and may diminish or nullify a person's response to this medication. As discussed in previous chapters, both intravenous and intranasal drug use have been associated with the transmission of both hepatitis B and C.

Tobacco and Liver Disease

Cigarette smoking may induce certain cytochrome P-450 enzymes in the liver, thereby increasing the susceptibility of smokers to the potentially hepatotoxic effects of some drugs, including acetaminophen. Smoking may also diminish the liver's ability to detoxify dangerous substances, and it may affect the dose of medication required to treat a particular liver disease. Furthermore, cigarettes may worsen the course of alcoholic liver disease. Also, cigarettes have been associated with a possible increased incidence of liver cancer. And, as noted above, cigarettes may increase the risk of hepatotoxicity of certain drugs, such as NSAIDs. Therefore, people with liver disease should refrain from cigarette smoking.

There is no conclusive evidence that other forms of tobacco use, such as pipe and cigar smoking or the use of chewing tobacco, have an adverse effect on the liver. However, it is likely that these forms of tobacco have effects on the liver that are similar to those from cigarette smoking. Therefore, it is recommended that people with liver disease refrain from using these forms of tobacco as well.

PREVENTION OF LIVER DISEASE

People living with liver disease must address two separate issues regarding prevention. The first concerns preventing the spread of a potentially infectious liver disease—namely, viral hepatitis—to others. Fortunately, the hepatitis A and B vaccinations are available and are an effective means of preventing a person from becoming infected with these types of viral hepatitis. The second issue concerns the importance of preventing additional liver diseases in people already living with liver disease. People with chronic liver disease often experience a severe if not life-threatening course of disease when infected with acute hepatitis A. And some people who have had a liver transplant are at risk for developing hepatitis B, which could lead to dysfunction of the transplanted liver, fulminant hepatitis, and/or cirrhosis. It is of utmost importance that all people with chronic liver disease receive the immunizations for hepatitis A and B. The following discusses the importance of vaccination, both for people living with or in close contact with someone who has viral hepatitis and for all people with chronic liver disease of any type. Also discussed are some general preventive strategies that all people with liver disease, their loved ones, and their friends should be aware.

Hepatitis A Vaccination

The hepatitis A vaccination was first approved by the FDA in 1995. Originally manufactured by SmithKline Beecham, this vaccination is called HAVRIX. In 1996, the FDA approved VAQTA, a hepatitis A vaccination manufactured by Merck and Company, Inc. As such, there are currently two hepatitis A vaccinations available, and they are equally effective. The hepatitis A vaccination is made by growing the hepatitis A virus (HAV) in a cell culture and then killing the virus with a toxic substance known as formalin. A vaccine manufactured in this method is known as a formalin-inactivated vaccine.

The hepatitis A vaccination is given via an injection into the shoulder muscle. This is known as an intramuscular (IM) deltoid injection. Side effects from the vaccination are rare. If experienced, they may include mild soreness at the site of the injection, a headache, and a low-grade fever. When a person receives the vaccination, her body's immune system will manufacture protective antibodies that guard her against a future hepatitis A infection. Because the HAV in the vaccination is dead and therefore incapable of multiplying or causing disease, inoculation with the hepatitis A vaccination cannot possibly cause a person to become infected with HAV nor can it make one capable of transmitting HAV to others.

Within two weeks of receiving the hepatitis A vaccination, 80 percent of people develop the hepatitis A antibody (HAV Ab). And within one month of receiving the vaccination, 95 to 99 percent of people develop immunity to hepatitis A. An additional dose of the hepatitis A vaccination is given six to twelve months after the initial injection. This second injection has the effect of extending the duration of protection. After receiving both doses of the hepatitis A vaccination, a person is totally protected against future hepatitis A infections. This protection lasts at least ten years, if not longer.

Although HAV does not cause chronic liver disease, infection with this virus can make a person quite ill (see chapter 8). In fact, some people are ill for as long as six months. Moreover, approximately 100 to 150 people die each year from fulminant liver failure caused by hepatitis A. It has been recognized that older people are especially likely to suffer a poor outcome when infected with HAV. In fact, as compared with people under the age of fifty, those over fifty years old are five to ten times more likely to die if infected with hepatitis A. In addition, people with chronic liver disease, particularly those with hepatitis B or C, may be more likely to experience a poor or fatal outcome when additionally infected with hepatitis A. Therefore, it is essential that all people with chronic liver disease, especially those over fifty years old, receive the hepatitis A vaccination. The hepatitis A vaccine should be administered to all people with chronic liver disease as early as possible and prior to the development of cirrhosis and liver failure— since among people with advanced liver disease the efficacy of the hepatitis A vaccine is diminished. It is further recommended that all people who are awaiting a liver transplant or who have received a transplant be vaccinated. The vaccination of food handlers and day-care-center workers should also be considered.

Other groups of people who are at increased risk for hepatitis A and who should therefore receive the hepatitis A vaccination include:

- People traveling to or working in areas of the world where hepatitis A infection is common

- Men who have sex with men

- People who use intravenous drugs

- People with blood-clotting-factor disorders

- People who work with nonhuman primates

- Laboratory workers handling hepatitis A–contaminated blood or stools

Children have the highest rate of hepatitis A, and they typically have a silent course of disease. This makes children a hidden reservoir for infection to adults who are not immune. Therefore, routine inoculation of children older than two years old with the hepatitis A vaccination was approved in 1999 for states with a consistently high incidence of hepatitis A (20 people per 100,000 population). Known as "high-rate communities," they include Arizona, Alaska, Oregon, New Mexico, Utah, Washington, Oklahoma, South Dakota, Nevada, California, and Idaho. "Intermediate-rate communities," including Missouri, Texas, Colorado, Arkansas, Montana, and Wyoming, where the incidence of hepatitis A falls between 10 people per 100,000 population (the national average) and 20 people per 100,000, do not mandate childhood hepatitis A vaccination but would be wise to enact such a mandate. Certain states have enacted immunization programs on a targeted basis. Texas, for example, requires vaccination in high-rate counties or when an outbreak has occurred. Mandatory hepatitis A vaccination for all children could make hepatitis A a disease of the past, or at least significantly decrease the incidence of hepatitis A in the United States. Hopefully, future policy changes will be directed toward accomplishing this goal.

If a person has already had hepatitis A or has been exposed (contact with the hepatitis A virus to a degree sufficient to cause the body to produce the hepatitis A antibody [HAV Ab]) to HAV at any time in the past, she is protected from reinfection lifelong. Past exposure can be detected by obtaining a blood test for the hepatitis A antibody (HAV Ab). If a person tests positive for HAV Ab, there is no reason to get the vaccination because it will not provide any additional benefit.

(If the hepatitis A vaccine is administered to a person positive for HAV Ab, no harm will be done, however.) The hepatitis A vaccination will not protect a person from hepatitis B or C or from any form of hepatitis or liver disease other than hepatitis A.

Immune Globulin (IG) for Hepatitis A

Prior to 1995, when the hepatitis A vaccination first became available in the United States, an injection of immune globulin (IG) was the only way to protect a person who had been exposed to someone with acute hepatitis A. IG is a preparation composed of multiple antibodies (immunoglobulins). It is made from human plasma that has been pooled from many people. This plasma is sterilized and must test negative for other infectious diseases. (All IG administered in the United States has tested negative for hepatitis B, hepatitis C, and HIV.)

Since the hepatitis A vaccine does not provide immediate protection against acute hepatitis A, IG continues to be an important form of protection for people who have recently been exposed to HAV. IG is typically given as a single intramuscular injection and is effective only if it is administered within two weeks of one's exposure to HAV. While IG provides immediate protection against hepatitis A, its beneficial effects are strictly short-term. The protection from HAV that IG provides usually lasts no more than three to five months. Therefore, a person who received IG more than five months ago and is exposed to someone with acute hepatitis A again will be at risk for infection. Although IG cannot prevent infection in a person who already has acute hepatitis A, it may reduce the severity of the disease.

Hepatitis B Vaccination

The development of the hepatitis B vaccine represents one of the most important advances in medicine. This is the first and only vaccine in history that can simultaneously prevent liver cancer, cirrhosis, and a sexually transmitted disease—namely hepatitis B. The FDA approved the hepatitis B vaccine in 1981, and it became commercially available in 1982. The original hepatitis B vaccine was made from the plasma of people chronically infected with hepatitis B. While this version of the vaccine is still available, it has been phased out in the United States beginning in 1986, when the FDA approved Recombivax, an improved version of the vaccine. Recombivax, which is manufactured by Merck, Sharp and Dohme, is made from common baker's yeast.

There are currently two separate hepatitis B vaccines in use, Recombivax and Engerix-B. Engerix-B, which is manufactured by GlaxoSmithKline, was approved by the FDA in 1989. A person cannot develop hepatitis B infection as a result of receiving the hepatitis B vaccine, nor can she transmit the virus to others by receiving the vaccine. The vaccination is administered via an intramuscular injection in the shoulder muscle, and it rarely produces side effects. Side effects, when experienced, can include mild soreness at the site of injection, headache, and low-grade fever.

Adults are given three separate injections—the initial injection, a second injection one month after the initial one, and a third one, six months after the initial one. Approximately 95 to 99 percent of adults are protected against hepatitis B as a result of receiving the three injections. Protection is manifested on blood work by a hepatitis B surface antibody (HBsAb) titer of greater than 10 IU/ml. When such a lab value appears on blood work, this signifies that a person is completely protected against a future hepatitis B infection for at least ten years and possibly lifelong. Additional hepatitis B injections are normally not necessary, with the exception of two circumstances—for people with poor immune systems, such as people with AIDS, and for people whose HBsAb levels are lower than 10 IU/ml.

Hepatitis B can lead to cirrhosis, liver failure, and liver cancer. Since the hepatitis B vaccine prevents hepatitis B infection from occurring, it is crucial for all people at risk for hepatitis B to obtain this vaccination. In fact, the hepatitis B vaccine has now been incorporated into the immunization programs of more than eighty countries. In 1991, the Advisory Committee on Immunization Practices (ACIP) mandated routine universal hepatitis B vaccination of all newborns in the United States. Routine prenatal screening of all pregnant women for HBsAg is now the standard of care. It is safe to administer the hepatitis B vaccine to a pregnant women if needed. Infants born to HBsAg positive mothers should receive both the hepatitis B vaccination and the hepatitis B immune globulin (HBIG; see below) within twelve hours of birth.

It is currently recommended that children receive the vaccination at age eleven or twelve if they did not receive it at birth. Many states have laws or regulations requiring the administration of the hepatitis B vaccination to children prior to their beginning day care or school.

Other groups of people who are at increased risk for hepatitis B and who therefore should receive the hepatitis B vaccination include:

- People of any age who have multiple sex partners (more than one sex partner within a six-month period)

- People with a sexually transmitted disease

- Immigrants from geographic areas in which high HBV is endemic—Asia, Sub-Saharan Africa, the Middle East, Amazon basin

- Children born in the United States to a person from an HBV-endemic area

- Adopted children from HBV-endemic areas

- Men who have sex with other men

- People who use intravenous drugs as well as their sex partners

- People with blood-clotting-factor disorders

- Those who have intimate or household contact with a person who is a hepatitis B carrier (HBsAg positive)

- People who work in healthcare

- Public-safety workers who may come into contact with blood

- People receiving hemodialysis

- People who live or work in an institution for the developmentally disadvantaged

- Prison inmates

- Alaskan Natives and Pacific Islanders

It is also advisable for any person with chronic liver disease to obtain the hepatitis B vaccination. These patients should receive the vaccine upon diagnosis, as the efficacy of the hepatitis B vaccine is decreased in people who have already progressed to advanced cirrhosis. Successful immunity to hepatitis B after receipt of the hepatitis B vaccination will eliminate the risk of acquiring hepatitis B through a liver transplant. It will also increase the number of potential donor livers available to a person awaiting transplant, because it will enable the use of a liver from an HBcAb positive donor. Finally, since it appears that coinfection with both HBV and HCV greatly increases a person's chance of developing liver cancer, obtaining the hepatitis B vaccination is crucial for people with chronic hepatitis C. Patients with chronic hepatitis C may have some difficulty attaining immunity (becoming HBsAb positive) from the hepatitis B vaccine. Thus, some experts suggest that the HBsAb titer be tested in patients with chronic hepatitis C. For those with an HBsAb titer of less than 10, an additional booster is recommended.

If a person has been exposed to hepatitis B at some time in the past, the vaccination will not afford them any benefit. Therefore, there is no reason for a person who is HBcAb or HBsAb positive to receive the hepatitis B vaccination, although it will not cause them any harmful effects if received. The hepatitis B vaccine will not protect a person against hepatitis A or C, and it will not protect a person against any form of hepatitis or liver disease other than hepatitis B.

Hepatitis B Immune Globulin (HBIG)

Hepatitis B immune globulin (HBIG) is made from plasma that has been pooled from people with high levels of the hepatitis B surface antibody (HBsAb). HBIG provides immediate but temporary protection to people who have been exposed to someone with infectious hepatitis B and to those who have accidentally been exposed to the blood or body fluids (for example, in a needle-stick injury or blood-splashing accident) of someone with infectious hepatitis B. Therefore, within two weeks of contact, HBIG should be administered to any person who has had exposure to hepatitis B–infected blood or who has had close or intimate contact with someone with infectious hepatitis B. As previously noted, infants born to mothers who are HBsAg positive should receive HBIG within twelve hours of birth. These infants must also obtain the hepatitis B vaccination. The hepatitis B vaccination may be obtained at the same time as HBIG. However, when the two are administered at the same time, they should not be injected into the same shoulder.

Combination Hepatitis A and B Vaccination

In May 2001, the FDA approved a hepatitis A and B vaccination. The vaccine, known as Twinrex, consists of the inactivated hepatitis A virus, and the recombinant hepatitis B surface antigen. As with the individual hepatitis A and B vaccines, it is impossible for a person to develop either hepatitis A or B infection, or to transmit these infections to others, as a result of receiving Twinrex. While Twinrex can prevent infection from the hepatitis A, B, and D viruses, it cannot prevent infection from the hepatitis C virus.

Approximately 95 to 99 percent of adults will be protected against both hepatitis A and B as a result of receiving this combined vaccine. It is recommended to administer Twinrex on a zero, one-, and six-month schedule (like that of the hepatitis B vaccine). Side effects are rare; when they do occur, they include soreness at the injection site, headache, and fatigue.

If a person has been exposed to hepatitis A and B at some time in the past, Twinrex will not afford them any benefit. Therefore, there is no reason for such a person to receive Twinrex, although it will not cause them any harmful effects if received.

Hepatitis C Vaccination

The development of a vaccination against HCV is being doggedly researched. Yet this challenging quest faces some considerable obstacles. One of the major barriers to the development of a vaccine involves the complex population of mutant strains of the hepatitis C virus, known as quasispecies, that can exist in a person infected with hepatitis C. The existence of quasispecies is also a factor responsible for the failure of so many people to respond to antiviral therapy. And it is one of the reasons why so many people relapse after initially responding to antiviral therapy. During treatment, mutant strains that are resistant to further therapy often emerge. Thus, to be effective, a vaccine would need to protect a person against many different HCV variants. Preliminary research on insect cells that are capable of generating "hepatitis C–like particles" (HCV-LPs) has some promise and may be helpful in creating a vaccine. The results of further research are being anxiously awaited. Indeed, if and when an effective, safe vaccination against HCV is produced, it would rank as one of the all-time great advances in the annals of medicine.

Immune Globulin for Hepatitis C

It has not been convincingly demonstrated that immune globulin can protect a person who has been exposed to hepatitis C from getting infected with the virus. Therefore, it is not recommended that a person in this situation obtain an immune globulin injection.

Hepatitis D Vaccination

There is presently no vaccine available against the hepatitis delta virus (HDV), nor is there an immune globulin available that can combat this virus. However, the hepatitis B vaccination will effectively prevent the occurrence of hepatitis D in a person who did not have hepatitis B at the time she was vaccinated. For people who already have chronic hepatitis B, obtaining the hepatitis B vaccination will not provide any protection against becoming additionally infected with HDV. Research being conducted on animals has shown some promising results as to the creation of a vaccine. In those animals experimentally vaccinated, although infection with HDV was not prevented, the resultant liver disease was less severe than usual. Further investigation needs to be conducted in this area.

General Preventive Strategies

Even though some liver diseases are impossible to prevent, there are many strategies that people can adopt to protect their livers and to maximize their health. All people—especially women—should consume alcohol only in moderation. People with liver disease should eliminate alcohol from their lives altogether. People with a family history of hemochromatosis or primary biliary cirrhosis should have blood work performed regularly to test for these liver diseases. If either disease is found to be present, treatment should be started as soon as possible. For the best results to be achieved, treatment should begin during the earliest stages of the disease before any symptoms develop. As a general rule, all people should attempt to maintain a normal weight and keep their diets low in saturated fats. This can reduce the likelihood of developing nonalcoholic fatty liver disease (although other factors may have a role in the development of this disease). As much as possible, all hepatotoxic medications should be avoided. Cigarette smoking should be terminated, as it has been linked to the development of liver cancer and may enhance the hepatotoxicity of some medications.

The hepatitis A virus can be killed by boiling infected foods for three minutes and by disinfecting surfaces infected with the virus with bleach. It is best to avoid eating raw or partially cooked mollusks (clams, oysters, mussels, and scallops), as these fish often live in HAV-contaminated rivers and seas. When traveling to areas of the world known to have a high incidence of hepatitis A, it is especially important to eat well-cooked foods and to drink only bottled water. Sanitizing diaper-changing tables is also important, as hepatitis A–infected infants are typically a silent source for the spread of hepatitis A infection. Meticulous hand washing is of a great importance after using the bathroom, before eating a meal, and when preparing food for others.

Not engaging in unprotected sex will greatly reduce the likelihood of infection with HBV. Placing a barrier such as a condom, dental dam, female condom, and finger cots between you and another person's body fluids and blood will decrease the risk of transmission and acquisition of HBV. While the risk of sexual transmission of HCV is rare, protected sex is recommended if a person engages in anal sex, has multiple sexual partners, has frequent prostate infections, has open cuts or sores on the genitalia, or is menstruating. People with hepatitis B or C should avoid sharing anything that may contain even the tiniest amount of their blood, including toothbrushes, razors, and nail clippers.

In order to further reduce the likelihood of spreading hepatitis B and C, people who are using injection drugs should never share needles with others or inject themselves with a used needle. A drop of blood so minuscule that it cannot be detected by the human eye may contain hundreds or even thousands of hepatitis B and/or C particles. Even meticulous cleaning may not totally eradicate the virus from a needle. If a person needs unused needles but cannot obtain them, she should seek out a needle-exchange program. Alternatively, needle use can be limited to autodestruct syringes. These needles are nonreusable. They are designed to self-destruct after one use so that they cannot be reused or shared with others. Of course, the best advice for a person who continues to actively use illicit drugs is to discontinue this activity immediately and seek help at a drug rehabilitation center. Also, anyone who intends to get a tattoo or have a body part pierced should make sure that they deal only with establishments that are clean and that adhere to meticulous sterilization practices.

Finally, while the risk of transmission of hepatitis B and C through a blood transfusion is extraordinarily low, if a person will be undergoing surgery and may need a blood transfusion, she may wish to donate her own blood or to select a specific person (usually a relative) to donate blood to her. These are known, respectively, as autologous blood and directed blood donation. If this route of blood donation is desired, it should, if possible, be planned out well in advance of surgery.

CONCLUSION

Hopefully, this chapter has shed some light on many significant issues that involve the daily lives of all people with liver disease. Issues regarding pregnancy and sex, medications and their effects on the liver, the importance of obtaining the hepatitis A and B vaccinations, and how to prevent the spread of liver disease were all discussed. However, the key point of this chapter is that most people with liver disease can enjoy a good quality of life, but they must make certain modifications in their lifestyles in order to maximize their chances of achieving this goal.

Glossary

This glossary should be used as a guide to assist you in defining words used throughout this book and words commonly used by doctors when they refer to hepatitis and liver disease. Refer to the appropriate chapters for detailed discussions on each of these topics.

abdomen. The part of the body below the rib cage and above the pelvis; does not include the back of the body.

acute hepatitis. Hepatitis with a course of six months or less.

acute liver failure. The rapid development of liver failure associated with coagulopathy.

adhesions. Scar tissue commonly resulting from prior abdominal surgery (but also has many other causes).

adipose tissue. Fatty body tissue.

alanine aminotransferase (ALT or SGPT). One of the transaminases (only found in the liver); high levels may indicate inflammation and/or injury to liver cells.

albumin. A protein produced by the liver. A low level is an indicator of poor health and nutrition and/or a poorly functioning liver.

aldosterone. A steroid hormone that regulates salt and water balance in the body.

alkaline phosphatase (AP). One of the cholestatic liver enzymes found primarily in the liver and the bones but may also be found in the intestines, kidneys, and placenta.

alpha-fetoprotein (AFP). A tumor marker often indicative of liver cancer when levels are very elevated.

ALT. See alanine aminotransferase.

alternative medicine. Any therapy used to treat an illness that is not within the realm of conventional and/or accepted medical therapies.

amenorrhea. A lack of menstruation.

amino acids. The building blocks of protein.

ammonia (NH_3). A product of amino acid breakdown that is often elevated in people with encephalopathy.

ampulla (of vater). A tiny opening in the duodenum that leads to the common bile ducts.

ANA. See antinuclear antibody.

analgesic. A medication or substance used to control pain.

analogue. A compound that resembles another compound in structure and function.

androgen. A steroid hormone responsible for masculine traits.

anemia. A condition in which the blood is low in red blood cells.

angiogenesis. The development of new blood vessels.

anicteric. Not icteric or not jaundiced; bilirubin level normal.

antibody (Ab). A protein of the immune system that fights against foreign substances (antigens) with the goal of destroying and eliminating them from the body.

antifibrotic. The ability to reduce scarring (fibrosis, not cirrhosis).

antigen (Ag). A substance foreign to the body, capable of stimulating an immune response, noted by the formation of antibodies.

anti-inflammatory. Capable of reducing inflammation.

antimitochondrial antibody (AMA). An autoantibody occurring in most people with primary biliary cirrhosis.

antinuclear antibody (ANA). An autoantibody produced in most people with autoimmune hepatitis.

antioxidants. A group of enzymes and/or other substances, some of which are produced by the body as a defense against free radicals, specifically oxygen free radicals.

antipyretic. A medication or substance used to control fever.

antirejection immunosuppressive substances. Medications or other substances that stifle the actions of the immune system.

antitumor. Able to fight cancer.

antiviral. Able to fight viruses.

AP. See alkaline phosphatase.

arrhythmia. Irregular heartbeat.

arteriogram. An X ray of an artery after the injection of dye.

arthralgias. Joint aches.

ascites. The accumulation of fluid in the peritoneal cavity; the most common complication of portal hypertension.

aspartate aminotransferase (AST or SGOT). One of the transaminases; high levels may indicate inflammation and/or injury to liver cells; also found in other organs, such as the kidneys and heart.

AST. See aspartate aminotransferase.

asterixis. An uncontrollable flapping of the hands that occurs with encephalopathy.

asymptomatic. Having no symptoms of disease.

autoantibodies. Antibodies produced by the immune system targeted against a person's own organs or tissues.

autoimmune reaction. A condition in which the body's immune system attacks its own organs and tissues as it identified them as being foreign or intruders.

barbiturate. A central nervous system depressant medication.

benign. Noncancerous; harmless.

bile. A bitter, greenish mixture of acids, salts, pigments, cholesterol, proteins, and electrolytes produced by the liver cells and stored in the gallbladder, which aids in the digestion of fats and is a neutralizer of poisons.

bile acid. A major component of bile closely involved in both the production and elimination of cholesterol.

bile ducts. Ducts that carry bile into the intestines and the gallbladder from the liver.

bile ductules. Small bile ducts.

biliary colic. Pain typically associated with an attack of gallstones characterized by right upper quadrant pain radiating to the right shoulder or back.

bilirubin. A yellow-colored pigment produced by the liver when it recycles old red blood cells; a component of bile, responsible for its yellow color.

biopsy. See liver biopsy.

blanch. To turn white with the application of light pressure.

BMI. See body mass index.

body mass index (BMI). A way to define obesity utilizing a person's weight in kilograms divided by the height in meters squared.

bruit. See hepatic bruit.

calcinosis. Abnormal deposits of excess calcium in parts of the body.

caput medusa. Dilated blood vessels that snake out from the umbilicus in people with massive ascites.

carbohydrate-deficient transferrin (CDT). A blood test that may be an indicator of excessive alcohol use.

cardiomegaly. Enlargement of the heart.

cardiomyopathy. Enlargement of the heart due to a chronic disorder of heart muscle.

CAT (CT) scan. See computerized axial tomography.

CBC. See complete blood count.

CDT. See carbohydrate-deficient transferrin.

celiac sprue. An autoimmune disorder characterized by gluten intolerance.

chelation therapy. A form of iron-reduction therapy involving infusion of an iron-binding drug either into a vein or beneath the skin, which promotes the elimination of iron from the body.

chelator. A binding agent.

cholangitis. An infection in the bile ducts that can occur in a person with gallstones or primary sclerosing cholangitis, for example.

cholecystectomy. Surgical removal of the gallbladder.

choledocholithiasis. Gallstones in the bile duct.

cholestasis. Impairment or failure of bile flow, manifested by elevated levels of GGTP and AP.

cholestatic liver enzymes. See alkaline phosphatase (AP); gamma-glutamyl transpeptidase (GGTP).

cholestatic liver injury. Liver injury in which there is an impairment or failure of bile flow within the bile ducts.

chromosome. A substance containing most or all of the deoxyribonucleic acid (DNA) or ribonucleic acid (RNA) composing the genes of an individual.

chronic hepatitis. Hepatitis occurring for longer than six months.

cirrhosis. Severe scarring of the liver that is sometimes irreversible.

claudication. A lack of arterial blood flow to the muscles, usually calf muscles, resulting in limping.

coagulopathy. A disorder of clotting, causing a tendency to bleed, manifested by a prolonged prothrombin time of greater than three seconds; indicative of severe liver damage or liver failure.

cocarcinogen. A substance that when combined with another carcinogenic factor hastens the progression to cancer.

cocktail therapy. Combining more than one drug with different modes of action to treat a virus.

coenzyme. An enzyme helper.

coinfection. Infection with two viruses (such as HBV and HDV) at the same time.

collateral shunts. The formation of alternative passageways for blood flow due to portal hypertension; also called collaterals.

colonoscopy. A procedure in which a flexible tube with a light at the end of it is used to evaluate the lower intestines (colon).

combination therapy. Therapy with more than one drug at the same time to treat a disease.

compensated cirrhosis. Cirrhosis without the development of complications, such as internal bleeding, jaundice, ascites, and encephalopathy.

complete blood count (CBC). A blood test that includes the levels of the white blood cell count, the red blood cell count, and the platelet count.

compound pharmacist. A pharmacist who prepares, mixes, assembles, packages, and labels medications from scratch.

computerized axial tomography (CAT or CT scan). An imaging study that uses gamma-radiation to transmit an X-ray beam through an organ.

congestive gastropathy. Buildup of pressure in the stomach due to cirrhosis, which can lead to inflammation and bleeding; also known as portal hypertensive gastropathy.

contagious. The capability to transmit infections to others.

contraindicated. Inadvisable to use.

CREST syndrome. An autoimmune syndrome characterized by calcinosis, Raynaud's phenomenon, esophageal dysmotility, sclerodactyly, and telangiectasias.

cytochrome P-450 system. A complex group of specialized enzymes within the liver that are responsible for the conversion of fat-soluble drugs or substances to water-soluble drugs or substances.

cytokines. Substances secreted by cells of the immune system involved in regulating the intensity and duration of the immune response.

cytoprotective agents. Medications or other substances that can protect cells.

decompensated cirrhosis. Cirrhosis accompanied by complications that include internal bleeding, jaundice, encephalopathy, and/or ascites.

deoxyribonucleic acid (DNA). A component of chromosomes that carries genetic and hereditary information.

diuretic. A water pill.

DNA. See deoxyribonucleic acid.

duodenum. The first part of the small intestine.

Dupuytren's contracture. A puckering of the palm that prevents a person from totally straightening his or her hand; common in people with alcoholic cirrhosis.

dysphagia. Trouble swallowing.

edema. Fluid accumulation commonly in the legs around the ankles. See also pedal edema.

electrolyte. Any compound that in solution conducts electricity and is decomposed (electrolyzed) by it. Sodium chloride (salt), calcium, and potassium are examples of electrolytes.

ELISA. See enzyme-linked immunosorbent assay.

encephalopathy. Altered or impaired mental status occurring in people with cirrhosis, which can lead to coma.

endemic. A disease prevailing continually in a restricted region.

endoscope. A tube with a light at the end of it that is used to visualize internal organs, including the esophagus, stomach, duodenum, and large intestine.

endoscopic retrograde cholangiopancreatography (ERCP). A special endoscope used to visualize the bile ducts and pancreatic ducts.

endoscopy. Examination of internal organs using an endoscope.

endotoxin. A poisonous substance in the cell wall of certain bacteria.

enteric route. Introduced into the body by way of the digestive tract.

enzyme. A protein that induces chemical changes in other substances while remaining unchanged by the process.

enzyme-linked immunosorbent assay (ELISA). A laboratory technique used to determine the presence of an antibody (such as the hepatitis C antibody) in the blood.

ERCP. See endoscopic retrograde cholangiopancreatography.

erectile dysfunction. The decreased ability to achieve and maintain an erection.

erythropoietin. A protein made by the body that can stimulate the formation of new red blood cells.

esophageal dysmotility. Abnormal movements of the esophagus.

esophageal varices. Enlarged blood vessels or varicose veins in the esophagus.

esophagitis. Inflammation of the esophagus.

esophagus. Food pipe; the portion of the digestive tract located between the pharynx and the stomach.

estrogen. A steroid hormone responsible for feminine traits.

exacerbation. Worsening.

excoriations. Severe scratch marks associated with breaks in the skin that often bleed.

extrahepatic. Outside the liver.

extrahepatic cholestasis. Bile duct blockage or injury occurring outside the liver.

fast. Abstain from eating or drinking.

fatigue. The most common symptom of liver disease, characterized by a diminished ability to exert oneself, usually associated with a feeling of being tired, sleepy, bored, weak, and/or irritable.

fenestrations. Wide-open holes in the blood vessels of the liver.

ferritin. The storage form of iron.

fetal-alcohol syndrome. A number of abnormalities that may occur in infants born to women who drink alcohol excessively during pregnancy.

fetor hepaticus. A foul, sweetish, or feceslike smell on the breath; often can be a sign of either acute or chronic liver failure and often precedes encephalopathy.

fibrosis. The initial stage of the formation of scar tissue in the liver.

FIBROSpect. A blood test that can differentiate among degrees of liver scarring in people with hepatitis C.

finger clubbing. A sign of liver disease, occurring especially in people with primary biliary cirrhosis, manifested by the enlargement and rounding of the tips of the fingers.

flatulence. Increased gas production.

focal fatty infiltration. Fat deposits in the liver concentrated in one area.

focal nodular hyperplasia (FNH). A benign liver tumor made of liver cells that have multiplied numerous times around an abnormally formed hepatic artery.

free radicals. Toxic, highly reactive compounds that are naturally produced by the body.

fulminant hepatitis. A particularly serious form of acute hepatitis associated with jaundice, coagulopathy, and encephalopathy.

fulminant liver failure. Acute liver failure accompanied by the development of encephalopathy within eight weeks of onset of symptoms or within two weeks of the onset of jaundice.

gallbladder. A pear-shaped organ located beneath the liver. Its main function is to store and concentrate bile.

gallstones. Stones that form in the gallbladder.

gamma-glutamyl transpeptidase (GGTP). One of the cholestatic liver enzymes, which is found predominantly in the liver and is, therefore, a sensitive marker for certain liver disorders.

gastric varices. Enlarged blood vessels or varicose veins in the stomach.

gastritis. Inflammation of the stomach.

genotype. The genetic makeup of the different HBV or HCV mutants in the hepatitis B or C viral population of an individual.

GGTP. See gamma-glutamyl transpeptidase.

Gilbert's syndrome. A benign familial disorder of bilirubin metabolism, manifested by an elevated level of bilirubin on blood tests.

glucose. A carbohydrate molecule; sugar.

glutathione peroxidase. An antioxidant enzyme produced by the liver that protects the liver from free-radical damage.

gluten. A protein found in wheat, rye, oats, and barley.

gluten intolerance. The inability to absorb gluten.

glycogen. A form of carbohydrate stored in the liver.

gout. A disease characterized by painful inflammation of joints and an elevated uric acid level in the blood.

granulomas. Nodules filled with a variety of inflammatory cells.

gynecomastia. Breast enlargement.

HCC. See hepatocellular carcinoma.

hemangioma. The most common benign tumor of the liver, often referred to as a blood tumor.

hematemesis. Vomiting of bright-red blood, often due to bursting of esophageal varices.

heme. Blood.

hemodialysis. A medical procedure used to treat people with kidney failure involving the removal of blood from an artery, cleaning the blood, and then replacing it in the person through a vein.

hemoglobin. An iron-containing protein, which is part of a red blood cell that carries oxygen to other organs and tissues.

hemolysis. Red blood cell (RBC) destruction.

hemolytic anemia. A low red blood cell count due to hemolysis.

hepatic. Pertaining to the liver.

hepatic adenoma. A benign liver tumor composed of liver cells (hepatocytes).

hepatic artery. The artery that carries blood to the liver.

hepatic bruit. A harsh, musical sound heard when a stethoscope is placed over the liver; suggestive of liver cancer.

hepatic vein. The vein that carries blood away from the liver.

hepatitis. Inflammation of the liver.

hepatocellular carcinoma (HCC). A primary malignant tumor of the liver (liver cancer); also known as hepatoma.

hepatocellular liver injury. Inflammation and/or injury to liver cells; typically indicated by elevated levels of ALT and/or AST.

hepatocytes. Cells that make up the liver.

hepatoma. See hepatocellular carcinoma.

hepatomegaly. Enlargement of the liver.

hepatorenal syndrome (HRS). Progressive deterioration of kidney function, leading to kidney failure, occurring in a person with liver failure.

hepatotoxic. Harmful or damaging to the liver.

herbs. Plaints or plant parts that are used for healing purposes.

heterozygote. A person who has inherited one gene for a genetic disease.

HFE. The gene for hereditary hemochromatosis.

HIPAA. Health Insurance Portability and Accountability Act. A law enacted in 1996 designed to protect the security and confidentiality of patients' protected health information (PHI).

hirsutism. Excessive hair growth.

HLA. See human leukocyte antigen.

homozygote. A person who has inherited two genes for a genetic disorder.

HRS. See hepatorenal syndrome.

human leukocyte antigen (HLA). A special antigen located on chromosomes that is believed to be a factor in the hereditary predisposition of people to different diseases.

hyperinsulinemia. A condition marked by an overabundance of insulin in the blood.

hyperlipidemia. Elevated levels of lipids (triglycerides and cholesterol) in the blood.

hyperpigmentation. Increased pigment or melanin in the skin, causing a bronze appearance.

hypersomnia. Excessive sleeping.

hypertension. High blood pressure.

hyperthyroidism. A disorder that occurs when the thyroid produces too much thyroid hormone, speeding up the body systems; an overactive or fast thyroid.

hypervitaminosis A. A toxic overload of vitamin A that can lead to cirrhosis.

hypogonadism. Impaired production of the sex hormones.

hypokalemia. A low potassium level.

hypothyroidism. A disorder that occurs when the thyroid produces too little thyroid hormone, slowing down the body systems; an underactive or slow thyroid.

idiosyncratic drug reaction. An abnormal, unexpected hypersensitivity to a normal dose of a drug.

immunity. The state of being immune or incapable of further infection.

immunocompromised. Having a poorly functioning immune system; also known as immunosuppressed.

immunoglobulins. Proteins associated with the immune system, some of which are made by the liver. Antibodies are examples of immunoglobulins.

immunomodulatory. Having the ability to regulate and stimulate the immune system.

immunosuppressed. See immunocompromised.

incubation period. The time between the entrance of the virus into the body and the initial appearance of symptoms and signs of the disease.

induction therapy. Daily dosing of a medication, such as interferon, during the initial treatment period (one to three months) usually at higher than normal doses.

infectious. Contagious; the capability to transmit infection to others.

infectious disease specialist. An internist who has completed a specialty fellowship in infectious diseases of all types.

infectious hepatitis. The old name for hepatitis A.

injection-site reaction. Mild pain, redness, itching, and swelling that occurs at the site of an injection.

insomnia. The inability to sleep.

insulin. A hormone made by the pancreas that controls sugar (glucose) levels.

insulin resistance. Unaffected by the insulin.

interferons (IFNs). A family of proteins that are made naturally by the body and that have antiviral, antitumor, and immunomodulatory activity; also manufactured synthetically.

interleukin. A natural protein made in the body that can regulate the intensity and duration of the immune response.

international ratio (INR). A formula that adjusts for the variation among different laboratories for measuring the prothrombin time (PT).

intractable. Incapable of being relieved.

intrahepatic. Within the liver.

intrahepatic cholestasis. Bile duct blockage or injury within the liver.

intramuscular (IM). Into or within the muscle.

intravenous (IV). Into or within the vein.

investigational drug. A drug that is considered experimental and is not yet approved by the FDA. It is only available to people who voluntarily enter a clinical drug trial, which involves the evaluation of the drug's effectiveness and potential side effects.

iron studies. Blood tests that show levels of iron, ferritin, and transferrin saturation percent; also known as iron profile.

jaundice. Yellow discoloration of the skin and eyes due to a buildup of bilirubin.

laparoscope. A thin, lighted tube inserted through a small incision in the abdominal wall in order to directly view the liver or other organs.

leukocytes. White blood cells (WBC).

LFTs. See liver function tests.

libido. Sex drive.

lipid. Fat.

lipid peroxidation. Iron-induced oxidation of cellular membranes.

liver. A wedge-shaped gland located on the upper right side of the body, lying beneath the rib cage; the largest organ in the body with numerous functions.

liver-assist device. A form of temporary dialysis for the liver involving removal of toxins from the blood of people with liver failure.

liver biopsy. The removal of a tiny piece of liver tissue using a special needle; performed for the purpose of examination under a microscope by a pathologist to determine the presence and extent of liver inflammation or damage.

liver cancer. See hepatocellular carcinoma.

liver failure. Cessation of normal liver function.

liver function tests (LFTs). Blood tests that give some indication of, although are not diagnostic of, what is going on inside the liver by measuring the levels of liver enzymes, bilirubin, and liver proteins.

liver-kidney-microsomal antibody (LKM-Ab). An autoantibody that occurs in people with type II autoimmune hepatitis.

liver palms. See palmar erythema.

liver spots. Brown spots most commonly located on the back of the hand that occur with aging and are not related to liver disease.

living donor transplantation. A procedure in which part of the liver from a suitable donor (such as a relative or other person with the same blood type) is transplanted into the patient.

LKM-Ab. See liver-kidney-microsomal antibody.

lymphoma. A malignant tumor of lymph tissue.

macrocytosis. Large red blood cells.

magnetic resonance imaging (MRI). An imaging study that utilizes electromagnetic radiation to create a picture.

malabsorption/maldigestion. Impaired or inadequate absorption or digestion of foods.

malignant. Cancerous.

MCV. See mean corpuscular volume.

mean corpuscular volume (MCV). The volume of the average red blood cell in a sample of blood.

melanin. Dark brown to black pigment in the skin.

melatonin. A hormone produced by the pineal gland that is involved in the sleep cycle.

MELD. See model for end-stage liver disease.

melena. Black, foul-smelling stool indicative of upper intestinal bleeding.

metabolic syndrome. A syndrome associated with obesity, hyperinsulinemia, insulin resistance, diabetes, hypertriglyceridemia, and hypertension. Also known as "syndrome X."

metabolism. The sum of the changes of the buildup and breakdown occurring in tissues of living organisms.

metastasis. The spread of tumor cells from the organ of origin to another organ, most commonly the liver.

metastasize. The spread of tumor cells to other organs.

mineral. A substance that originates in the soil and water and eventually becomes incorporated into all animal and plant life through the food chain.

Model for End-Stage Liver Disease (MELD). A scoring system for evaluation for liver transplantation.

monotherapy. Treatment with only one drug or agent.

MRI. See magnetic resonance imaging.

mucositis. Painful, burning, excessively dry or ulcerated mouth that may occur while on interferon therapy.

muscle wasting. Loss of muscle mass, most prominent in the arms and upper body; associated with cirrhosis and general poor nutrition.

mutation. A permanent alteration of genetic material.

myalgias. Muscle aches.

mycophagist. An expert mushroom picker.

myoglobin. A protein responsible for delivery of oxygen to muscles.

myopathy. Sore, swollen muscles.

NANB. See non-A non-B hepatitis.

neutropenia. A decreased white blood cell count.

neutrophils. Special white blood cells that are the body's first line of defense against infections.

nodular regenerative hyperplasia (NRH). A condition in which normal liver tissue is totally replaced by nodules of regenerating liver cells.

non-A non-B hepatitis (NANB). The old name for hepatitis C.

noninvasive. No surgery required.

nonresponder. A person with hepatitis C whose transaminase levels do not normalize and who continues to have detectable levels of HCV RNA in the blood while on therapy.

nonsuppurative. Not pus-producing.

nucleoside/nucleotide. Compounds that form the building blocks of DNA and RNA.

oral hypoglycemic. Sugar-lowering medication taken orally.

osteomalacia. A softening of the bones.

osteoporosis. A decrease in bone quantity.

overdiuresis. The excessive use of diuretics.

oxidative stress. Oxygen in a deformed toxic state due to alcohol consumption.

palmar erythema. Bright red coloring of the palms, particularly at the base of the thumb and pinky; often a sign of chronic liver disease; also called liver palms.

pancreatitis. Inflammation of the pancreas.

paper money skin. A condition in which the upper body is covered with numerous thin blood vessels that resemble the silk threads on a U.S. dollar bill.

paracentesis. The removal of large amounts of ascitic fluid through a needle inserted into the abdomen.

paraneoplastic syndrome. The manifestation of tumor symptoms in other parts of the body.

parenterally. Introduced into the body by any way other than via the intestinal tract.

parotid gland enlargement. A condition in which the parotid gland enlarges, causing the earlobes to protrude at right angles to the jaw; often a sign of alcoholic cirrhosis.

PCR. See polymerase chain reaction.

pedal edema. Swollen ankles.

PEG. Polyethylene glycol.

PEG-interferon. An interferon requiring only a once-a-week administration.

pegylation. A process that involves attaching a large substance known as polyethylene glycol (PEG) to a protein.

percutaneous route. Through the skin.

perinatal transmission. Transmission of disease during childbirth.

peritoneal cavity. The space between the abdominal organs and the skin.

peritonitis. An infection of abdominal fluids.

PHI. Protected health information. Any information that a doctor's office possesses about the patient.

phlebotomy. Removal of blood through a vein; often used as a form of iron-reduction therapy.

physician extender. A doctor's representative such as a nurse, physician's assistant, or medical assistant, who may provide follow-up care for a patient.

placebo. An inert, harmless substance that has no actual medical effect on a person's illness, but is identical in appearance to a medication under investigation.

placebo effect. Improvement in the condition of a person in response to treatment that is due to a "dummy drug" or "sugar pill" and not to the active ingredient of the substance being tested.

platelets. Blood cells that promote blood clotting.

polymerase chain reaction (PCR). A laboratory test used to detect hepatitis C virus RNA levels in the blood.

polypeptide. A group of amino acids linked together.

portal hypertension. High blood pressure in the liver and the portal circulation commonly due to cirrhosis.

portal hypertensive gastropathy. See congestive gastropathy.

portal vein. The vein that carries blood to the liver.

portal vein thrombosis. A blood clot in the portal vein.

precore mutation. The failure of the hepatitis B virus to make the hepatitis B "e" antigen (HBeAg).

primary organ. Organ of origin.

prognosis. The anticipated course of a disease without treatment.

prophylactic therapy. A type of therapy that acts to prevent a disease.

protein. The basic element of living tissue essential for the growth and repair of tissues; composed of amino acids.

prothrombin (factor II). A protein produced by the liver that is involved in the process of blood clotting.

prothrombin time (PT). A blood test that measures the time it takes blood to clot; prolonged in liver failure.

pruritus. Medical term for itching.

pseudotumor. A fake tumor.

pyruvate dehydrogenase. An enzyme involved in carbohydrate metabolism; a component of the major antigen against antimitochondrial antibody (AMA).

quasispecies. Genetic variations of the hepatitis C virus due to mutations of the virus.

Raynaud's phenomenon. A rheumatic disorder characterized by the fingertips turning blue and numbness upon excessive exposure to cold weather or emotional stress.

RBCs. See red blood cells.

recidivism. Relapsing back to old negative behavior, such as drinking alcohol.

recombinant immunoblot assay (RIBA). A laboratory technique used to detect antibodies to hepatitis C in the blood.

red blood cells (RBCs). Cells in the blood that carry oxygen to organs and tissues.

reference range. A standardized set of normal testing values obtained from the laboratory test results from a healthy group of people. Also known as reference interval.

refractory ascites. Ascites that do not respond to treatment with dietary restrictions and medications.

relapse. The recurrence of disease after a period of improvement.

relapser. A person with hepatitis C who initially responded to therapy but when taken off therapy, HCV RNA again becomes detectable in the blood and transaminase levels again become elevated.

resection. Surgical removal of part of an organ or tissue.

responder. A person with hepatitis C who normalizes transaminase levels and eradicates HCV RNA while on therapy.

RIBA. See recombinant immunoblot assay.

ribonucleic acid (RNA). A component of chromosomes that carries genetic and hereditary information.

ribozyme. A type of RNA molecule with the unique ability to cut targeted genetic material.

right upper quadrant pain or tenderness (RUQT). Pain or tenderness over the liver; occurs most commonly in the acute stages of liver disease, due to acute inflammation, irritation, and distension of the liver's surface.

RNA. See ribonucleic acid.

RUQT. See right upper quadrant pain or tenderness.

salt. Sodium chloride.

sampling error. The uncommon occurrence of a liver sample taken during a liver biopsy looking better or worse than the rest of the liver.

sarcoidosis. A disease characterized by the formation of granulomas in the lungs, skin, lymph nodes, liver, and bones.

SBP. See spontaneous bacterial peritonitis.

scleral icterus. Yellow discoloration of the sclera (whites of the eyes).

sclerodactyly. Scleroderma of the fingers and toes.

scleroderma. An autoimmune disease characterized by a thickening and hardening of the skin and internal organs due to excessive collagen deposits.

sclerotherapy. The injection of a clotting agent directly into a bleeding varix to stop hemorrhage.

serology. The measure of either antigens or antibodies in the blood.

serum hepatitis. The old name for hepatitis B.

shunt. A surgical procedure performed to decrease portal hypertension in the liver and portal circulation by creating an alternative passageway for blood. Portal systemic and splenorenal shunts are two examples.

signs. Physical clues or findings of a disease.

Sjögren's syndrome. An autoimmune disorder characterized by xerophthalmia and xerostomia, which often occurs in people with primary biliary cirrhosis.

SLE. See systemic lupus erythematosus.

SMA. See smooth muscle antibody.

smooth muscle antibody (SMA). An autoantibody produced in some people with type 1 autoimmune hepatitis.

sonogram (ultrasound or sono). An imaging study done by a radiologist by a technique that uses sound waves to produce an image.

spider angiomatas. Enlarged blood vessels found on the upper chest, back, face, and arms, resembling little red spiders.

spleen. An organ lying directly opposite the liver under the ribcage on the left side of the body; plays a role in the storage of platelets.

splenomegaly. An enlarged spleen.

spontaneous bacterial peritonitis (SBP). An infection of ascitic fluid (ascites).

steatohepatitis. Fatty liver accompanied by inflammation.

steatonecrosis. Fatty liver accompanied by scarring.

steatorrhea. Loose, frothy, light-colored stool due to fat malabsorption.

steatosis. The medical term for fatty liver.

subcutaneous (SQ). Beneath the skin.

superinfection. Infection with a virus (such as HDV) in a person who already has a chronic viral illness (such as chronic hepatitis B).

sustained responder. A person with hepatitis C who has eradicated the virus for more than six months beyond the date when therapy was discontinued.

symptom. Any abnormal sensation experienced by a person that is indicative of a disease or disorder.

syndrome X. See metabolic syndrome.

synergistic. In union with; complementary.

systemic lupus erythematosus (SLE). An autoimmune disease affecting multiple organs characterized by fever, skin rash, and arthritis.

telangiectasia. Small, thin, red spots on either the skin or mucous membrane.

teratogenic. Capable of causing birth defects.

Terry's nails. A condition in which the normal pinkish color of the nail bed turns completely white and the half-moon circles at the base of the nails disappear; usually a sign of cirrhosis.

testicular atrophy. A condition in which the testicles shrink; usually a sign of cirrhosis.

testosterone. A sex hormone responsible for masculine traits.

thrombocytopenia. A low platelet count; lower than 150×10^3/microliter.

thrombocytosis. Elevated platelet counts.

thymosin. A hormone involved in the immune system; produced by the thymus gland.

thymus gland. A gland in the neck that produces thymosin.

TIPS. See transjugular intrahepatic portosystemic shunt.

transaminases. See alanine aminotransferase (ALT or SGPT); aspartate aminotransferase (AST or SGOT).

transferrin. A protein made in the liver that transports iron through the body.

transferrin saturation percent. The percentage of transferrin that is saturated with iron at any given time.

transjugular intrahepatic portosystemic shunt (TIPS). A procedure that creates an alternative passageway in the liver between the portal and hepatic veins in an attempt to reduce portal hypertension.

treatment naive. A person who has never been treated, for example, with interferon for chronic hepatitis C.

treatment refractory. A person who does not respond to therapy; a nonresponder.

triglycerides. The form of fat stored in the liver.

truncal obesity. Excessive fat around the midsection.

tumor. A mass that may be either benign or malignant.

tumor marker. A blood test that is indicative of, but not diagnostic of, cancer.

ulcerative colitis. An inflammatory disease of the colon.

ultrasound. See sonogram.

umbilical hernia. A protrusion of the umbilicus (belly button), often due to massive ascites.

upper endoscopy. A procedure in which a tube with a light at the end is inserted through a patient's mouth and passed into the esophagus, stomach, and duodenum.

varices. Enlarged, distended blood vessels that result from the formation of collateral shunts in people with portal hypertension; usually located in the esophagus and stomach.

varix. A dilated blood vessel usually located in the esophagus and stomach.

vascular. Full of blood vessels.

vasculitis. Inflammation of blood vessels.

veno-occlusive disease. Blockage of the hepatic vein leading to a lack of supply of blood to the liver.

vertical transmission. Transmission of disease during pregnancy.

viral load. The amount of viral particles per milliliter of blood.

virus. A tiny microorganism whose main activity is to reproduce more viruses.

vitamins. Organic substances that come from plants and animals.

vitiligo. An autoimmune skin condition manifested by smooth nonpigmented patches on various parts of the body.

Wilson's disease. A genetic disorder of copper overload, which leads to an accumulation of copper in the liver, eventually resulting in cirrhosis.

xanthalasmas. A yellow nodule or patch on the eyelids associated with high cholesterol levels; occurs in people with primary biliary cirrhosis.

xanthomas. An irregular yellow nodule or patch, usually on the elbows and knees, associated with high cholesterol levels; occurs in people with primary biliary cirrhosis.

xenotransplantation. The use of organs from animals for transplantation into humans.

xerophthalmia. Dry eyes.

xerostomia. Dry mouth.

Index

About the Author

Melissa Palmer, M.D., is an internationally renowned hepatologist who maintains a private practice devoted to liver disease. Dr. Palmer graduated from Columbia University with a B.A. and obtained her medical degree from Mount Sinai Medical School. After training in internal medicine at Beth Israel Hospital, Dr. Palmer completed a hepatology fellowship at Mount Sinai Hospital. She then went on to complete a gastroenterology fellowship and is currently board-certified in both internal medicine and gastroenterology.

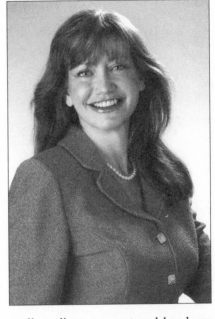

Dr. Palmer has authored numerous scientific publications in the field of hepatology. She is frequently called upon by the media for her opinion on various topics related to liver disease. Dr. Palmer has appeared many times on television as a liver disease expert and has been quoted in such publications as *TIME* magazine, *Cosmopolitan* magazine, *Prevention* magazine, the *Los Angeles Times,* and *Newsday.* She also has appeared in videos and CD-ROMs aimed at educating the public about hepatitis C.

Dr. Palmer lectures to the medical and general public on liver disease–related topics on a regular basis. She also serves as a liver consultant to five major pharmaceutical companies. In addition, Dr. Palmer sits on the medical advisory board of the New York chapter of the American Liver Foundation (ALF) and on the nutrition education subcommittee of the national chapter of ALF.

Dr. Palmer has performed trials on various experimental medications for the treatment of hepatitis. She is currently conducting research on new therapies for liver disease, specifically in the area of hepatitis C. She maintains a popular Internet website, liverdisease.com. Dr. Palmer currently treats patients with both liver and digestive problems in her two offices located on Long Island, New York.